BIOETHICS

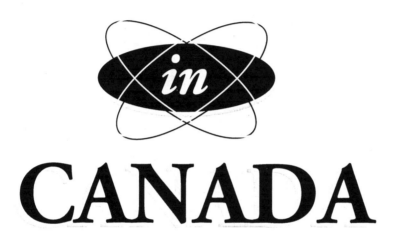

CANADA

DAVID J. ROY
*Center for Bioethics, Clinical Research Institute of Montréal
Faculty of Medicine, University of Montréal*

JOHN R. WILLIAMS
*Department of Ethics and Legal Affairs
Canadian Medical Association*

BERNARD M. DICKENS
*Faculty of Law
Faculty of Medicine
Centre for Bioethics
University of Toronto*

Prentice Hall Canada Inc.

Canadian Cataloguing in Publication Data
Roy, David J., 1937-
Bioethics in Canada
ISBN 0-13-328097-7
1. Bioethics - Canada. I. Williams, John R.
(John Reynold), 1942- . II. Dickens, Bernard M.,
1937- . III. Title.
R724.R68 1994 174'.9574 C93-094565-4

Prentice-Hall, Inc., Englewood Cliffs, New Jersey
Prentice-Hall International (UK) Limited, London
Prentice-Hall of Australia, Pty. Limited, Sydney
Prentice-Hall Hispanoamericana, S.A., Mexico City
Prentice-Hall of India Private Limited, New Delhi
Prentice-Hall of Japan, Inc., Tokyo
Simon & Schuster Asia Private Limited, Singapore
Editora Prentice-Hall do Brasil, Ltda., Rio de Janeiro

ISBN 0-13-328097-7

Acquisitions Editor: Marjorie Munroe
Developmental Editor: Lisa Penttilä
Production Editor: William Booth
Production Coordinator: Sharon Houston
Cover Design: Olena Serbyn
Page Layout: Jerry Langton

23 24 25 DPC 07 06 05

Printed and bound in Canada

Every reasonable effort has been made to obtain permissions
for all articles and data used in this edition. If errors or
omissions have occurred, they will be corrected in future
editions provided written notification has been received by the
publisher.

Contents

PREFACE

This book is written primarily for undergraduate students taking bioethics courses in health care programmes, including medicine, nursing, dentistry and health administration, in law, and in the social sciences and humanities, especially philosophy and religious studies. It discusses the principal ethical issues faced by professionals in these disciplines, and by patients and family members.

There are many different approaches to bioethics. The one that we take in this book has the following characteristics:

- It is primarily *descriptive* and *analytical*. We present the relevant scientific, medical, legal and ethical data on each issue in such a way that the strengths and weaknesses of the major competing positions on the issue are clearly identified. We generally do not argue for one position against the others.

- It is *pluralist*. We acknowledge the diversity of ethical viewpoints in a country such as Canada. On most issues we distinguish between *personal* ethics, *public* ethics and *social* ethics. We argue that different approaches to contentious issues should be respected as much as possible, although sometimes the requirements of an institution or of society will result in a limitation of personal freedom. For example, euthanasia may be justifiable on a personal level in some cases, but that does not necessarily mean that it should be tolerated in a particular hospital, or by society in general, for instance through the law.

- It is *historical*. Although the emphasis in this book is on the contemporary state of the bioethics debate, we contend that the present can only be understood if we know what happened in the past. All bioethical issues, even those that arise from new developments in medical technology, must be considered within their social context, and this context has a particular history, which varies from one country to another.

- It is *Canadian*. This book discusses the bioethical issues that arise within, and are determined by, the health care system of this country. This system is, in turn, the product of Canadian culture, broadly understood. It is governed by legislation passed by the federal and provincial/territorial governments, and by the decisions of our courts. It incorporates several important cultural features that distinguish Canada from other countries, such as a peculiar, and precarious, balance between centralized authority and decentralized decision-making, and a commitment to equal treatment of all citizens in need of health care, while respecting their ethnic and linguistic differences. The book also emphasizes the contributions of Canadian authors, organizations and courts to the discussion of bioethical issues.

Our approach to bioethics is developed more fully in the first five chapters of the book, which provide essential background information for the discussion of specific issues that makes up the major part of the text. Each of the remaining chapters deals with one important bioethical issue, or set of related issues.

The many chapters of this book, though covering the most diverse of issues, are bound together by a single central question; a question emerging inevitably from the history of science in this century — a century that has demonstrated the intimate link between scientific knowledge and technological power. The three major scientific revolutions of this century — in physics, in information and computer science, and in molecular biology — have delivered greater technological power into the hands of human beings than the scientific activity of all the other centuries combined. The central ethical question of this book is: how can we maintain democracy and civilization, when great and innovative power is bound into the knowledge upon which everyone depends and only the few possess?

We would have been unable to write this book without the superb administrative support of Electa Baril; the painstaking manuscript preparation and reference verification of Susan Lebel; the documentary assistance of Carole Marcotte; the persistent literature search and retrieval of Richard Carpentier, Louis Chauvin, Elizabeth Brown, and Lynn Pierce; the journal-managing skill of Suzanne St-Amour that gave one of us (DJR) sufficient free time to work on this book. To all these persons, our warmest thanks.

We also express our appreciation to Dr. Laurent Larouche, University of Sudbury, Ontario for inviting two of us (DJR, JRW) several years ago to prepare a distance course for his college. That invitation led to the idea of this book.

That we could write this book at all is greatly due to the steady financial support of one of the Center for Bioethics' most generous benefactors, who prefers to remain unnamed. We express our thanks publicly.

DJR
JRW
BMD

P A R T 1

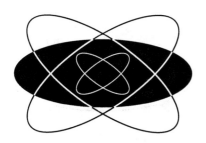

FRAMEWORK

1

BIOETHICS: PAST AND PRESENT

Bioethics today is a "growth industry." There are courses offered in philosophy and religious studies departments and faculties of medicine and nursing in almost every university in Canada and the United States. At least fifteen research centres have been established in Canada, to investigate bioethical problems and offer advice to policy makers and practitioners in the health field. Every institution that carries out medical research has a research ethics committee, to evaluate project proposals according to established standards of ethical behaviour. An increasing number of Canadian hospitals are setting up clinical ethics committees, to prepare policy documents and give advice to patients, families, physicians, nurses and other health professionals on ethical aspects of medical care. Legislatures and courts are having to deal more and more with legal problems in health care. And the media have discovered that there is tremendous public interest in such bioethical issues as abortion, the reproductive technologies, organ transplantation and euthanasia.

The extent of this activity is all the more remarkable if we consider that, twenty-five years ago, the word *bioethics* did not exist. It was only in 1971 that this term first appeared, in the title of a book by the American physician, Van Rensselaer Potter. The book was *Bioethics: Bridge to the Future*, and in it Potter states:

"I ... propose the term *Bioethics* in order to emphasize the two most important ingredients in achieving the new wisdom that is so desperately needed: biological knowledge and human values" (p. 2). Although Potter's own use of the term pointed in the direction of what is now called environmental or ecological ethics, the word "bioethics" quickly became identified with all academic and professional efforts to address the ethical issues posed by developments in the biological sciences, and their application to medical practice.

Despite the novelty of the term *bioethics*, its roots reach far back into history. For more than two thousand years, the ethical aspects of medical practice have been subjected to close scrutiny by physicians, philosophers, and religious scholars and authorities. To a large extent, modern bioethics is only the latest phase in the development of this reflection. However, just as the practice of medicine has been drastically altered by recent developments in scientific research and technology, as well as by significant changes in society and the economy, so too has ethics had to expand its horizon and deal with problems that were never even imagined in previous times.

Modern bioethics, therefore, is a combination of the old and the new. Much recent bioethics literature tends to emphasize the latter and neglect the former. We are convinced that this is a mistake; those who ignore history not only deprive themselves of the wisdom of past generations, but also fail to appreciate the deep roots of cultural attitudes towards health, sickness, suffering and death that influence, often very subtly, bioethical discussion and debate on specific issues. Consequently, we begin this book with a brief history of ethics in medicine, and in subsequent chapters we provide an historical perspective wherever it is relevant.

The plan of this chapter is as follows: first we will present an overview of how ethical issues in medicine were dealt with before the rise of modern bioethics in the 1960s; next we will describe the major factors in the emergence of bioethics; we will then examine the principal manifestations of bioethics in institutional, legal and academic settings; the following section will analyse these developments in terms of a challenge and response; and finally, a brief conclusion will introduce Chapter 2.

THE ROOTS OF MODERN BIOETHICS

Every culture has had to deal with ethical problems related to the practice of medicine. In this chapter, we shall focus on the discussion of these issues in North America and Western Europe (the "Western world"). We shall examine three types of ethical analysis which, in one way or another, have influenced the development of modern bioethics. These are: medical ethics, philosophical ethics and religious ethics.

Medical Ethics

Medical ethics can be defined as the study of physician morality; that is, the behaviour and decision-making of physicians in their relations with patients, other physicians, other health care workers, and society in general. The best-known person in the history of Western medical ethics is undoubtedly Hippocrates, a Greek physician who is believed to have lived in the fifth century B.C.E.[1] Little is known about his personal life. However, from the fourth century B.C.E. onwards, he was regarded as the author of numerous treatises on medical practice, as well as the famous Hippocratic Oath. The latter is widely regarded as the foundation of Western medical ethics. It consists of four parts: (a) a preamble, which includes the actual swearing of the oath; (b) a covenant, which mentions the duties of medical students to their teachers, and their obligations regarding the transmission of medical knowledge to others; (c) the ethical code, which involves, among other things, prohibitions against dispensing poisons, performing abortions, having sexual relations with patients, and revealing to others details of a patient's private life; and (d) a prayer, wherein speakers express their hope that they will be rewarded for keeping the oath (Carrick 1985, 69-70). This oath, somewhat revised, is regarded even today as one of the foundational statements for the ethical practice of medicine.

For many centuries, the teachings of Hippocrates were not widely followed by physicians in the Greek and Roman empires. The practice of medicine was not regulated, either by physicians themselves or by the state. There were no medical schools and no licensure; potential physicians either learned their craft from someone else or were self-taught, and they were free to practise where and how they wished. The standards of medical ethics, as enunciated by Hippocrates and others, such as Galen (second century C.E.), were ideals, not requirements.

Despite this "do-it-yourself" character of ancient medicine, the role of the physician gradually acquired a certain uniformity, as medicine developed into a profession. This movement began around the beginning of the Christian era. At first, its major stimulants were the teachings of Hippocrates and of Stoic philosophers. Several centuries later, it was greatly influenced by Christianity. During the Middle Ages (approximately 500-1500 C.E.) the Hippocratic ideals were combined with Christian teachings to provide a basic ethics for physicians, which consisted of virtues that medical practitioners should possess and rules for their interactions with patients (MacKinney, 1977, 200-201).

The religious domination of medical ethics lasted until the sixteenth century, when the breakup of Christianity into Protestant and Catholic denominations allowed physicians the freedom to devise their own rules for professional

---

[1] B.C.E. is an abbreviation of "Before the Common Era." It is used in place of B.C. (Before Christ), in order not to offend non-Christians. Similarly, C.E. refers to the Common Era, which Christians identify with A.D. or *Anno Domini* ("In the Year of the Lord").

behaviour. By this time, the medical profession had been organized into guilds and other associations: these were accorded certain privileges by civil or ecclesiastical authorities, in exchange for their maintenance of high standards of competence and ethics. In England, the guilds of physicians and barber-surgeons eventually gave way to the Royal College of Physicians (1518), the United Company of Barbers and Surgeons (1540), the Apothecaries Society (1617), and the Royal College of Surgeons (1800). Similar institutions emerged in Scotland and Ireland. Instead of allowing church authorities, theologians and philosophers to set ethical standards for them, physicians themselves increasingly began to take over the field of medical ethics.

In the eighteenth and nineteenth centuries, the writings of the British physicians John Gregory (1724-1773) and Thomas Percival (1740-1840), especially the latter's *Medical Ethics* of 1803, provided the field with systematic interpretations of medical morality from the physician's point of view. Percival's book served as the basis of various codes of medical ethics, including the one adopted in 1847 by the newly formed American Medical Association. The Canadian Medical Association adopted an almost identical code one year after its establishment in 1867 (Burns, 1978). These codes, and other writings of physicians on ethics, displayed relatively little knowledge of, or interest in, ethics as a philosophical or theological discipline. They dealt primarily with practical matters, and their precepts were usually derived from common sense (the physicians' version) rather than by any explicit reasoning process.

During the nineteenth century, Henri Dunant created the Red Cross organization and a new health care profession, nursing, began to emerge. A decisive step in its development was the establishment by Florence Nightingale of the first school of nursing, at St. Thomas' Hospital in London, England. The British approach to professional training of nurses spread to many other countries, and in 1899 the International Council of Nurses (ICN) was formed. Nine years later, in 1908, the Canadian Nurses Association (CNA) was established. Although these groups were concerned with ethical issues from early on, many years passed before they adopted a code of ethics (1953 for the ICN; 1954 for the CNA). In the meantime, a number of books had appeared, which dealt with nursing ethics. Most of these were written for, rather than by, nurses; Catholic moral theologians figured prominently among the authors.

During the first half of the twentieth century, medical ethics remained under the domination of physicians. The codes of ethics of the Canadian and American Medical Associations underwent periodical revisions, but they continued to represent the point of view of the medical profession, rather than those of other health care professionals and patients. It was only in the 1960s that this situation began to change, as medical ethics was faced with a formidable competitor, in the form of bioethics.

Philosophical Ethics

The second principal influence on modern bioethics is philosophical ethics. The interest of philosophy in the ethical aspects of medical practice extends back at least as far as Aristotle, the last of the great trio of Athenian philosophers, whose other members were Socrates and Plato. Aristotle, who lived from 384-322 B.C.E., distinguished two types of knowledge: theoretical (e.g., geometry) and practical. The latter is further divided into technical knowledge (how to do things, such as fixing a broken table) and prudence or practical wisdom (the Greek term is *phronesis*). Ethics is an exercise of this practical wisdom. It requires the use of judgment in the application of general principles to specific cases. The task of the ethicist is "to show what kinds of procedures reasonable human beings use in facing problems, exchanging opinions, advancing relevant considerations and arriving at well-argued resolutions of their problems...." (Jonsen, 1988, 72). Although Aristotle's practical understanding of ethics did not receive immediate acceptance, and for many centuries was overshadowed by Plato's more theoretical approach, it did emerge into prominence in thirteenth-century Europe and was one of the dominant ethical theories for several hundred years.

Like medical ethics, philosophy was overshadowed by religion during the Middle Ages, and only began to regain its independence after the Protestant Reformation. During the seventeenth and eighteenth centuries, the religious foundations of Western culture and civilization began to crumble. Religious authority, now seriously divided within Christianity among Protestants and Catholics, was rejected by many of the intelligentsia in favour of the authority of human *reason*, and philosophers began to challenge theologians as the champions of truth. It soon became evident, however, that "reasonable" individuals, including philosophers, could not agree on moral issues, and the Western world gradually became accustomed to ethical pluralism.

The Enlightenment, a European intellectual movement based on the supremacy of human reason, which lasted from about 1650 to 1800, had important consequences for medical ethics. First of all, the religious basis for determining appropriate conduct in medical matters was rejected in favour of a rational, and especially a "professional," standard, the latter meaning that an action is morally right if it is how physicians usually act. Secondly, philosophers began to desert the field of practical ethics, including medical ethics, in favour of ethical *theory*, which they considered to be a more worthy object of rational inquiry.

This preoccupation of philosophers with theory lasted well into the twentieth century. They were more concerned with clarifying issues than deciding them, and they concentrated on defining terms such as "value," "right," "good," etc., establishing rules for argumentation, and debating the relative merits of ethical systems, such as utilitarianism, deontology, and intuitionalism.

According to Stephen Toulmin, by the 1960s "the central concerns of the philosophers had become so abstract and general — above all, so definitional or analytical — that they had, in effect, lost all touch with the concrete and particular issues that arise in actual practice, whether in medicine or elsewhere" (Toulmin, 1982, 749). For philosophers to play a role in the development of bioethics, they had to reject this approach to ethics in favour of the Aristotelian concern with practical reasoning, a movement which was not to begin until the late 1960s.

Religious Ethics

The third main source of Western medical ethics is the biblical-faith traditions of Jews and Christians. Although these two religions came to differ in many respects, their approaches to moral behaviour and decision-making had much in common in the first few centuries of the common era. They both taught that the overriding criterion for determining right from wrong is the will of God, as revealed in the Scriptures and interpreted by religious authorities. Whereas for Greek philosophy, virtue was to be determined by *reason*, for Jews and Christians virtue was first and foremost *obedience* to God's will.

Christians and Jews also differed from the Greeks on many specific moral issues. The former valued individual human life very highly, and condemned infanticide, abortion and non-procreative sexual practices. They also believed in the fundamental moral equality of all human beings, which entailed an obligation to assist the poor and otherwise disadvantaged.

Although the Bible contains no medical ethics as such, it does teach that all that occurs on earth, including sickness and disease, is under God's control. Prayer and trust in God, by both the patient and the physician, are important elements in the care of the sick. But God makes use of human efforts to implement his will, and so the knowledge, skill and devotion of physicians are necessary for health care. Physicians and other caregivers are required to practise their art for the good of others and not just for themselves, since they are engaged in a fundamentally religious endeavour — the care of the sick.

While Christianity was becoming the dominant religion in Europe, Islam was spreading even more rapidly, from its source in Arabia both west and north around the Mediterranean and eastwards into Asia. From its earliest years, Islam devoted considerable attention to medicine, including both the physical and the spiritual dimensions of health care. Muslims were several centuries ahead of Christians in establishing medical schools and writing textbooks and treatises on medical subjects, including ethics. The principal authority for Islamic medical morality was Hippocrates, and it was usual for the Hippocratic oath to be sworn by doctors beginning their practice. Muslim scholars, such as Ibn Sina (980-1037), wrote treatises on philosophy and medicine which were greatly influenced by the ancient Greeks and which, in turn, were widely used by Christian thinkers in Europe as sources for their own teachings on medicine, ethics and philosophy.

Although Jews were a small minority in Muslim and Christian territories during the Middle Ages, they made important contributions to the development of medical ethics. Unlike the followers of other religions, Jews never adopted the Hippocratic Oath. They relied instead on the teachings of the Bible, and especially on rabbinic interpretations of these teachings (*responsa*) for guidance on how to behave, in medical matters as in other areas of life. The most influential Jewish teacher in the Middle Ages was Moses Maimonides (1135-1204). A physician as well as a philosopher and legal scholar, he was the author of ten medical works, in addition to an important summary of Jewish law.

Throughout the Middle Ages, many Christian teachers used the writings of Hippocrates, along with those of Muslim and Jewish scholars, as the basis of their medical ethics. They saw no conflict between these writings and their own religious beliefs. As moral theology began to flourish in the twelfth and thirteenth centuries, under the leadership of such famous scholars as Peter Abelard and Thomas Aquinas, the practical norms of Hippocrates were given considerable theoretical explanation and justification. Aquinas addressed such issues as whether the physician is morally obliged to treat the poor without charge (his answer was "yes," if the patient would die without treatment) and whether euthanasia is sometimes acceptable ("no").

More important than the answers to specific questions that Aquinas provided was the *method* of ethical reflection that he helped to develop. Following Aristotle, he emphasized the practical character of ethics and the need to exercise judgment in applying general moral rules (such as "thou shalt not kill") to particular cases and issues (e.g., capital punishment and self-defence). Aquinas argued that this approach to ethical decision-making was consistent with the Bible, but other Christian authorities and scholars felt that he was allowing too much liberty to individual conscience, and that obedience to the rules of the Church was the best way to make moral decisions.

The method of Aquinas was further developed from the fourteenth to the eighteenth centuries, and became known as *casuistry*, or the study of cases. Casuistry proved very useful to Catholic priests in the sacrament of confession, where they had to determine whether certain actions were sinful or not. Since physicians and patients sought guidance on the moral acceptability of various medical procedures, casuistry played an important role in the development of Catholic medical ethics during this period.

The above-mentioned rejection of religion in favour of reason by Enlightenment thinkers led to a rejection of reason in favour of faith by many religious authorities; in the Catholic church this resulted in the demise of casuistry and a resurgence of ethical authoritarianism, in which difficult ethical issues were resolved not by the individuals concerned, but by bishops or the Pope. In many Protestant churches the result was Biblical fundamentalism, which held that the answers to all moral problems could be found somewhere in the Bible.

In contrast to philosophers, religious scholars and officials never abandoned the world of practical issues in favour of a preoccupation with ethical theory. Throughout the nineteenth and twentieth centuries, there was a continuing interest in medical ethics among religious scholars, especially Roman Catholics. In North America, Catholic moral theologians worked closely with health care professionals to prepare ethical directives for church-affiliated health care institutions. The U.S. Catholic Hospital Association issued such a document in 1949; a Canadian equivalent appeared in 1955. Theologians also published numerous books and articles on medical ethics, and offered courses on ethics in Catholic university medical and nursing schools (McFadden 1946; Kelly 1949; Ford 1964). During the 1950s, there were stirrings of interest in this field in other religious traditions. The American Protestant theologian, Joseph Fletcher, published a book entitled *Morals and Medicine* in 1954, and Rabbi Immanuel Jakobovits's *Jewish Medical Ethics* appeared in 1959. Although these books were to exercise considerable influence on the later development of bioethics, they lacked some of the identifying characteristics of bioethics, as will be discussed in the next chapter, especially applicability in non-religious settings.

At the beginning of the 1960s, there were signs that a new wave of interest in medical ethics might be approaching. But no one could have predicted what was to happen in this field during that decade, much less what has taken place since then. A bioethics revolution is well and truly underway; we do not know when it is going to end, but in what follows we will see how it began.

THE EMERGENCE OF MODERN BIOETHICS

The transition from traditional medical ethics, largely the preserve of physicians, to the new field of bioethics, in which physicians are only one group of participants, along with other health care professionals, patients and their families, theologians, philosophers, social scientists, lawyers, judges, and legislators, occurred largely within a single decade, beginning in the mid-1960s. The major factors that brought about this virtual revolution in ethics can be classified under two headings: medical/technological and societal.

Medical Science and Technology

During the 1960s, rapid advances were made in the understanding and treatment of a broad range of diseases that hitherto were untreatable. One of the first ethical issues to be faced by researchers was the use of human subjects for testing their new discoveries. Many of the new pharmaceuticals turned out to be of great benefit to humankind (e.g., vaccines for polio and other diseases, and oral contraceptives). Others produced disastrous results in some patients (e.g., thalidomide caused serious birth defects when taken by pregnant women). Often, the only way to determine the effects of new drugs was to test them on humans. In 1966, a Harvard Medical School professor, Henry Beecher, published an article that described numerous abuses in human experimentation (Beecher, 1966). As a result, the scientific community and regulatory bodies were called upon to examine closely the ethical questions raised by medical experimentation, and to produce detailed regulations for protecting research subjects from harm (Rothman, 1991).

Once treatments were proven to be effective, a further ethical problem sometimes had to be resolved. When first approved, some treatments were in very short supply, and not all patients in need could be accommodated. An early example was the kidney dialysis machine, which, when first introduced in the 1960s, provided life-saving treatment for patients with terminal kidney failure. However, there were not nearly enough machines to service all patients with this disease, and so it was necessary to establish procedures for choosing which patients would receive the treatment and which would be left to die. Similar decisions had to be made for access to other scarce medical resources, such as organs for transplantation.

The development of transplantation technology raised a further ethical issue. The removal of organs from recently deceased persons required a new definition of death, since by the time death could be verified according to the traditional definition ("the permanent cessation of breathing and blood circulation"), the organs of the deceased would no longer be suitable for transplantation. The process of redefining death, which has occupied medical researchers, ethicists and legislators since the late 1960s, is just one example of how developments in medical technology have produced significant changes in how we think about life, death, health and sickness.

One important, and unintended, result of medical progress in the 1960s was a breakdown of the traditional physician-patient relationship. Both doctors and health care institutions became increasingly more specialized, in order to cope with the rapid growth of medical knowledge, and in the process they began to lose their familiarity to patients. As doctors became strangers and hospitals strange places, they gradually lost the confidence of many of their patients. There developed a widespread feeling that doctors needed to be regulated, in order to protect patients from thoughtless or unscrupulous behaviour. Medical ethics itself became suspect, because it was controlled by physicians. It seemed to be in need of radical change, which would involve, at the very least, greater participation by non-physicians in determining the rules for medical research and practice.

Societal Changes

The 1960s were a period, not only of rapid scientific progress, but also of enormous social change in the Western world. Three indicators of change are of particular relevance for the development of bioethics: moral pluralism, the human rights movement, and attitudes towards death.

The so-called "sexual revolution" of the 1960s is just one example of the breakdown of the traditional social, legal and religious consensus regarding moral standards in most Western countries. At the same time as medical technology was providing the means to greater sexual freedom — the birth-control pill and other contraceptive devices — legislators were removing legal barriers to the exercise of this freedom by reforming laws restricting divorce, contraception, and abortion. The close relationship between sexuality and medical practice meant that physicians, nurses and other health care professionals were faced with such ethical issues as how to respond to requests for contraceptives and abortion, and when to respect confidentiality in these matters, especially for adolescents.

The 1960s and 1970s saw a great increase in concern for individual rights on a wide range of issues. One manifestation of this concern was the consumer movement, which rejected the traditional approach of "Let the buyer beware" in the relationship between manufacturers (especially the automobile companies) and purchasers. Under pressure from consumer groups, governments passed consumer protection legislation in many countries. This movement soon turned its attention to the field of health care, where its opponents were not only large corporations (in this case, especially the drug companies), but also hospitals and the medical profession. The tradition of medical paternalism, or "doctor knows best and patients should do what they are told," came under serious criticism as consumers of health care began to assert their claim to decision-making authority in matters affecting their own persons. The ethical arguments for patient autonomy were supported by important legal judgments in Canada and the U.S.A., all of which provided bioethics with a fresh new approach to the ethical issues in the physician-patient relationship.

The third major societal factor in the development of bioethics was a radical shift in attitudes towards death in the Western world, particularly in North America. For much of the twentieth century, death had been avoided in medical education and practice. Physicians were taught to conquer death, and when this was not possible, as in the vast majority of cancer patients, they tended to deny the reality of death, by refusing to tell patients the truth about their condition and by avoiding dying patients altogether. This denial of death was mirrored throughout society in many ways: very few people died at home; funeral practices, especially embalming, attempted to disguise the fact of death; and common language employed euphemisms such as "pass away" and "the departed" in place of "die" and "the dead."

In the late 1960s, two woman physicians were largely responsible for bringing about a more positive attitude towards death in Western society. In England, Dr. Cecily Sanders began the modern palliative care movement, which emphasizes *care* rather than *cure* of terminally ill patients. In the U.S.A., Dr. Elizabeth Kübler-Ross introduced medical students and then the general public to a new understanding of the special needs of dying patients. With death becoming a socially respectable topic, the door was opened for a rapid increase in public and professional attention devoted to the many ethical issues in the care of dying persons, such as the termination of treatment for seriously ill newborns, the application of "do not resuscitate" orders, and euthanasia.

THE MANIFESTATIONS OF MODERN BIOETHICS

Institutional Responses

To provide answers to the many ethical questions that arose from all these changes in medicine and society, a wide range of organizations has been established or remandated during the past two decades. These include bioethics research centres, public commissions, professional associations, and international groups.

Bioethics Research Centres

In 1969, The Institute of Society, Ethics and the Life Sciences was established in the small town of Hastings-on-Hudson, NY, not far from New York City. Now known as The Hastings Center, its purpose is to study and make recommendations on a wide variety of bioethical issues, with input from many different professions and academic disciplines. Two years later, the Kennedy Institute of Ethics was established at Georgetown University in Washington, DC. In addition to research, it offers a graduate programme in bioethics and shorter courses for teachers and health care professionals. In 1976, the Clinical Research Institute of Montréal created the Center for Bioethics, the first in Canada. These three centres have been joined by many others during the past two decades, including fifteen in Canada and a large number in Europe, Australia, and several other countries. Together they represent a major resource for the research, publication, and teaching activities of bioethics, which have expanded exponentially during this period.

Public Commissions

When governments are faced with difficult bioethical issues, they often appoint public commissions to study the issues and make recommendations for their resolution. One of the first such bodies was the U.S. National Commission for the Protection of Human Subjects of Biomedical and Behavioral Research, which operated from 1974 to 1978, and produced reports on numerous aspects of research with human subjects. In 1978, a new American organization, the President's Commission for the Study of Ethical Problems in Medicine and Biomedical and Behavioral Research, was created to continue and expand the work of its predecessor. By the time it was wound up in 1983, it had published reports on many contentious bioethical questions, including the definition of death, decisions to forgo life-sustaining treatment, genetic experimentation, and access to health care.

In Canada, there have been at least thirty commission inquiries into bioethical issues since 1970 (Williams, 1989). Some of these were created by the federal or provincial governments to study particular issues, such as the non-medical use of drugs, the workings of the 1969 abortion law, and the new reproductive technologies. After making their reports, these bodies cease to exist. There have also been some longer-serving commissions, such as federal and provincial Law Reform Commissions, which have dealt with a series of issues related to bioethics. Many of their reports are discussed in other chapters of this book.

Numerous other countries have used public commissions to help formulate policies on bioethical issues. In France, a National Ethics Consultative Committee for the Life and Health Sciences was formed in 1983. Its purpose is to give advice on bioethical issues and to educate politicians, health professionals and the general public about these matters. In Australia, Great Britain and Germany, national and state commissions have studied the ethical and legal aspects of the new reproductive technologies. In Japan, the national government has recently set up a special research committee for brain death and organ transplantation. It is likely that this approach to dealing with bioethical issues will continue to be favoured, especially by governments.[2]

Professional Associations

The rise of modern bioethics has convinced many physicians that their traditional approach to dealing with ethical issues in medicine is no longer adequate. As a result, many of their professional associations have established or remandated committees to examine these issues and to recommend new ways of dealing with them. In Canada, the Royal College of Physicians and Surgeons of

---

[2] A useful source of information and analysis of many national commissions is the special issue on "Bioethics Commissions: International Perspectives" of *The Journal of Medicine and Philosophy* 1989;14/4.

Canada created a Biomedical Ethics Committee in 1977. It has organized symposia and produced numerous discussion papers for the membership of the College, which includes all medical specialists in this country. The Canadian Medical Association recently expanded its ethics activities by setting up a Department of Ethics and Legal Affairs, staffed by a professional ethicist and two lawyers. The staff assists the Association's Ethics Committee in preparing position papers on ethical issues for Canadian doctors. Certain medical specialty societies, such as the Canadian Paediatric Society, the Canadian Andrology and Fertility Society and the Society of Obstetricians and Gynaecologists of Canada, as well as the College of Family Physicians of Canada, have committees for dealing with the bioethical issues that are specific to their members' practice.

In the U.S.A., the American Medical Association has a Council on Ethical and Judicial Affairs, which publishes occasional "current opinions" on important bioethical issues. As in Canada, certain U.S. medical specialist organizations, such as the American Academy of Pediatrics, have their own bioethics committees. The British Medical Association and the Royal College of Physicians are two physicians' organizations in the U.K. that are active in the field of bioethics, and there is increasing interest in this field among comparable groups in other countries.

Since 1970, many national and provincial associations of nurses have examined how developments in medicine and society present them with ethical dilemmas in the course of their work. The Canadian Nurses Association revised its *Code of Ethics* in 1973, 1980, 1985 and 1991, in response to changes in the role of the nurse, vis-à-vis doctors on the one hand and patients on the other. The Québec government enacted a *Code of Ethics* for the Québec Nursing Association in 1976, and the College of Nurses of Ontario adopted its *Guidelines for Ethical Behaviour in Nursing* in 1980. These documents reflected the increasing professionalization of Canadian nurses, who were no longer content to function as doctors' servants. Many nurses began to see themselves as advocates for patients, especially for those whose rights were being infringed by paternalistic physicians or faceless hospital bureaucrats.

Another profession that has started to deal with bioethical issues is hospital administration. During the 1980s, the Canadian Hospital Association, which brings together hospital administrators and trustees to promote the interests of their institutions, identified bioethics as one of its top priorities. The development of hospital ethics committees was a particular concern. Another Canadian organization of health administrators, the Canadian College of Health Service Executives, adopted in 1991 a new set of *Standards of Ethical Conduct for Health Service Executives*, which are designed to eliminate conflict-of-interest situations and ensure that ethical values are respected throughout health care institutions.

In addition to the organizations whose membership is limited to a single profession or medical specialty, there are numerous interdisciplinary associations in the field of bioethics. In Canada, two such groups were created in 1986: the Canadian Society for Medical Bioethics, which was supported by several physicians' organizations, and the Canadian Society of Bioethics, which included members from a broad range of disciplines and professions. In 1988, these groups joined together to form the Canadian Bioethics Society.

International Groups

Since many bioethical issues are not limited to national boundaries, a number of international organizations have begun to exchange information and set general standards for ethical behaviour in medicine and the life sciences. The Council for International Organizations of Medical Sciences, which was established jointly by the World Health Organization and UNESCO in 1949, has produced numerous reports on issues related to experimentation with human subjects and, more recently, with animals. The World Medical Association, an international physicians' organization, has likewise dealt with varied topics in bioethics, and has prepared an international code of ethics for doctors everywhere.

In Europe, the Council of Europe has been dealing with bioethical issues through a Committee of Experts on Progress in the Biomedical Sciences, consisting of up to three representatives from each member country (scientist, jurist and ethicist). Its recommendations for common European standards on such issues as genetic engineering and the reproductive technologies have been considered by the Council's Committee of Ministers and by the European Parliament. Another European organization in this field is the European Association of Centres of Medical Ethics, which brings together members from at least ten different countries to share information and resources.

Several other international associations of bioethicists have been established or are in the planning stages. These developments provide convincing evidence that bioethics has become a major institutional force within the world of medical science and practice.

Legal Dimensions

Since its beginnings in the 1960s, modern bioethics has been closely associated with the law. In this section we will review some of the major legal events of the past twenty years that have greatly influenced bioethical reflection. The two main initiators of these legal activities have been the courts and legislatures.

Courts

The United States is undoubtedly the world leader in the legalization and the judicialization of medical practice. When disputes arise, Americans seem to have an innate tendency to seek a decision in the courts. The 1973 U.S. Supreme Court decision in the case of *Roe v. Wade* established a legal standard for abortion in that country, and thereby framed the subsequent debate over the morality of this act. The case of Karen Ann Quinlan, which was considered by two New Jersey courts in 1976, oriented all future reflection on the ethics of withdrawing treatment from terminally ill or permanently unconscious patients. Many other bioethical issues have been influenced by U.S. court decisions, including informed consent, confidentiality, surrogate motherhood, and the treatment of severely handicapped newborns.

In other countries, there has been much less recourse to the courts in matters of medical research and practice. Nevertheless, in some jurisdictions there have been legal decisions which, as in the U.S.A., exercise a significant influence on bioethics. In Canada, the Supreme Court has issued judgments on sterilization of mentally handicapped women, abortion and informed consent. In England, there have been decisions on informed consent, birth control for minors, sterilization of mentally handicapped women, and withholding of life-saving treatment for handicapped children. It remains to be seen whether the pace of litigation in these countries will increase under the influence of the U.S.A., or whether other ways of dealing with disputes will prevail.

Legislation

The second principal means of legal influence on bioethics is through legislation, which is a product of the political process of law-making. Here again, the U.S.A. has been very active, especially in the state assemblies. American legislators have shown a great interest in medical issues, and have introduced proposals for laws to govern a wide range of practices, from abortion to the determination of death. Some initiatives, such as those that would legalize active euthanasia, have never been accepted, but many others, including those that regulate abortion and the determination of death, are in effect now, and new ones are constantly being introduced.

In Canada, legislators have shown a great reluctance to deal with laws regulating health care. Abortion is one of the very few bioethical issues that have been the subject of federal legislation during the past twenty years. The proposals of the former federal Law Reform Commission for new laws concerning the definition of death, euthanasia, and protection of human research subjects have been neglected by successive federal governments. Provincial governments have been equally reluctant to enter this field, when it is within their constitutional power to do so, with the remarkable exception of Québec which, as far back as 1971, legislated in the *Civil Code* on research on human beings and on disposal of human tissues and organs.

Outside North America, legislation is generally a more acceptable means of regulating bioethical disputes than is recourse to the courts. Most countries have abortion laws, and many others have recently introduced, or are considering, legislation to deal with other bioethical issues, such as the protection of human research subjects, assisted reproduction, organ transplantation, living wills and euthanasia. As noted above, there is an active movement, especially in Europe, to standardize the laws of various countries on such matters in accordance with universal human rights.

Academic Bioethics

In addition to its institutional and legal aspects, bioethics has also developed as a major academic enterprise. This is evident in two principal areas of academic activity: teaching, and research leading to publication.

Teaching

In the 1970s, courses in bioethics began to proliferate in university departments of religious studies and philosophy, and faculties of medicine and nursing. At first it was not easy to find qualified teachers for these courses, since the combination of expertise in both ethics and medical science was quite rare. Gradually, however, theologians and philosophers who specialized in ethics began to acquire a familiarity with medicine, and some physicians and nurses began to study ethics. As faculty resources increased and new courses were offered, students responded in great numbers, and soon courses in bioethics were among the most popular ones offered in philosophy and religious studies departments. The progress of such courses in medical and nursing faculties has been slower, due to the heavy emphasis on scientific and clinical knowledge and the lack of time in the curriculum for additional subjects. Nevertheless, most North American universities now offer instruction in bioethics to students in the health professions, at least at the undergraduate level (Williams, 1986). An increasing number of postgraduate programmes are being developed for health professionals, as well as for those with other backgrounds.

Research and Publication

As mentioned above, the first book with the word *bioethics* in its title was published in 1971. However, the previous year had seen the appearance of several important books in this field, including Paul Ramsey's *The Patient as Person* and Daniel Callahan's *Abortion: Law, Choice & Morality*. From that time on, there has been an exponential growth in the number of books, articles and reports in this field. The first journal devoted primarily to this subject, the *Hastings Center*

Report, started publication in 1971. By 1978, the field was sufficiently advanced to support a four-volume *Encyclopedia of Bioethics*. Numerous other journals and newsletters have appeared since then, as has the first computerized database for bioethics, *Bioethicsline*.

For many years, the writings in this field dealt primarily with issues and cases. The 1970s saw a proliferation of textbooks that treated a standard set of issues from abortion to euthanasia. During this decade, only a few topics, notably abortion, received individual attention in book-length monographs and collections of essays. During the 1980s, however, a large number of books were published on specific issues or areas of bioethics. These included discussions of specialized topics, such as the treatment of severely handicapped newborns, the new reproductive technologies, AIDS, and the medical care of elderly persons, as well as issues in particular areas of medicine, such as paediatrics and genetics. Many of these works are referred to in later units of this manual. The 1980s also saw the development of a large body of writings in nursing ethics.

As the 1980s progressed, the concentration on issues and cases proved unsatisfactory to some scholars in this field, because their work was not producing any resolution of contentious issues, such as abortion and active euthanasia. In order to understand the source of these enduring conflicts, these scholars began to investigate more closely the theoretical foundations of bioethics as a field of study and practice. For some of them, the result of this analysis was a return to the historical origins of Western civilization, namely Greek philosophy and Judaeo-Christian religion. The state of the current debate about the nature of bioethics will be discussed in Chapter 2.

Competition in Bioethics

The transition from traditional medical ethics to modern bioethics has been marked by a power struggle among disciplines and professions for control of the field. During the first six decades of the twentieth century, the only groups, besides doctors, who were interested in the ethical aspects of health care were nurses and theologians. As we have noted, each of these groups was active in the development of bioethics, which began in the 1960s. At the same time, the influence of physicians declined, as they came to realize that their approach to ethical issues was no longer adequate in the face of major changes in medical science and societal attitudes.

As bioethics rapidly developed into a major academic enterprise, it began to attract the participation of disciplines that had shown little interest before then, especially philosophy. During the 1960s, some philosophers reacted against the abstract focus of their discipline, and began to apply their skills to such emerging issues as human rights and the legitimacy of certain wars (especially American involvement in Vietnam). As more and more public attention became focused on problems in medical science and practice, it was natural for philosophical ethicists to take up these issues, especially since there was enormous interest on the part of the rapidly expanding student population at the time. So enthusiastically did philosophers embrace the newly emerging field of bioethics that they soon came to dominate it, at least in North America. Physicians and, to a lesser extent, nurses were made to feel that they were not qualified to analyse ethical issues that arise in their practice, precisely because these were *ethical* in nature, and therefore required an academic background in philosophical ethics for their resolution. Theologians, too, began to consider themselves inadequate in this field, unless they had philosophical training and did not allow their religious convictions to influence their approach to bioethical issues. In short, during the 1970s philosophers and philosophy rapidly took over bioethics in North America.

This state of affairs, however, was not to last. During the 1980s, members of the health care professions, especially physicians and nurses, began to reassert their claim to expertise and authority in regard to the ethical issues that affect members of their professions. Other disciplines, too, entered the field, notably law, sociology, anthropology, and even economics. The results of all this interest and involvement are mixed. On the one hand, there has been some competition for leadership, which can result in mutual suspicion and non-cooperation. On the other hand, there has emerged a widespread realization that bioethics is a truly interdisciplinary field, which requires the input and participation of all the relevant disciplines and professions if it is to succeed. Even where a cooperative attitude prevails, however, it is yet to be determined how the interdisciplinary character of bioethics can best be realized in practice.

BIOMEDICINE AND BIOETHICS: CHALLENGE AND RESPONSE

Arnold Toynbee, the famous historian, organized his account and interpretation of the rise and fall of civilizations in terms of challenge and response. The earliest civilizations sprang forth from the original responses some audacious peoples in primitive societies managed to mount against changes in the physical, geographical environment that threatened their habitual way of life. To survive and to thrive, they had to move, change their way of life, their often centuries-old way of life, or both. Later civilizations came into existence primarily out of responses to challenges from the human environment. When dominant minorities ceased to lead and became oppressive, people responded by breaking away from the failing civilization and founding a new one (Toynbee, 1947, 569-570).

The Late-Twentieth-Century Environmental Challenge

The events in the former Soviet Union, over the last decade or so, illustrate how a civilization can fail and fall apart when people are challenged to respond to autocratic and directionless governing minorities. People across the planet, late in this century, are also facing powerful environmental challenges to their habitats, to their ways of life, and some are now facing environmental challenges to their lives. One need only think for a moment of the thousands of people in Southern regions of the planet who die yearly, because they cannot mount adequate responses to the devastating challenges of drought, crop-failure, incompetent local governments, and exploitation of their resources by powerful corporations and states of the planet's Northern regions.

The environmental threats that challenged early peoples to mount civilization-building responses came from natural changes in the environment, such as those that followed upon the end of the Ice Age. The devastating environmental threats characteristic of this late period of our century, quite to the contrary, come from a continuing stream of provocations mounted by human beings against the environment. The human environment has become the major threat to the geographical environment. The current environmental threats to human life and to ways of life have been caused largely by the way industrial and technological activities have damaged, and are still damaging, local environments and the global ecology. This challenge to ecological integrity, coming from the human environment, is calling forth a human response in the form of a large and growing movement, the movement of environmental and ecological ethics. These are integral dimensions of bioethics, but are not the subject of this chapter or this book. However, we shall return briefly to the question of ecological ethics, when we examine the current limitations of bioethics later in this chapter.

The Biomedical Challenge

In this work, we centre attention on bioethics as a response to a related, but different, challenge. Like the late-twentieth-century threat to ecological integrity, the challenge upon which we concentrate now comes from the human environment. This challenge is ambivalent, because the activities and advances from which it arises present simultaneously both a threat to human integrity, and an emancipation from some of the suffering inherent in the human condition.

A new word, *biomedicine*, names the *source* of the challenge. This composite word mirrors the conjunction or close interaction of the biological sciences and medicine, and of biomedical science and technology. A new conjunction of deepening scientific insight into the nature of living things, and of growing technological power over life, came to the fore of public attention after research in the basic and clinical sciences of medicine, and especially in genetics, reproductive biology, molecular biology, and the neurosciences, began to expand and intensify in the decades following World War II.

To capture the *magnitude* of the challenge, authors warned that a *biomedical revolution* was underway. The term *revolution* suggested that biomedical advances would occasion major changes that would, in a relatively short time, potentially affect everyone. The biomedical technologies, unlike the technologies with which people were familiar in industry — physics, chemistry, engineering, and electronics — would deliver power to modify components of the human organism — from genes to brain — and not only power over objects external to human beings themselves. Human nature, then, would fall within the *scope* of the biomedical challenge.

The biomedical challenge is many-faceted. The *ambivalence* of the challenge appears in frequently used couplings of words, such as "peril and promise," "glory and threat," "dangers and benefits" of the biomedical sciences and technologies. P.B. Medawar, the Nobel-laureate immunologist, said that the great glory and the great threat of science is that everything that is, in principle, possible can be done, if the intention to do it is strong enough. He thought that scientists tended to stress the glory of science, and ordinary people, mid-way in the twentieth century generally cowered at the threat of science. (Medawar, 1990, 15)

Bioethics: The Response

However, we are no longer in the middle of the twentieth century, a moment when Medawar's words may have held true. As we enter the last decade of this century, so-called ordinary people are much less likely to cower at the threat of science, and scientists are much more at the forefront of critical reflection on science since the rise of bioethics two decades ago. People have awakened to the challenge to devise alternatives to the notion that power is its own ethics.

The challenge of the biomedical revolution is directed to the foundational beliefs and values of a society. Should everything that is, in principle, scientifically possible be done, or even tried, if these projects were to bring into question human heredity, human reproduction, and human integrity? Yet, the projects also promise remedies for ancient unconquered sufferings. Both the promises and the perils of the biomedical sciences and technologies are powerful, new, and deeply ambiguous. Where should limits be set on what should be done or tried, among all the new things that are, day by day, becoming scientifically possible? The answer is not immediately obvious, but it soon became quite clear that the issues emerging from the biomedical challenge are not just a set of moral puzzles that can be solved by the traditional deductive modes of moral reasoning.

The more recent roots of contemporary bioethics can be traced to writings at the turn of the century, such as V. Veressayev's *Memoirs of a Physician*, which warned of dangerous abuses perpetrated by medical scientists who used their fellow human beings like guinea pigs in medical research (see Chapter 13). However, that kind of abuse was recognized as evil, and could be contained and managed, by appeal to the ethics human beings had been using for centuries. The *Nuremberg Code* (again, see Chapter 13) is a specification and expression of that ethics. One should realize that, at the time of the Nuremberg trial, biomedical science as we now know it had not really begun to blossom. For example, molecular biology, shortly after World War II, was still in an embryonic stage: what genes are made of had not been determined. The structure of DNA had not been worked out, and the genetic code had not yet been deciphered.

Abuse of human beings, of the kind performed by some physicians in the Nazi period, or by medical scientists in their research on venereal diseases at the turn of the century, would by itself most probably not have provoked the development of bioethics as we know it today. The vast panoply of thinkers, institutes, and governmental commissions, and the complex network of interdisciplinary reflection, mobilized over the past twenty years to carry out the work of bioethics, exhibits a magnitude and complexity of responses far in excess of what would have been required to control flagrant abuses of human beings in the kinds of medical research carried out prior to the Second World War.

A qualitatively new ethical response had to be mounted to match the power, the range, and the moral ambiguity of projects released by biomedical advances after the war. The *way of doing ethics* had to change. The initiators of bioethics sensed that ethical thought, as it had been carried out in the philosophical and theological modes of the past, could not match the new and ambiguous challenge of the biomedical sciences and technologies. Ethical reflection, unless anchored in new biomedical knowledge and technology, and if not intimately familiar with the methods of biomedical discovery, would, it was sensed, always arrive too naïve, too out of touch with the real issues, and too late to do its work.

There are two basic reasons why biomedical advances were a challenge to develop a new way of doing ethics.

The first reason derives from a breakdown in the classicist notion of culture. In the classicist notion of culture, there is one set of beliefs, ideals, and norms, and these are the standard of thought, word, and act for all human beings in all places and all times. The scope of human duty and obligations, and of reprehensible behaviour, is readily accessible to, and comprehended by, the cultivated mind. This is what Voltaire meant when he said that it took centuries for human beings to acquire knowledge of even a small sector of nature's laws; but a day is enough for a man of wisdom to know what the duties of man are (Voltaire, 1879, 195-196).

The breakdown in this classicist notion of ethics was not a once-and-for-all event in history. The breakdown has been going on for centuries, as some cultures continue to adhere to the classicist idea, others abandon it, and still other cultures return to some version of it. The biomedical challenge emerged within, and contributed to, an historically particularly striking transition of Western societies into a post-classicist culture. Within this culture, ethics is not a ready-made achievement, stored for all time in great books and great minds, and waiting for universal application (Lonergan, 1988, 241). In Western society, we find ourselves in the difficult situation of having to strive and to struggle together to construct the standards and norms that can enable us to distinguish right from wrong, when we differ as extensively as we do on the level of beliefs and values.

There is a second reason why the biomedical challenge is a provocation to devise a new way of doing ethics. Within a classical notion of culture, traditional method in ethics, whether ethics was done in the philosophical, theological, or religious mode, distinguished right from wrong on the basis of explicit or tacit appeal to notions, however diverse, of human nature and the human good. *Traditional ethics assumed three stabilities*: the unchangeability of the human condition; wide consensus on specifications of the human good; and geographical-temporal limits on the reach and consequences of human action (Jonas, 1974, 3).

These stabilities no longer hold. Human nature, for the biomedical sciences and technologies, is no longer simply the fundamental and comprehensive principle governing human action, as it was in traditional ethics. Human nature is also an unanswered question and an unfinished project. There is also now widespread dissent on what is good and what is bad for human beings, at least in regard to applications of the biomedical technologies to human life. We shall consider many examples of this dissent in later chapters. Lastly, technologically empowered human action can now exert an impact on people around the globe, and upon distant future generations.

Environmental threats challenged earlier people to change their place, their pace, and their ways of life. The promises and threats of the biomedical revolution are challenging people in late Western civilization to find a new way of doing ethics. Bioethics is a response to that challenge about how to do interdisciplinary and intercultural ethics in highly pluralistic societies.

CONCLUSION

Despite all the activity that has taken place in bioethics during the past twenty-five years, this field is still quite young and relatively underdeveloped. For some issues (e.g., informed consent), there has emerged a considerable degree of consensus about what should be done and what should be avoided. On other matters (e.g., abortion), the questions are clear but there is no agreement on the answers. Finally, there are certain new issues for which even the appropriate questions have not yet been devised.

Before we begin our examination of specific bioethical issues, we need to have a general understanding of bioethics as a field of study and practice. The following chapter will provide such an overview. It will become clear that the nature of bioethics is as contentious as are many of the issues to be discussed later in the book. You should not be disappointed if you do not find general agreement on any of these matters. In its present state of development, bioethics is not capable of providing such agreement. What it lacks in certainty, however, bioethics makes up for in excitement. We hope that you will share in this excitement as you work through this book.

REFERENCES

Beecher H.K. "Ethics and Clinical Research." *The New England Journal of Medicine* 1966;74:1354-1360.

Burns C.R. "History of Medical Ethics: North America: Seventeenth to Nineteenth Century." In: W.T. Reich, ed. *Encyclopedia of Bioethics.* New York: The Free Press, 1978, 963-968.

Carrick P. *Medical Ethics in Antiquity.* Dordrecht/Boston/Lancaster: D. Reidel, 1985.

Ford J.C. and **Kelly G.** *Contemporary Moral Theology.* Westminster, MD: Newman Press, 1964.

Jonas H. *Philosophical Essays. From Ancient Creed to Technological Man.* Englewood Cliffs, New Jersey: Prentice Hall, 1974.

Jonsen A.R. and **Toulmin S.** *The Abuse of Casuistry: A History of Moral Reasoning.* Berkeley: University of California Press, 1988.

Kelly G. *Medical-Moral Problems.* St. Louis: Catholic Health Association, 1949.

Lonergan B. "Dimensions of Meaning." In: F.E. Crowe and R.M. Doran. *Collected Works of Bernard Lonergan.* Vol. 4. Toronto: University of Toronto Press, 1988.

MacKinney L.C. "Medical Ethics and Etiquette in the Early Middle Ages: The Persistence of Hippocratic Ideals." In: C.R. Burns, ed. *Legacies in Ethics and Medicine.* New York: Science History Publications, 1977, 178-203.

McFadden C.J. *Medical Ethics for Nurses.* Philadelphia: F.A. Davis, 1946.

Medawar P. *The Threat and the Glory. Reflections on Science and Scientists.* New York: HarperCollins, 1990.

Rothman D.J. *Strangers at the Bedside: A History of How Law and Bioethics Transformed Medical Decision Making.* Basic Books, 1991.

Toulmin S. "How Medicine Saved the Life of Ethics." *Perspectives in Biology and Medicine* 1982;25/4:736-750.

Toynbee A.J. *A Study of History.* Abridgement of Volumes I-VI by D.C. Somervell. New York, London: Oxford University Press, 1947.

Voltaire *Dictionnaire philosophique IV.* In: *Oeuvres complètes de Voltaire.* Paris: Garnier Frères, 1879.

Williams J.R. *Biomedical Ethics in Canada.* Queenston, Ontario: Edwin Mellen, 1986.

Williams J.R. "Commissions and Biomedical Ethics: The Canadian Experience." *The Journal of Medicine and Philosophy* 1989;14/4:425-444.

2

BIOETHICS: ISSUES, FIELDS, AND METHOD

The preceding historical overview carried three messages. The first is that bioethics is rooted in centuries of Western thought on medical, philosophical, and theological ethics. The second is that bioethics cannot be totally identified with, and is not simply a smooth continuation of, any one of the past ways of doing ethics in earlier or more recent periods of the Graeco-Roman and Judaeo-Christian traditions. The third is that bioethics, though representing a transformation of traditional ways of doing ethics, nevertheless mirrors the tensions and divergences within and among the traditions of the West about how ethics should be done.

THEME AND TASKS OF THE CHAPTER

The messages of the opening chapter set the questions for this chapter. What distinguishes bioethics, as it has developed since the late 1960s, from morality, and from philosophical, theological, and professional ethics? We shall answer this question in the light of the unifying theme of this book (developed in Chapter 1), namely, that bioethics has developed as a transformation of traditional ways of doing ethics, and has done so as a response to a double challenge. That double challenge may be summarized in terms of a *breakthrough* and a *breakdown*:

multiple, cumulative, and utterly new *breakthroughs* in the biomedical sciences delivering the power to do things that never could be done before, at roughly the same time as increasing *breakdowns* were occurring in the moral stability and homogeneity of Western society, following upon this century's two World Wars.

The challenge is reflected prismatically in the panoply of issues that have generated work in bioethics over the past twenty-five years. So we examine the structure of these issues, and it is in this context that we will discuss how bioethics, as ethics, differs from, and yet stands in interdisciplinary relationship to, other ways of doing ethics. We shall then consider the fields of bioethics, and offer notes about the method of bioethics in relationship to each of its fields.

Bioethics is still evolving, and encloses within its ill-defined borders many different directions of ethical thought and method. If this chapter attempts to find some pattern, some order in the way bioethics has developed, it would be erroneous to suggest that this pattern tells the whole story. It could not, in part because we are trying to describe a moving target. The development of bioethics is far from finished and, as we shall discuss in the last chapter, the limitations of contemporary bioethics are simultaneously directions for continuing development.

THE FOUR OUTCOMES OF A BIOETHICAL ANALYSIS

Bioethics requires a shift from theoretical reason to practical judgment. And these judgments, whether they focus on individual cases or on policies covering categories of cases, centre upon choices, decisions, and actions. The outcomes of bioethical analysis are practical judgments about what is mandatory, what is permissible, what can be tolerated, or what must be prohibited among all the new and often untested things that can be done to and for human beings, as a result of advances in medicine and the life sciences.

An in-depth discussion of each of these outcomes, and of their differences, would involve us in a course in metaethics (see below). Since that would exceed the scope of this chapter, a few words of explanation may be enough to clarify the meaning of these four outcomes.

Fundamental rights are one arena in which we encounter practical judgments that something is mandatory, or is to be prohibited. There are few rights recognized as more fundamental than the right to life. Linked to this fundamental right is the right to the necessities of life. Recognition of these rights is the basis for two practical judgments of policy: one is a prohibition, the other an obligation. The prohibition is on any policy that would allow people to die, simply because they cannot pay for the medical or hospital care they need. The converse of this prohibition is the judgment that some form of guaranteed access to necessary care, some form of national health insurance, is mandatory.

Judgments of permissibility, namely that something is neither mandatory nor to be prohibited, occur in the arena of human liberties. One may, for example, agree to participate in a properly designed medical research project. Participation is neither mandatory nor subject to prohibition.

Judgments of tolerability occur in the arena of constraints on choice and freedom. Something judged wrong and as meriting prohibition in normal circumstances may have to be tolerated when people have little choice open to them, other than a choice between the lesser of two or more evils. Judgments of tolerability rest upon the assumption that right and wrong, good and evil, exhibit gradations. Some evils are worse than others. So judgments of tolerability span the spectrum from what is permissible to what has to be prohibited.

BIOETHICS: TWO FUNDAMENTAL QUESTIONS

One of the early authors in bioethics stated that we must all get used to the idea that biomedical technology makes possible many things we should never do (Kass, 1971, 787). The many professions, disciplines, and organizations introduced in Chapter 1 as main actors in bioethics have all been working, individually and in consort, to answer two fundamental questions hidden within that statement. The two fundamental questions are:

First,*what* must we do, what should we permit, what can we tolerate, and what must we prohibit among all the new things that biomedical science and technology now enable us to do with human beings and other forms of life on this planet?

Second, *how* do we determine what is mandatory, what is permissible, what is tolerable, or what must be prohibited when new powers enable us to do things that could never be done before?

In the central part of this book (chapters 6-18), the first of these two questions, the *what* question, will predominate in the analysis of fourteen important areas of research with human beings, of medical and nursing practice, and of applications of biomedical technology to human life. This chapter, and the following chapter on bioethics and law, will examine more explicitly the various approaches adopted to answer the closely related second fundamental question, the *how* question. We must consider how bioethics differs from, and yet is related to, law and morality and to philosophical, theological, and professional ethics, in determining the scope of justifiable constraints on choice, decision, and action.

THE STRUCTURE OF ISSUES IN BIOETHICS

Bioethics has been "issue oriented" since its inception. The two fundamental questions of bioethics stated above are not just questions; they are *issues*, because the answers proposed to date are uncertain or conflicting. These questions are *ethical* issues, because the questions bear upon the rights and wrongs of human behaviour. They involve conflicting beliefs about how human beings should live, about the values individuals and groups should uphold, and about the values that may be sacrificed when all values in a situation cannot be honoured and maintained. These questions are issues in *bioethics*, because they centre upon right and wrong decisions, policies, and acts in medicine and in the uses of biomedical science and technology.

An issue, then, involves conflict and controversy. The two fundamental questions of bioethics, the *what* and the *how* questions, return over and over again, in the vast array of specific issues linked to questions about interventions and acts that span the alphabet: from abortion to experimental manipulation of zygotes. Because the answers to these questions are so often diverse and conflicting, the questions become or generate issues. But issues are not all of one kind. In this section, we examine how issues differ in bioethics, according to the varied kinds of conflict they involve.

Since the way to resolve one kind of issue will often not work for issues involving conflicts of quite different kinds, it is essential to recognize precisely what kind of conflict we are dealing with, when people strongly disagree about what should or should not be done in medicine and in applications of the life sciences and technologies to human life.

In the following subsections, we shall characterize each of the various kinds of conflict implicated in the issues of bioethics, offer examples of each, and close each discussion with a practical observation about a strategy to resolve the conflict. We shall return to these strategies later in this chapter, in the section on fields and method, since the strategies, taken together, are the anatomy of method in bioethics. It may not be obvious, so we draw attention to the fact that some of the issues in bioethics involve several kinds of conflict simultaneously. If these issues are to be resolved at all, then certainly one strategy alone will not suffice.

Conflicts Based on Insufficient Evidence and Experience

Some of the issues of bioethics involve conflicts that can only be solved empirically. What is needed is an accumulation of fresh data, decisive evidence, or the weight of experience that will support one view, show others to be either mistaken or exaggerated, or eliminate still others from serious discussion. This kind of conflict, of course, is not peculiar to bioethics or ethics.

For example, years of experience with artificial or donor insemination have produced no evidence to support the position that would condemn artificial insemination as unethical, *because* it supposedly causes greater stress on marriages, or greater damage to a child's development than can be seen in families using natural insemination. Of course, some people oppose artificial insemination on the basis of principles and beliefs, and not on the basis of any empirically detectable consequences. We shall consider conflicts of this kind below.

Controversies over recombinant DNA in the 1970s (see chapter 18) offer a second example. Some people wanted to block all gene-splicing experiments, because they feared that new hybrid forms of life created by gene-splicing would lead to epidemics of uncontrollable infection. The weight of years of experience with recombinant DNA experiments has resolved that conflict in favour of allowing recombinant DNA work, now a standard part of molecular biology, under appropriate laboratory conditions.

We make a practical observation about a strategy to follow in resolving issues rooted in insufficient evidence or experience.

When the social consequences are difficult to foresee and are uncertain, new developments need a trial run under close monitoring until a sufficient accumulation of knowledge and experience reveals whether limits, restrictions, and protective barriers have to be established. It is difficult to judge new developments adequately by using thought experiments alone.

Conflicts Based on Partial Perceptions

A second type of conflict occurs when persons possessing limited information, like the fable's blind men touching different parts of the elephant, reach divergent or contradictory descriptive or evaluative views about a phenomenon as a whole. This kind of conflict, and the mistake of taking a part to be the whole, can easily occur when people are facing a new and socially complex phenomenon.

Consider surrogate mothering, as an example. Some of the early positions in favour of, and some of the positions against, surrogate mothering were based on partial perceptions and limited information. Some people looked upon this new reproductive arrangement only from the point of view of an infertile couple's desire for a child. Others directed their attention primarily to the large sums of money being offered to women to be surrogate mothers, and they saw exploitation of poor women. Still others concentrated only on the tragic cases that did not work out and had to be adjudicated in the courts, with media attention given to the emotional turmoil of all involved. These are only a few instances of the many partial perceptions of surrogate mothering that need to be considered and integrated, to obtain a balanced view of the whole phenomenon.

We close this discussion with a *practical observation about strategy* in resolving conflicts rooted in partial perceptions.

Conflicting positions based on partial perceptions and limited information can usually be resolved when the parties in conflict can be brought to accept information about the total phenomenon; and when they can come to adopt a higher viewpoint that will integrate and balance the partial perceptions. Conflicting positions based on partial perceptions and limited information are rarely intractably opposed.

Conflicts Arising from a Restricted Value-Focus

A third kind of conflict arises when individuals or groups restrict their attention, concern, and allegiance to one value. Restricted focusing on one value causes another to appear as a threat. Threats provoke defensive postures, people adopt adversarial strategies, and both sides of the value conflict can become increasingly blind to the values their adversaries are trying to defend and protect.

During the early debates on recombinant DNA in the 1970s, some scientists were concerned with protecting the scientific enterprise as a whole from what they saw as the destructive meddling of outside non-scientifically trained persons and groups. They focused on the protection of *scientific autonomy*. Others, a number of scientists included, feared that science was proceeding in a manner that would be detrimental to human life and other forms of life on the planet, and especially to future generations of human beings. They wanted to protect *human integrity* and the *integrity of the biosphere*.

The conflict in the recombinant DNA controversy that was based on a restricted value-focus, and other conflicts of this kind, suggest another *practical observation about strategy* in the resolution of issues.

An issue rooted in conflicts based upon a restricted value-focus can hardly ever be resolved unless each party to the conflict acquires an understanding of, and respect for, the values the other party is trying to protect. That is unlikely to happen without interdisciplinary, interprofessional and intercultural collaboration.

Conflicts Deriving from Unexamined Assumptions

In our choices, decisions, actions, and policies, we all use a great number of ideas that we take to be solid and true without having the time, or being able to take the time, to check them out and test them critically. If we had to test every idea we need, we could hardly ever get to decide or do anything. Such ideas, the ideas we take for granted, are called assumptions. But there are quite different kinds of assumptions, and the ethical issues that arise when people hold conflicting assumptions differ accordingly. So also do the strategies to resolve these issues differ.

There are conflicts based upon assumptions of fact, on assumptions of principle, and on assumptions of belief. And assumptions of belief may involve instrumental beliefs or world-view beliefs. In this section, we concentrate on ethical issues arising from conflicting assumptions of fact and conflicting assumptions of instrumental belief. In the next section, dealing with conflicts of ethos, we shall consider ethical issues arising from conflicts of world-view beliefs; and conflicting assumptions of principle will come up for discussion in the section below devoted to conflicts on the level of morality.

Assumptions of Fact

A team of cancer specialists published a study several years ago, in which they claimed that 50% or so of the 120 dying patients they treated experienced such severe pain in the last days of their lives that, to control the pain, it was necessary to put them into a deep state of unconsciousness with high doses of sedatives prior to their deaths. Palliative care and cancer experts in other parts of the world strongly disagreed with the idea that it was necessary and right to sedate dying cancer patients in the last days prior to death.

Whether or not dying patients should be so deeply sedated is certainly an ethical issue, indeed, a deeply agonizing one. But the issue here arises from conflicting assumptions of fact about whether cancer patients experience a final crescendo of pain immediately before death. Perhaps some do, and others do not. It may depend on the kind of cancer and the site of the tumor in the body. It may depend on the kinds of medication being used and the way they are administered. Patients with similar kinds of cancer may experience pain differently in different cultures, or at different ages in life. These are multiple questions of fact, and the resolution of the ethical issue regarding deep sedation depends largely upon how the questions of fact are answered.

The strategy, then, for resolving ethical issues that arise from conflicts of assumptions of fact, is to conduct more comprehensive and methodologically sound research. Conflicts about matters of fact cannot be resolved by argument. For conflicts of this kind, comprehensive, rather than partial, data constitute the court of appeal.

Assumptions of Instrumental Belief

The store of our beliefs covers more than the beliefs we commonly call religious or moral. The inventory of that store covers the whole of human experience, and contains whatever we know on the basis of what others have told us. Every human being has a store of knowledge that far exceeds what he or she has acquired through immediate personal experience, personal insight, personal research, and personal contributions to the advance of knowledge and science. A large part of our knowledge comes from our decision to believe what others, working in areas where we have no experience or expertise, tell us they have discovered.

We call these beliefs *instrumental* because they enable us to get on with the task of achieving the goals of work and life we have chosen to pursue. *Instrumental beliefs* are to be clearly distinguished from *world-view beliefs*, which are more fundamental and more comprehensive. *World-view beliefs* open the horizon within which we can see and determine the goals of work and life to which we want to dedicate ourselves.

Ethical issues may arise because people are assuming conflicting instrumental beliefs. But instrumental beliefs can be simply mistaken.

An instrumental belief may be mistaken because it rests upon an unjustifiable generalization. The conflict mentioned above, between those who believe there is and those who believe there is not a final crescendo of pain in the last days of terminal cancer, will only be resolved by finely tuned and comprehensive research that distinguishes different kinds of cancer, different kinds of patients, and different kinds of palliative care. Each of the currently competing beliefs may be partly true, and yet mistaken precisely as a generalization encompassing all dying cancer patients.

An instrumental belief may also be mistaken because it is based upon faulty, biased, or incomplete research. Examples abound in the development and evaluation of new drugs and surgical operations. The thalidomide tragedy illustrates a mistaken belief, namely, that this drug was a safe treatment for nausea in pregnancy, that was based on utterly inadequate research.

An instrumental belief, thirdly, may be mistaken because it rests upon an unquestioned, oft-repeated view, coming from persons who have little or no direct experience with the reality upon which they are issuing pronouncements. For example, many people have said that giving free or low-cost needles to intravenous drug users will not reduce the frequency of their infection-prone needle-sharing behaviour. This belief, though strong in certain quarters, has been shown to be mistaken, at least for some IV drug users in certain countries, and in cities of our own country.

The resolution of an ethical issue based upon a conflict of instrumental beliefs requires the unmasking of the mistakes in one or the other or in both beliefs. These mistakes may not be easily detectable by simple observation, and their unmasking may well require well-organized research.

Conflicts on the Level of Ethos

An ethos encompasses the governing beliefs we have about the status, destiny, and meaning of human life, or about the order of society and the purposes and roles of societal institutions in maintaining human community. The conflicts in a number of highly important and socially prominent issues in bioethics are rooted in profoundly differing beliefs of this sort. They are conflicts on the level of ethos. Abortion, research with the human embryo, euthanasia, and national health insurance are foci for striking conflicts on the level of ethos.

An ethos is a world-view belief. Such beliefs are fundamental and comprehensive, and they bear a religious, moral, or philosophical character. These beliefs cannot easily be changed or shaken by accumulations of data, facts, or information, because they are the field, the lighted space, or the horizon within which data, facts, and information are interpreted and acquire their meaning and their value.

Ethical issues involving a conflict between world-view beliefs cannot be simply resolved, particularly if "resolved" means attainment of widespread consensus. The resolu-

tion, if ever attainable, requires, on the part of one or many groups or individuals, a change of belief so profound that the change involves a personal or community conversion. In these situations, the best attainable solution is often a political accommodation, such as we find in many abortion laws and laws barring discrimination against people because of their sexual orientation, that maintains the coherence of a society, fosters the process of moral and philosophical discourse and debate, supports respect for personal conscience, and protects minorities (whether they be religious, cultural, or moral) from subjection to the dictates of majorities without justifying cause.

Conflicts on the Level of Morality

An ethos is a foundation for moral life. It partially determines the principles and the hierarchy of values in the light of which positions are taken about what human behaviours are imperative, permissible, tolerable, or need to be prohibited. We do not all share the same principles or identical hierarchies of value in our highly pluralistic societies. We often do differ quite sharply about what is of greater or lesser importance, even if we are not always able to express clearly why we differ. The issue then involves a conflict on the level of morality, a conflict about which values may be sacrificed and which may not, when two or more values cannot be honoured or achieved in a given situation.

A study several years ago of the comparative safety and efficacy of a surgical, versus a medical, approach to the treatment of a condition called morbid obesity offers an example. The researchers perceived the value of adequately informed patient consent to be irreconcilably in conflict with the value of enrolling enough patients into the clinical trial to obtain a reliable answer to the study question. In the researchers' view, one value or the other had to be sacrificed. They sacrificed adequately informed consent, so that the number of people who would agree to participate would be sufficient for the study to reach a scientifically valid conclusion.

The issues to be studied in later chapters, particularly the chapters on abortion, sterilization, genetic counseling, prenatal diagnosis, life-prolonging treatment, and limited resources, will offer abundant examples of what we call conflicts on the level of morality. These are conflicts about which principles must be honoured, and which may be set aside; about which values may be sacrificed and which may not — in situations where conflicting principles and values cannot be all simultaneously honoured and maintained.

How are issues involving conflicts on the level of morality to be resolved? The strategy, in its first instance, focuses on conflicts of principle. For example, some doctors believe that saving life is the highest principle of medical practice. Is it? Does the principle of saving life have priority over the principle of respecting a patient's liberty, when she refuses respirator support because she no longer wants to live as a totally paralysed person? Or when a patient refuses blood transfusions because of her Jehovah's Witness belief?

The resolution of conflicts of principle requires two approaches. First, rigorous clarification of arguments about the foundation, implications, scope, and interrelationship of principles. This is the work of philosophical and theological ethics, as we shall discuss below. Second, when the arena of clinical care is the place where principles are in conflict, the strategy requires sensitive attention to the patient's body and biography, so that the patient governs resolution of the conflict and is not used as a battleground for conflicting philosophies or theologies. This is the work of clinical ethics, as we shall discuss later in this chapter.

The strategy, in its second instance, focuses on conflicting hierarchies of value. *Value* is a word for what is important, for what is cherished in life. Though many things are important and cherished, they are not all equally so. Value hierarchies vary, depending on a person's ethos and culture.

Issues rooted in conflicting hierarchies of value can rarely be resolved to everyone's satisfaction. What appears right and good to one group committed to one hierarchy of values will appear wrong and bad to those who hold to an inverse value hierarchy.

These issues cannot be simply resolved, if resolution means a decision or policy with which everyone in society can wholeheartedly agree. In these morality-conflict situations, the most practical and civilized strategy aims at a compromise. A policy is sought which sets the conditions under which a morally disputed behaviour will be at least socially tolerated by most people, even if it may not be socially championed by many.

Bioethics as public ethics employs this strategy, and its policies may at times need to be buttressed by law. We shall consider this strategy in greater detail later in this chapter, again in Chapter 3, and examples will be considered in the chapters of this book dealing with specific issues.

Conflicts and Confusion on the Level of Ethics

Bioethics, as early noted, is a composite word, made up from the Greek word for life (*bios*) and a traditional word for the study of right conduct. Within the limits of this book, bioethics, then, is the study of right conduct in medical and biomedical interventions into life; into human life in particular. But bioethics, if we return to earlier statements in this chapter, is not just study. It is practical study, or *analysis*, of real-life medical and biomedical issues, leading to practical judgments and policies about decisions and actions. *So bioethics is ethics, and ethics, as we shall use the term, is the working out of the judgments that have to be made, the compromises that have to be struck, and the guidelines and policies that have to be devised when individuals and groups in a pluralistic society clash on the levels of ethos and morality regarding matters of medicine and the life sciences. It is in this sense that bioethics is ethics.*

Now there is some conflict, and perhaps more confusion than conflict, about how bioethics is being, or should be, done. This is a confusion about bioethics as ethics. There is no space here, and this is not the place, either, to tell the whole story. So our more limited objective at this point is to use the above definition of bioethics to clarify at least how we, in this book, see bioethics working as ethics. To achieve that clarification, we will use the following six sections to explain that bioethics is not a morality, or a professional ethics; that bioethics is not to be identified with theological, philosophical or feminist ethics; and lastly that bioethics is not applied ethics.

BIOETHICS IS NOT MORALITY

A morality, we have already suggested in the above brief discussion of conflicts on the level of morality, is a set of positions about which values may be sacrificed and which may not, when all values cannot be simultaneously maintained or honoured in given situations. A morality, then, expresses, and is based upon, a hierarchy of values that determines which values, if any, must be maintained at all costs. The maintenance of values is not just in thought, but more crucially, in choice, decision, and act. So a morality is also a set of positions — sometimes more, sometimes less, systematically elaborated — about the justifiability of various human behaviours, including behaviours in medicine and the life sciences. A morality, with its hierarchy of values and its normative system of positions on behaviour, is rooted in a set of world-view beliefs of the type mentioned earlier, in the discussion of conflicts on the level of ethos (Frankena, 1980, 16-40).

A pluralistic society is pluralistic, in part, because it houses and exhibits several, or even many, quite divergent moralities. The position of Roman Catholic morality, for instance, on abortion and on experimentation with the human embryo, is based upon a hierarchy of values and upon a belief about the personhood of the human embryo: a hierarchy and a belief that are not shared by a number of other moralities in our society. The Jehovah's Witness morality holds a distinctive position on blood transfusions, and that position is based, among other things, upon a belief about how the Scriptures should be interpreted, a belief that is not shared by the other Judaeo-Christian moralities. These are only two examples, among many other possible illustrations, of how the term *a morality* is being used in this book. It is important to emphasize that the set of world-view beliefs upon which different moralities are based, and differ, need not be only world-view beliefs of a religious sort. Moralities may also differ profoundly because of the very divergent and conflicting philosophical world-views in which they are rooted.

The important idea we are emphasizing here is that *bioethics is neither a morality nor a substitute for a morality.*

Bioethics is not a substitute for a morality, because a morality encompasses much more than bioethics has ever claimed, or is prepared, to offer. A morality offers a more or less unified version and vision of a way of living a good human life. Bioethics has a more limited and instrumental focus. It is the work of determining the decision and policies that are reasonable and justifiable in a pluralistic society, when divergent moralities clash on matters of medicine and the biomedical technologies. For this reason, the converse of the above leading statement is also true: a morality is no substitute for bioethics.

The positions of the various moralities on controversial issues in medicine, and in the applications of the biomedical technologies to human life, are the starting point of bioethics. These conflicting positions enter into the structure of the issues bioethics attempts to resolve.

BIOETHICS IS NOT PROFESSIONAL ETHICS

In this book, we also distinguish bioethics from medical ethics, nursing ethics, and the ethics of the other health professions. These different forms of ethics are not to be confounded, even if they often do intersect on a wide range of issues, such as cessation of treatment, resuscitation, or euthanasia. We understand "medical ethics" and "nursing ethics" to be two forms of professional ethics, and medical ethics will serve as our point of reference to explain why bioethics is not the ethics of a profession. The other side of this distinction also needs emphasis. When physicians, nurses, and others are involved in clinical ethics, which is a field of bioethics, they are doing something quite different from resolving issues solely by appeal to the dictates of the ethics of their profession.

A profession is an occupation, and a professional ethics is the system of obligations and responsibilities binding on those who practice the occupation. Needless to say (but it is better to say it), a profession is not just any kind of occupation, but an occupation marked by certain specific social characteristics. There are core characteristics and derivative characteristics. The core characteristics are: autonomy of the members of a profession in determining what its work should be, and how it should be done; prolonged specialized training, to assure that people entering the profession possess the required competence to do the work; and socially highly valued service, designed to meet important needs shared by the society as a whole. Professions, as a consequence of these core characteristics, usually set their own standards of practice and of training, control the issuance of licence to practice, and exert considerable influence on any legislation regulating their occupational activities (Freidson, 1970, 71ff). Some professions, notably medicine, have also worked out a code or system of ethics.

Medical ethics, as the ethics of the profession, shares some features in common with a morality: it encompasses an ethos, a value system, and a normative system of positions on ethically correct and ethically reprehensible behaviour. The central point is that responsibilities, and in their light, right, wrong, and tolerable behaviour, are determined by reference to the values, acts, and relationships that are intrinsic to the practice of medicine.

A medical ethics, structurally, has five major dimensions or interrelated components: an ethos or foundation; a system of values; a normative set of responsibilities; a set of practical maxims about right and wrong behaviour in specific situations; and, particularly characteristic of contemporary medical ethics, an evolving body of doctrine about how specific ethical issues along the entire front of medical practice are to be resolved.

Physicians, in collaboration with their more philosophically inclined colleagues, and in consort with philosophers of medicine, have written many volumes to elucidate the foundations, values, and responsibilities of the profession. We need not discuss this massive and on-going work, which is summarized in existing codes and manuals of medical ethics, such as the Canadian Medical Association *Code of Ethics*, the World Medical Association *Declaration of Geneva*, or the *Ethics Manual* of the American College of Physicians. Few would confuse these dimensions of medical ethics with the work of bioethics.

It is at the level of its evolving body of doctrine about how the specific ethical issues of everyday clinical practice are to be resolved that traditional medical ethics intersects with the field, or specialization, of bioethics that we call clinical ethics (to be discussed in greater detail below). This chapter holds a thesis about that intersection, and this thesis is one of the guiding assumptions of this book. The thesis is that clinical ethics, a field of bioethics, is a distinct activity that cannot be reduced to traditional medical ethics. Clinical ethics is not just the ethics of the medical profession. Clinical ethics surely involves physicians, but when physicians are doing clinical ethics, they are resolving ethical dilemmas at the bedside in an interdisciplinary and intercultural fashion. The practical judgments they reach, in collaboration with patients, families, and persons from other disciplines, are not based solely on appeal to the ethics of their profession.

Bioethics, as explained in the preceding section, is not a morality, nor is it a substitute for a morality. Conversely, a morality is not a substitute for bioethics. A similar conclusion applies to medical ethics. Bioethics, as clinical or research ethics, is not the ethics of the medical profession, nor is it a substitute for a medical ethics. But, in the contemporary world, the converse is also true. Medical ethics, understood as the ethics of the medical profession, is not a substitute for clinical ethics or for bioethics in its other fields of research ethics and public policy ethics.

BIOETHICS IS NOT THEOLOGICAL ETHICS

Some of the most prolific and influential writers in the early period of contemporary bioethics were theologians or religious scholars (Walters, 1985). They took a lead in confronting the emerging issues of the biomedical challenge, and bridged a transition from the quite closely church-based moral theologies dealing with issues of medical ethics in the 1950s and 1960s, to the pluralistic and practical bioethics of the 1980s and 1990s.

It is no slight on the tremendous and lasting importance of the work of these pioneers in bioethics to claim, as we do in this book, that bioethics is, and cannot be, a theological ethics. These authors themselves implicitly distinguish theological ethics from bioethics, when they take pains, as they have in recent years, to describe the contributions theological ethics has made, or can make, to bioethics (McCormick, 1989). A theological ethics may consider and pronounce on all of the same issues handled in bioethics, but it does so from a perspective, with a method, and for immediate objectives that are quite different from those characterizing bioethics.

A theological ethics, first of all, is not simply a code of religiously motivated behaviour. Neither is a theological ethics simply identical to a religious or ecclesiastical morality. A theological ethics is the intellectual explication and defense of a religious morality, a morality that flows from, and expresses, a faith or religious belief. Theology, going back to a phrase of Anselm of Canterbury, is faith seeking an understanding of itself (*fides quaerens intellectum*). But people, even within one religious community, may differ quite significantly about how their common faith is to be understood, and we can find quite different theologies and forms of theological ethics within the same community of faith. Obviously, there are many quite different faiths, and these contribute to a considerable pluralism within theological ethics itself. There is even a specialization within theology, called ecumenical theology, that has this pluralism between religious communities, including the pluralism of theological ethics, as its object of study.

If we attend only to this pluralistic aspect of theological ethics, we have reason enough to claim that bioethics is not, and cannot be, a theological ethics. A theological ethics, even one working on the issues of the biomedical challenge, serves the function of determining how these issues can be resolved in harmony with the belief and morality of a faith community. Bioethics, however, seeks to formulate the decisions and policies that can be accepted and defended within a pluralistic society, where the pluralism arises in part from the divergent moralities and competing forms of theological ethics in society.

BIOETHICS IS NOT FEMINIST ETHICS

It has been observed that the rise of feminism has coincided with the rise of bioethics (Sherwin, 1992), and that the two movements overlap, insofar as feminism is concerned with, and derives much of its modern dynamic from, medical and health care experiences. Abortion, the new reproductive technologies, and nurses' inferior role in health service delivery are common focal points of feminist discourse. Feminist consciousness extends far beyond medicine, health care and the pursuit of biological science, however, to address fields such as psychology, sociology, history, anthropology and jurisprudence.

Feminism has been alienated from sources of traditional ethics, meaning medical, philosophical and religious ethics. Women were long precluded from qualification and membership in the medical profession, the societies and universities in which philosophy was pursued, and the religious institutions and hierarchies of the Judaeo-Christian and Islamic worlds. The relatively recent rise in respect paid to equal opportunities for the sexes has sensitized many people, both women and men, to the contribution that women's insights and perspectives can make, and should be able to make, to understanding. In quite recent times, the higher rate of admission of women to professional schools has led to descriptions of the impending feminization of medicine and feminization of law in North America. Indeed, in 1991, three of the nine judges of the Supreme Court of Canada were women. Not all women are feminists, however, and not all feminists are women.

It has been observed that *"feminism* is the name given to the various theories that help reveal the multiple, gender-specific patterns of harm that constitute women's oppression. It is also the term used to characterize the complex, diverse political movement to eliminate all such forms of oppression"(Sherwin, 1992, 13). Like theological and philosophical ethics, feminism is internally varied. The movement includes such divergent and, at times, opposing strains as liberal feminism, socialist feminism, radical feminism, cultural feminism, postmodern feminism, ecofeminism, psychoanalytic feminism, feminist spirituality and feminist aesthetics. Major contributions to modern feminist ethics come from the fields of philosophy and of bioethics, which have conditioned such concerns as feminist practical reasoning. Feminist jurisprudence is now represented in most law schools, and contributes significantly to feminist analysis (MacKinnon, 1987, 1989).

Feminists want to intensify bioethical concerns with questions of gender and power, and to expose frequently subtle oppression of women, which is unlikely to be discerned unless an explicitly feminist analysis is adopted. For instance, the leading cases in which disabled patients' preferences for terminal care have been considered unreliable or not rational have concerned women (Miles, 1990).

Susan Sherwin has claimed that feminism expands the scope of bioethics, in demanding that ethical evaluation of medical and health care practices focus on structures of oppression and on the patterns of discrimination, exploitation, and dominance that condition the way services and care are given in our society (Sherwin, 1992, 4-5).

Bioethics, in each of its three fields, will inevitably intersect with feminist ethics, as it must also intersect with the various moralities, and with professional, theological, and philosophical ethics. This intersection implies differentiation, not indifference, and requires both a division of labour and interdisciplinary collaboration.

Differentiation means that bioethics, as we understand its functions and methods, is not feminist ethics. But bioethics is not professional, theological, or philosophical ethics, either. Division of labour implies, among other things, that we should not overestimate what bioethics can and should achieve. Bioethics is not the whole of ethics. To do its work well, bioethics must not attempt to do the work of the other ethics disciplines, feminist ethics included. Interdisciplinary collaboration, with feminist ethics as with other disciplines, is the cardinal principle of method in bioethics. There is no other viable way to achieve practical resolution of issues, whether at the level of judgments in particular cases, or at the level of public policy.

It is probable, in its field of public ethics, that bioethics will intersect most productively with feminist ethics, for any policy in medicine, health care, and the biomedical technologies cannot long survive, or be justified, if it harbours and perpetuates, let alone enhances, discrimination and oppression.

BIOETHICS IS NOT PHILOSOPHICAL ETHICS

Contemporary philosophical ethics comprises three principal levels of work: metaethics, normative ethics, and applied ethics. It is a thesis of this chapter, and of this book, that bioethics is not metaethics (and few would claim that it is); nor is bioethics involved in doing what philosophers do when they construct normative theories or systems of ethics (and few would claim that it is); nor is bioethics applied ethics (which many claim is precisely what bioethics is).

In this section, we shall discuss each of these levels of philosophical ethics briefly, and focus our attention in the next section on an explanation of why bioethics is not applied ethics. We emphasize this issue in particular because, while recognizing the value and utility of philosophical applied ethics for bioethics, we disagree with the prevalent view that applied ethics is the method bioethics uses in its three fields of research ethics, clinical ethics, and public policy ethics.

Metaethics

Metaethics, sometimes called the epistemology of ethics, or the logic of ethics, focuses attention on the concepts, languages, modes of reasoning and argumentation, and, finally, the ways of knowing or kinds of knowledge exhibited in normative and applied ethics. Bernard Lonergan's discussion of ethics in his book *Insight* is one example of work on the level of metaethics. He is not constructing a normative theory, a system of principles, governing right or wrong behaviour. Much less is he applying any one normative theory to reach practical conclusions about specific right and wrong decisions or acts in concrete situations. Rather, he sketches the anatomy of the fundamental notions used in ethical discourse: the notion of the good, of value, of freedom, of responsibility. He presents a position on method in ethics, and discusses the nature of practical insight and practical reflection, and offers a decision theory and elements of a theory of action. He distinguishes the rationality of knowledge judgments from the rationality of practical judgments and the act of deciding (Lonergan, 1957, 595-633). This is part of the work of metaethics.

It is also the work of metaethics to analyse, criticize, and correlate various normative theories of ethics. When Paul Ricoeur tries to demonstrate that Aristotle's ethics of virtue and Immanuel Kant's ethics of duty are complementary and not incompatible, he is working on the level of metaethics (Ricoeur, 1987).

We have given only a couple of examples to suggest what work on the level of metaethics involves. Metaethics will quite surely gain increasing relevance over the next several years, for understanding, criticizing, and systematizing the work actually being done in bioethics. But the work of metaethics is not the work of bioethics, as we have briefly defined it to be above. Producing practical judgments about the justifiability of specific acts in medicine and biomedicine, the work of bioethics, is not the work of metaethics.

Normative Ethics

Normative ethics has at least two different meanings. It can mean basing decisions and actions on a system of norms and principles. It is in this sense that Daniel Callahan, in an article written several years ago, contrasted normative ethics with an "ethics" that would distinguish right from wrong by appealing to spontaneous feelings, to majority opinion, or to statements from authorities (Callahan, 1972). It is also in this sense that we shall speak of applied ethics below, where we refer to two prominent authors who characterize their approach to biomedical ethics as being "applied normative ethics."

Normative ethics can also refer to the work of constructing a normative ethical theory. Many such theories have been worked out over the centuries of philosophical discourse. Some of the general theories of ethics, such as the deontological, consequentialist, and utilitarian theories, which have received at least summary discussion in nearly every book on bioethics published over the last fifteen years, are examples of normative theories of ethics.

A normative theory of ethics is a system of justification, consisting of an ascending order of rules, norms, and principles to which appeal is made in judging the rightness and wrongness of decisions and actions. The order is ascending, because more specific rules of action are based on more general norms that are, in turn, based upon more comprehensive principles.

When philosophers are working on this level of normative ethics, they are involved in determining what these rules, norms, and principles are, what they mean, what they imply, and how they are interrelated. To construct such a theory, to modify it, to work out its implications, to improve its consistency, to perfect it and defend it against critique is to do philosophical work in normative ethics.

Some of the leading philosophers of the past two centuries and the contemporary period, such as Immanuel Kant (deontological theory), John Stuart Mill (utilitarian theory), W.D. Ross (common-sense-based deontological theory), John Rawls (contract-based theory of justice), Robert Nozick (rights-based deontological theory), and others, too many to name here, have been involved in the construction of normative theories of ethics.

When philosophers are doing this work they are not doing bioethics; and the work of bioethics does not consist in the construction of normative theories, but rather in the construction of practical judgments.

Applied Ethics

There is an obvious link between normative ethics and applied ethics. The application takes the form of "because" reasoning, and consists in the construction of an argument for or against the rightness of an action by appealing to principles from one or another of the existing normative theories of ethics. The argument is a demonstration, usually a deductive demonstration, that the rightness or wrongness of a specific action is implied in the system's or theory's basic principles. An action is judged as wrong because it violates one or several of the theory's principles.

The rigor of this application process will vary considerably, depending on whether the theory being applied is anchored in one fundamental principle; or in a small number of principles hierarchically organized according to a priority of application; or in a plurality of principles that have no hierarchical order of priority.

Alan Donagan, following the Kantian tradition of deontological ethics, a duty-based theory of ethics, will trace judgments about the rightness or wrongness of actions back to the single fundamental principle, namely, that it is imperative to respect every human being, oneself and others, as a rational creature (Donagan, 1977, 76-81).

In John Rawls's theory of distributive justice, acts and policies must first of all satisfy the highest of the three principles in his system, the principle of equal liberty. If that principle is satisfied, then the second principle, the difference principle, can be applied. It states that the theory can permit unequal sharing of social and economic goods only if these inequalities will benefit everyone, and in particular, those who are most disadvantaged in society. These two principles have priority over the third principle, the principle of fair equality of opportunity (Rawls, 1971, 40-45, 60-67, 298-303).

Contemporary philosophers working in applied ethics are generally not inclined to trace their way through the levels of a tightly-knit normative theory, to demonstrate that their conclusions about right and wrong behaviour are ultimately based on the theories' highest principles. They rather tend to base their conclusions on a loosely connected set of more-or-less self-evident, commonly accepted principles of right conduct. W.D. Ross, for example, based his deontological theory on a set of duties generally recognized in society to be prevailing obligations, unless honouring these duties were to involve people in conflict with other obligations. Ross called such duties *prima facie* duties (Ross, 1930). A number of the duties Ross included in this set of *prima facie* duties correspond rather closely to the four cardinal principles widely used in American versions of applied ethics, namely, the principles of autonomy, beneficence, non-malficence, and justice.

These are the principles contemporary philosophers working in bioethics generally apply, to resolve issues in medicine and the life sciences. We must examine the thesis that bioethics is applied ethics.

IS BIOETHICS APPLIED ETHICS?

A number of influential authors have argued that bioethics is a special kind of ethics only insofar as it relates to a particular realm, the biomedical realm, of facts, concerns, and issues. Bioethics, according to this quite prevalent view, *does not employ* or represent a *unique* or *new ethical methodology*. Bioethics is just *applied ethics*, because it employs the same moral principles and rules used in ordinary circumstances.

According to this view, the ethics that is applied is an ethics based in rationality, and its basic rules are equally applicable to all people, at all times and places. The basic rules are universally applicable, but new scientific developments may require new derived rules, or middle principles, to arrive at correct ethical conclusions.

For example, if the principle of non-malficence (do no harm!) is a basic ethical principle, a new derived or middle principle, defining what is or is not harm, may be necessary as new medical technologies, unknown to earlier societies and philosophers, such as the life-prolonging technologies or the reproductive technologies, enter medical practice (Clouser, 1978). Is the use of respirators to prolong the lives of persons in a vegetative state harmful or beneficial?

The view that bioethics is methodologically indistinguishable from applied ethics, and is distinguished only by the kinds of medical and biomedical issues with which it deals, is quite prevalent and governs some of the leading textbooks of biomedical ethics used in North America (Beauchamp, 1989). We part ways with this thesis that bioethics is applied ethics for two reasons. First, the concept of applied ethics itself merits serious criticism. Second, applied ethics does not correspond to the way practical judgments and policies are attained in the three main fields of bioethics, to be discussed below.

The Concept of Applied Ethics: Its Difficulties

The concept of applied ethics, and the thesis that bioethics is simply applied ethics, rests upon a number of unexamined and very shaky assumptions. Because this is not the place to conduct a comprehensive critical analysis, we draw attention only to the following points.

First, the concept of applied ethics assumes that there is a set of basic moral principles that apply to all human beings, at all times, and in all places. The drive of philosophical applied ethics is to anchor conclusions about right and wrong action in these principles. But, as mentioned earlier, we live now in a post-classical world, and we can no longer assume the existence of a universally binding system of beliefs and values that would give this presupposed set of basic principles their meaning and obligation force. Any ultimate reason put forth by one thinker as *the* justification for an ethical conclusion can, and generally will be, questioned by people who are at home in a different philosophy or a different culture, or who are at home in no philosophy at all.

Second, the practical judgments and policies sought in work in bioethics require a strategy or method likely to bring about a convergence of minds. The approach of applied ethics leads in a quite different direction, the direction of divergence. How can people ever agree, by way of deductive demonstration about conclusions of applied ethics, if they fundamentally disagree on the meaning or ranking of the basic principles that serve as the premises for the deduction? The society in which we live is pluralistic precisely because we do not share a single philosophy.

Third, the adjective *applied* in applied ethics suggests that there is a solid, coherent structure of ethical theory that can be applied. But how can this be if there is not one, but many, and indeed conflicting, ethical theories available for application? If bioethics is applied ethics, does it not matter at all which of the ethical theories is being applied (Green, 1990)?

Philosophers using applied ethics in bioethics generally recognize this problem. They skirt the problem, however, by assuming that there is extensive convergence of the principles guiding behaviour, however wide the divergence may be regarding the foundations of the various conflicting ethical theories. So they start their work of application with these principles that they assume are widely accepted ethical guides for action. Bioethics done in this way runs the risk of becoming an exercise in "cookbook" ethics, little more than a rote application of principles that new generations of philosophically unsophisticated bioethicists do not really understand and master.

Fourth, the problem that those working in applied ethics generally leave in the wings needs to be brought to centre stage. Do right answers or solutions in applied ethics depend upon the choice of the theory (the correct theory?) to be applied? Deciding which of the many ethical theories is the correct one for applied ethics, or even deciding that an eclectic use of various theories will do just as well as slavish attachment to one theory, are *metaethical* questions, *not* questions of *applied ethics*. If these metaethical decisions are not made, and are not rationally defended, practitioners of applied ethics run the risk of using ethical theory as a mask for ethical prejudice, in the sense of a pre-judgment. Ethical theory in such a situation would be used not as a method for reaching an objective ethical judgment on a particular ethical issue, but as a tool of rationalization to defend a starting preferred position, or even just a "gut reaction" one would have on an issue before even beginning the work of ethical analysis (Holmes, 1990).

Those who hold that bioethics is applied ethics cannot escape the task of doing serious and sustained philosophical work on the theories and principles they presume to apply to ethical issues in medicine and the life sciences. That work, however useful and necessary, is not the work of bioethics.

Bioethics Is Not Applied Ethics

Bioethics, as we shall discuss in greater detail when describing its three main fields, does not employ the deductive approach of applied ethics to reach its practical judgments and policies for specific cases and situations. The order of principles, the normative order, underlying work in bioethics is, to borrow a distinction from David Bohm, an implicate order, not an explicate order (Bohm, 1980).

The normative order in applied ethics is assumed to be an *explicate order*: the principles of behaviour, their meaning and their relationships, are already worked out in normative theories, in advance of any application made of them. That order is explicate because it can be laid out, made explicit as a whole, and appeal is made to that order to justify conclusions about which behaviours are right and which are wrong. We have already raised some critical questions about the assumed explicate normative order of applied ethics.

An implicate order cannot be made explicit as a whole. It is manifested slowly and only partially, as it is expressed in one historical instance after the other. Personalities are examples of an implicate order. You only get to know who persons really are after seeing them in action in hundreds of different situ-

ations. The normative order of bioethics is something like that. The real principles of bioethics — their meaning and their relationships, what they command, permit, tolerate, and prohibit — are not all laid out as a whole in
advance of the practical judgments bioethics seeks to reach on issue after issue.
The real normative order of bioethics is still emerging, and will continue to
emerge slowly and partially in the case-by-case, situation-by-situation, practical
judgments and policies that are the responses of bioethics to the biomedical
challenge.

The normative order governing judgments of right and wrong in bioethics
cannot, then, be set out as a whole, ready-made for deductive application.
Bioethics does not proceed by deduction, as applied ethics does. Quite the contrary. The practical judgments of bioethics emerge out of a comprehensive and
detailed consideration of the full particularity of each ethically problematical
case and situation in medicine and the life sciences. The approach in bioethics is
inductive. The guidance for action that it can exhibit comes not from pre-
established principles, but rather from a comparison and a criticism of the practical judgments it has reached in cases of a similar kind.

THE FIELDS AND METHODS OF BIOETHICS

Bioethics has evolved, and is still developing, as a tree of branching specializations. We use the term *fields* to organize the various categories of specific ethical questions, the divisions of labour, and the specialized kinds of knowledge,
experience, and interdisciplinary collaboration required for the work of
bioethics. As a field develops, observations accumulate, new problems are
identified, concepts are refined, analyses deepen, a literature expands, and
heightened experience and knowledge are prerequisites for making an original
contribution to the field. The three main fields of bioethics are research ethics,
clinical ethics, and public policy ethics. Each of these main fields branches out
into more specific field specializations, according to the disease or condition
being studied, treated or remedied and the medical or biotechnologies being
applied.

Bioethics as Research Ethics

If bioethics is a tree of branching specializations, it is also a tree with many
roots. One of these roots reaches back to warnings published early in this century (see Chapter 13) that some doctors, in their conduct of medical experiments on human beings, failed to distinguish between their fellow human
beings and guinea pigs. The warning and the charge, documented in numerous
case examples, was that zeal for scientific progress led many prestigious and

respected physicians to imperil the health and lives of patients and to neglect grossly the requirements of respect for human liberty and dignity. Similar warnings were repeated shortly after the Second World War, and again in the three decades following the war.

The warnings led to the establishment of commissions and working groups to formulate principles, codes, regulations, and special review procedures, such as research ethics committees or institutional review boards (IRBs) designed to guide, and even govern, pharmaceutical, medical, and surgical research with human subjects.

Research Ethics: An Emerging Specialization

As already mentioned, research of all three kinds increased dramatically after the Second World War. Research projects increased in *number*; in *size*, with respect to the number of researchers, centres and human patients or subjects involved in any given project; in *scope*, embracing an ever wider range of diseases; in *objectives*, moving from research into the causes of disease on to the expanding frontier of research to develop and evaluate the safety and efficacy of new methods to diagnose, treat, and prevent disease and injury; and, lastly, in *complexity of research design* (see Chapter 13).

Research ethics, though a concern reaching back into the last century, came into its own as a specialization of bioethics because a division of labour, and the development and employment of distinct kinds of knowledge, interdisciplinary collaboration, and experience became increasingly necessary, to keep step with the expansion in scope and the increase of complexity of medical and biomedical research.

Rooted in early warnings of abuse of human beings in medical experimentation, research ethics has emerged, and is still developing, as a specialization of bioethics. The ethical issues specific to research ethics all demonstrate and express variations of three basic tensions or conflicts between:

- the welfare of individuals and the common good of society as a whole;
- a doctor's responsibilities as an individual patient's physician and a doctor's responsibilities as a scientist and clinical investigator; and
- patients' demand for rapid access to promising new treatments and the need (scientific, clinical, and economic) to evaluate new treatments rigorously with regard to safety, efficacy, and the cost-benefit ratio.

Method in Research Ethics

The difficult and unique ethical problems and dilemmas that appear in specific research projects and clinical trials cannot be resolved by simple appeal to, or deductive application of, existing ethical principles, codes, and guidelines. These principles set general moral perimeters, but they do not of themselves decide concrete cases. They do not of themselves determine whether a concrete project is within or outside the moral perimeter.

The ethics of research requires a continuous feedback between tailored ethical judgments on specific research projects and clinical trials on the one hand, and the principles and norms for the ethical conduct of research on the other. Working out the ethics of research, and the achievement of that feedback between judgments tailored to specific cases of research and broader ethical principles, require distinct kinds of interdisciplinary collaboration between scientists, clinicians, methodologists, biostatisticians, ethicists, and, depending on the research in question, representatives of other disciplines.

This interdisciplinary collaboration has given research ethics its own particular system of concepts and language to identify and analyse ethical problems in research, and has generated a distinctive and expanding body of literature. Competent work within research ethics presupposes special kinds of expertise, knowledge, and experience. In these senses, research ethics is a specialized field of bioethics.

Research Ethics: Sub-Specializations

Sub-specializations are now developing within research ethics in keeping with the differences of interdisciplinary collaboration, as well as the differences of knowledge and experience needed to work on ethical problems in quite different domains of pharmaceutical, medical, surgical, and biomedical research. For example, sub-specializations of research ethics are developing in relation to surgical research, to research on cancer, to research on HIV disease, and in relation to research with populations of persons who are incompetent to give consent, as opposed to those who are. Research with small children or with older persons affected by advanced dementia, poses ethical problems very different from those faced in research with competent adults.

We usually associate research with experimentation in laboratories. At some point, though, in the development of new treatments, research has to take place at the bedsides of patients, at times at the bedsides of very sick and dying people. Research here intertwines with compassionate care, and we enter the domain of clinical ethics, the second specialization of bioethics.

Bioethics as Clinical Ethics

Bioethics is also rooted in difficult decisions about cessation of treatment and the prolongation of life. Some of the earliest controversies in bioethics turned around the issues of whether or not to save the lives of severely deformed newborn babies; of whether or not to maintain respiratory support of comatose patients; of whether or not to resuscitate patients in various stages of advanced disease, or when outcome was very uncertain.

When there was little that medicine could do in these tragic circumstances, few decisions had to be taken. Patients simply died, and efforts were made to comfort the dying as much as possible. However, the times and the power of medical technology have changed. With the development of intensive care units, of new drugs and surgical operations, of new chemotherapeutic treatments, of new life-support technologies, of transplantation techniques, of new reproductive technologies, and of genetic counseling and prenatal diagnosis, the powers of medicine to affect life before birth, and after birth, and right up to the advanced stages of lethal disease have increased enormously. Diseases and conditions that could not be cured or treated in earlier times can now be managed — but not always to the satisfaction, and not always with the agreement, of all involved. As the powers of clinical teams have increased, so also have the number and the difficulties of the decisions that have to be taken. Ethical uncertainties, dilemmas, and controversies at the bedside are frequent in clinical practice. This is the domain of clinical ethics.

The Scope of Clinical Ethics

Clinical ethics covers the decisions to be made, and the uncertainties, value-conflicts, and dilemmas that may arise when physicians and clinical teams treat patients at the hospital bedside, in the operating theatre, in the office and clinic, or in the home.

The outcome of clinical ethics is a practical judgment about what should be done now, to help this particular person make those therapeutic choices that will best correspond to her clinical needs and total-life interests. At other times, the outcome is a practical judgment about how to help a gravely ill person die in a fashion that honours his dignity. These decisions, and the ethical conflicts associated with them, are highly focused, bounded as they are by the unique biology, clinical condition, needs, desires, life plans, hopes, sufferings, strengths, vulnerabilities, and limitations of particular human beings. The extent of these decisions and potential conflicts is as wide as the range of conditions and diseases encountered in clinical practice.

Method in Clinical Ethics

The issues of clinical ethics involve uncertainties and conflicts that are inextricably bound up with the unique circumstances of particular cases. Each clinical case, particularly those involving infertility, reproduction and parenthood, and those involving life-death decisions, brings thousands of years of cultural and moral tradition to bear upon a particular crisis. The principles of the great philosophers, the moral traditions of medicine and the world's religions, and the moral common sense of preceding generations pass more, or less, clearly through the prism of a small circle of people gathered around a particular sick person to illuminate the one governing question of the moment: what, among all the things that are clinically possible, is required, or prohibited, by this person's condition, suffering and dignity? Philosophical and moral traditions are challenged in the arena of clinical ethics to come down from the levels of abstract discourse, and to take a stand on what should be done now, when the decision is decisive for this patient's future and the consequences are, so frequently, irreversible.

In clinical ethics, *the patient is the norm* governing the decisions and practical judgments to be made. The patient's body and biography — his or her clinical course, relationships, life plans, and total-life interests — constitute this norm.

Clinical ethics works with *patients' biographies* to interpret the meaning of principles; that is, to determine what principles command, permit, tolerate, or prohibit for this particular patient. As such, clinical ethics is a *particular kind of inductive ethics*. In terms of clinical ethics, we do not know what our philosophical and moral traditions mean until we test them on a range of particular cases. We cannot simply pass each individual case through a grid of philosophical and religious moral principles, to reach a clinical ethical conclusion. We simultaneously have to pass these principles through the grid of individual cases, through a range of personal histories comforting the suffering of multiple loss, as well as the threat of personal disintegration and death.

Clinical ethics, then, *is not applied philosophy or theology*. Clinical ethics is an original, distinctive intellectual activity, not a derivative one. Ethical dilemmas will be misconstrued, if the clinical situation is not understood in all its subtle medical and human complexity. The maxim of method in clinical ethics is: each case contains its own resolution. Understand the patient, body and biography as comprehensively as possible, and the balance of elements required to resolve an ethical uncertainty, conflict, or dilemma will emerge.

However, communication is essential to reach a comprehensive description and understanding of a patient. Communication means attention to, and the mutually corrective interplay of, all informed and relevant points of view; primarily those of the patient, if conscious and competent, and the points of view also of the physicians, nurses, family members, consultants and other participants in the clinical drama.

Competence in clinical ethics presupposes the skill and the sensitivity to seek, and the ability to orchestrate, the contributions of many persons, to arrive at an adequate understanding of the patient and of what constitutes the patient's best interests. The challenge of clinical ethics is to construct this dialogue and sustain it, until the play of one view against another leads to a comprehensive grasp of the essentials and to a tolerable consensus on what should be done or avoided.

A tolerable consensus is often the most that can be achieved. Respect for the informed will of a patient may well require that one or several participants concur in a decision that is not fully consistent with their own moral perceptions or persuasions. When a tolerable consensus cannot be achieved, people may turn to the courts, and we shall consider the contribution of jurisprudence to clinical ethics in the next chapter, on bioethics and law.

Clinical Ethics: A Specialization of Bioethics

Clinical ethics requires its own distinctive kinds of interdisciplinary collaboration, and also quite variable kinds of knowledge and experience, depending upon the similarity or wide divergence among the diseases and the conditions giving rise to the issues it must resolve. Whereas the method of research ethics focuses on specific populations of patients and how they are affected by the unique problems of particular research projects and clinical trials, the method of clinical ethics bears directly upon individual patients and the particular cases of clinical practice.

As the range of ethical issues to be managed in clinical ethics has widened over the years, and as specialized knowledge and experience needed for the management of these issues has accumulated, a literature distinct to clinical ethics has grown. Specialized articles, books, and reviews mark off clinical ethics as a distinctive field of bioethics, and the role of clinical ethicist or of consultant in clinical ethics has crystallized as the focus of specialty training programmes.

While clinical ethics is still in the process of developing the full panoply of expertise, instruments, and activities characteristic of a disciplinary specialty, sub-specialties within clinical ethics are already coming into existence. This is particularly noticeable regarding the distinctive knowledge and experience required for the ethical issues in neonatal medicine, in the care or persons with neurological trauma, in transplantation, in the treatment of infertility, in palliative medicine, in the treatment of HIV disease, and in medical genetics.

Bioethics as Public Ethics

When existing law and conflicting moralities in a society are unable to deliver unambiguous guidance on novel practices affecting the entire community, people enter a period of moral searching and transition. At such a time, the values that silently guide a society come to clash openly in vibrant public expression: in television and radio programmes, in a continuous stream of newspaper and magazine articles, and in the reports of more formal and systematic discussion carried out in commissions, committees and working groups convened by professional associations, religious bodies, and governments in countries throughout the world.

The Context of Bioethics as Public Ethics

Since the early 1970s, one has been able to observe this exercise of public ethics taking shape as a response of bioethics to the biomedical challenge. Bioethics as public ethics emerged from warnings in the 1960s and 1970s that momentous advances were taking place on the frontiers of the life sciences. Scientists and scientifically literate philosophers, theologians and lawyers took up the responsibility of awakening an uninformed public to possible threats these advances could direct to the foundational values of society.

The central idea of bioethics as public ethics is that the common good, as potentially threatened or enhanced by biomedical developments, is too important to be left in the hands of any one elite group, or any collection of elite groups. It makes little difference whether these elites be groupings of scientists, technocrats, physicians, or ethicists. Robert Sinsheimer directed attention, in the late 1970s, to newly emerging threats to individuals and to society that could arise from the power that modern science can give to a small group, and from the power gained by any one group, when it can discover the control points of a society and thereby direct society's evolution (Sinsheimer, 1979, 63).

In the face of deep divisions about fundamental values, there is no viable substitute in open societies for the long process of civilized argument and persuasion. Compromises have to be struck; guidelines have to be drawn; policies have to be formed; and judgments have to be made about the choices that are consonant with a society's identity, about what behaviours can be tolerated, even if not endorsed, about where limits have to be set in liberty, and about which rights and values have to cede to others when all cannot be honoured.

Finding a common ground and achieving consensus and compromise as a basis for policy, when people are divided on issues of liberty, rights, and values, is the work of public ethics, and public ethics has been one of the most important fields of bioethics since the public debates on recombinant DNA in the mid 1970s. Many of the ethical issues that appear at the bedside and in the laboratory reach out beyond these confines into health care institutions as a whole, into the health care system, into government, and into society at large. This has been the case with abortion, euthanasia, the reproductive technologies, sterilization of the mentally disabled, HIV infection and AIDS, genetic testing and genetic therapy, research with the human embryo, and the allocation of limited resources. Each of these problematic areas involving medicine and the biomedical technologies has been a focus of bioethics as public ethics over the last three decades.

The Scope of Bioethics in Its Field of Public Ethics

To understand the place and scope of bioethics as public ethics, it would be useful to discuss the general relationships between social ethics and public ethics.

Each of these domains of ethics shares the goal of protecting and enhancing the common good. They differ, however, with respect to the scope of the common good with which they are concerned (Jonsen, 1975).

The common good encompasses many interrelated values. One of these, the most comprehensive, is the order of society as a whole. Social ethics deals with judgments about what is obligatory, permissible, tolerable, or totally unacceptable in social policies that serve to correct, stabilize, or advance the organization of society as a whole (Winter, 1968).

Public ethics is more restricted in scope, in two ways. First, public ethics centres, not on the order of society as a whole, but rather on the order of specific institutions within society. We use the word *institution* here, not in the sense of a building housing a societal function, but to name the function itself and the order without which it would not exist. In this broad sense, education, the media, the family, science, the economy, health care and the professions, such as medicine and law, are societal institutions. A society, as we now know it, could not exist without these functions. Public ethics focuses on the policies related to the maintenance and advance of the good of order of these functions or institutions.

There is also a second sense in which public ethics is more restricted than social ethics. Social ethics deals with the broad problems related to the purposes and structure of society as a whole, and its schedule of work stretches into the range of long-term goals and consequences. For example, to the extent that ethics was involved in the 1992 constitutional discussions about the future of Canada, it was social rather than public ethics that was at work. Public ethics is rather restricted to the domain of particular issues of public concern, issues involving particular segments of the common good, and issues that require resolution within a relatively short period of time. The schedule of public ethics covers short- and mid-term goals and consequences.

Bioethics, in its field of public ethics, is concerned with the policies (whether or not these take the form of law, regulation, or guidelines) covering segments of the common good affected by the biomedical challenge. For example, reproduction, parenthood, and the family are affected by developments in genetics and the reproductive technologies, and these two areas of biomedicine have been centres of intense activity in the public ethics field of bioethics over the last fifteen years. In the coming years, bioethics as public ethics will very likely find that the order of the health care system, which is part of the common good of the order of society as a whole, will become a centre of activity as intense as that required for abortion and the reproductive technologies over the last decade.

Method in Bioethics as Public Ethics

The analysis and resolution of bioethical issues in the field of public ethics requires the same kind of practical reasoning displayed in research ethics and clinical ethics. However, the kinds of interdisciplinary and intercultural collaboration needed for the resolution of public issues in ethics are more varied than those suited for resolution of conflicts of belief and value conflicts in the laboratory or at the bedside. Uniquely difficult ethical issues arise when biomedical challenges target institutions that implicate the welfare of an entire population in a highly pluralistic society. The resolution of these issues, as Daniel Callahan saw years ago, forces biomedical ethics to move into the mainstream of political and social theory, beyond the model of the individual decision-maker, and into the thicket of important vested and legitimate private and group interests (Callahan, 1980, 1233).

The goal of method in public ethics is to extricate ethics from the deadlock of interminable discourse about matters upon which people are likely never to agree. For this reason, the method of public ethics parts ways, as do the methods of research ethics and clinical ethics, with the thesis that bioethics is simply applied ethics.

This is the central insight Stephen Toulmin acquired from his experience while working with the United States National Commission for the Protection of Human Subjects of Biomedical and Behavioral Research. The members of the Commission, though representing quite different professions, disciplines, and philosophical outlooks on life, came to agreement on detailed recommendations, provided they considered one difficult kind of case and compared it in detail with other clearer and easier cases. Toulmin observed that he and other people could frequently agree on practical judgments about what should or should not be done, about what could or could not be tolerated, but they began to really disagree when each appealed to principles to explain why this or that practical judgment was justifiable. As Toulmin concluded, "They could agree; they could agree what they were agreeing about; but, apparently, they could not agree why they agreed about it." (Toulmin, 1981, 32)

When conflicts and controversies in bioethics are rooted in deep differences of belief and of values, it is extremely difficult to justify the claim that one single decision or position is reasonable and all the others involved in a conflict are unreasonable. The reasons brought forth for and against positions in deep moral controversies are shaped within very different world-views, which, when elaborated, produce a plurality of philosophies and moralities. Any attempt to base public ethics, not on practical judgments where people can agree, but on the basic reasons and arguments used to justify these judgments, will entrap public ethics in an ever more fragmenting process of divergent thinking. As emphasized earlier, we no longer live in a classical culture, where appeal could be made to a single universally binding world-view to ground practical judgments on morally controversial matters.

Bioethics in public ethics, as well as in research ethics and clinical ethics, is a matter of practical reasoning, and not the deduction of action conclusions from self-evident principles. Practical reasoning, first of all, requires comprehensive attention to the full particularity of specific cases and situations. Even if two cases or situations are similar in many respects, one cannot, if practical reasoning is correctly exercised, simply apply or transfer the judgment made in one case or situation to a new situation. There is, as Jonathan Dancy has observed, nothing available (and abstract principles certainly will not do) to drive us on rails from what needs to be decided in one case to the decision the next case or situation requires (Dancy, 1985, 147).

An example from clinical ethics will illustrate this point. Should one aggressively treat severe, nearly total body burns, when survival is likely, but blindness and paralysis of legs and arms is certain? Such burns were treated in one case, because the young man wanted to live at any and all costs. In a similar case, some while later in the same hospital, another young man was simply comforted and allowed to die, because he simply could not bear the thought of never being able to read, play sports again, or do any of the things that made his life worthwhile.

In practical reasoning, it is essential to determine carefully what each new case and situation is like and what it requires. The tendency of applied ethics, with its reliance on principles, is to exaggerate the similarity between cases and situations and to distract attention away from their uniqueness and their differences. Attention to this uniqueness may well necessitate decisions or policies that we cannot show to be consistent with principles or earlier decisions in similar situations. Insistence on consistency can prevent people from taking the decision or adopting the policy that a unique situation requires (Dancy, 1985, 153).

Second, practical reasoning emphasizes the central methodological importance of Aristotelian dialectic in bioethics as public ethics. Aristotle's method to arrive at the best ethical judgments possible in any given situation is based on the assumption that people need to learn what they really think about a specific issue. The method pits both the many and the wise, that is, ordinary people and experts, in discussion with each other. The aim is to unfold, to lay out, the values and judgments of people who come to an issue with definite intuitions and value commitments. The mutually corrective interplay of these different views, achieved as people work through alternatives in dialogue, is what Aristotle's dialectic involves. The goal of this dialectic is that the people exercising practical reasoning in dialogue will, both individually and in community with one another, arrive at a harmonious adjustment of their initial beliefs or starting positions (Nussbaum, 1986).

Practical reasoning, the method of bioethics in its three fields of research ethics, clinical ethics, and public ethics, is of central importance in all situations marked by the absence of indisputable truth or authority, as the standard for the justifiability of concrete decisions and policies. This, generally, is the situation in which we find ourselves in a post-classical world. Practical reasoning in bioethics, modeled on the method of Aristotle's dialectic, reveals the implicate ethical order (discussed above) contained in the community of people brought together in contemporary working groups and commissions. That ethical order, the governing practical judgments and policies, emerges as people mutually criticize, refute, and justify their views. This dialectical system is not the deductive system of applied ethics, but an open exploratory system of people who discover the ethical order they share, in the course of their discussion. The goal of practical reasoning in bioethics is the peaceful coexistence and collaboration of free and reasonable people in a pluralistic society (Perelman, 1968).

CONCLUSION

This chapter opened with the question of what distinguishes bioethics, as it has developed since the late 1960s, from morality and from professional, theological, feminist and philosophical ethics. Bioethics has been presented in this, and in the preceding, chapter as society's response to the biomedical challenge. That challenge, as Hans Jonas has said, has introduced into society power and actions of such moral scale, objects, and consequences that the framework of former ethics can no longer contain them (Jonas, 1974, 8).

This challenge forced bioethics to go to the root of ethics. But the root of ethics, as Bernard Lonergan has explained, is not found in sentences, propositions, principles, codes, or guidelines. The root of ethics is found in the unfolding of rational self-consciousness; the unfolding of the rational self-consciousness of many people, involved in mutually corrective deliberation to reach the best possible judgments for specific cases and situations. Existing persons, not pre-existing propositions about principles, are the real root of ethics (Lonergan, 1957, 604).

The method of bioethics proposed in this book is radical, in the Latin sense of the word. The method goes to the roots and origins of ethics in seeking to derive an ethical order, an order of value priorities and related practical judgments and policies, from the prudential deliberation, interdisciplinary and intercultural, of existing persons seeking to resolve specific issues. This is what Gordon Dunstan has called a new development in method (Dunstan, 1988, 6). Paul Ricoeur has reached back to Aristotle's term *phronesis*, to characterize this method as one based on practical wisdom, as a method based on the prudence of the many (*une phronesis à plusieurs*) (Ricoeur, 1991, 268).

It is this approach, this method, that distinguishes bioethics from morality and from professional, theological, and philosophical ethics.

REFERENCES

Beauchamp T.L. and **Childress J.F.** *Principles of Biomedical Ethics*. Third Edition. New York, Oxford: Oxford University Press, 1989.

Bohm D. *Wholeness and the Implicate Order*. London: Routledge and Kegan Paul, 1980.

Callahan D. "Normative Ethics and Public Morality in the Life Sciences." *The Humanist* Sept.-Oct. 1972;5-7.

Callahan D. "Shattuck Lecture - Contemporary Biomedical Ethics." *The New England Journal of Medicine* 1980;302:1228-1233.

Clouser D. "Bioethics." In: *Encyclopedia of Bioethics*. Vol. I. New York: The Free Press, 1978, 115-127.

Dancy J. "The Role of Imaginary Cases in Ethics." *Pacific Philosophical Quarterly* 1985;66:147, 153.

Donagan A. *The Theory of Morality*. Chicago: The University of Chicago Press, 1977.

Dunstan G.R. "Two Branches from One Stem." In: D. Callahan and G.R. Dunstan, eds."Biomedical Ethics: An Anglo-American Dialogue." *Annals of the New York Academy of Sciences*. Vol. 530. New York: The New York Academy of Sciences, 1988, 4-6.

Frankena W.K. *Thinking about Morality*. Ann Arbor: The University of Michigan Press, 1980.

Freidson E. *Profession of Medicine*. New York: Harper & Row, 1970.

Green R.M. "Method in Bioethics: A Troubled Assessment." *The Journal of Medicine and Philosophy* 1990;15:179-197.

Holmes R.L. "The Limited Relevance of Analytical Ethics to the Problems of Bioethics." *The Journal of Medicine and Philosophy* 1990;15:143-159.

Jonas H. *Philosophical Essays. From Ancient Creed to Technological Man*. Englewood Cliffs, New Jersey: Prentice Hall, 1974.

Jonsen A.R. and **Butler L.H.** "Public Ethics and Policy Making." *Hastings Center Report* 1975;5:19-31.

Kass L.R. "The New Biology: What Price Relieving Man's Estate?" *Science* 1971;174:779-788.

Lonergan B. *Insight. A Study of Human Understanding*. London: Longmans, Green and Co., 1957.

MacKinnon C. *Feminism Unmodified: Discourses on Life and Law*. Cambridge: Harvard University Press, 1987.

MacKinnon C. *Toward a Feminist Theory of the State*. Cambridge: Harvard University Press, 1989.

McCormick R. "Theology and Bioethics." *Hastings Center Report* 1989;19/2:5-10.

Miles S.H. and **August A.** "Courts, Gender and 'The Right to Die'." *Law, Medicine and Health Care* 1990;18:85-95.

Nussbaum M.C. *The Fragility of Goodness - Luck and Ethics in Greek Tragedy and Philosophy.* Cambridge: Cambridge University Press, 1986, 240-263.

Perelman C. "Le Raisonnement pratique." In: R. Klibansky, ed. *Contemporary Philosophy. A Survey.* Vol. I. Firenze: La Nuova Italia Editrice, 1968, 168-176.

Rawls J. *A Theory of Justice.* Cambridge, Mass.: Belknap Press of Harvard University Press, 1971.

Ricoeur P. "Lectures 1." *Autour du politique.* Paris: Éditions du Seuil, 1991.

Ricoeur P. "The Teleotogical and Deontological Structures of Action: Aristotle and/or Kant?" *Archivio di Filosophia* 1987;55:205-217.

Ross W.D. *The Right and the God.* Oxford: Oxford University Press, 1930, 16-47.

Sherwin S. *No Longer Patient: Feminist Ethics and Health Care.* Philadelphia: Temple University Press, 1992.

Sinsheimer R. "Technology Can Free, but It Can also Impose Its Own Constraints." *The Center Magazine* 1979:XII/2:61-63.

Toulmin S. "The Tyranny of Principles." *Hastings Center Report* 1981;11:31-39.

Walters L. "Religion and the Renaissance of Medical Ethics in the United States: 1965-1975." In: E.E. Shelp, ed. *Theology and Bioethics.* Dordrecht, Boston, Lancaster, Tokyo: D. Reidel, 1985, 3-16.

Winter G. *Social Ethics: Issues in Ethics and Society.* New York: Harper & Row, 1968.

3

BIOETHICS
AND LAW

Bioethics, law, and the various moralities in a pluralistic society intersect and interact, sometimes harmoniously, sometimes discrepantly, on all the issues we shall be discussing in this book. Since we have already explained that bioethics is not a morality, the main topic of attention in this chapter is the relationship of bioethics to the law, with an emphasis on the relationship as it has developed in Canada.

PURPOSE AND OVERVIEW OF THE CHAPTER

Both bioethics and law are concerned with determining the scope and limits of obligations, rights, responsibilities, and liberties regarding the powers and projects rendered possible by biomedical developments. How, then, does bioethics relate to law, and vice-versa, in determining what is mandatory and what is to be prohibited, what is permissible or tolerable, in medicine and the life sciences? This is the central question of the chapter, and we shall approach it in the following way.

Because the relationship of bioethics and law varies from country to country, depending on the differences between the various systems of law in each country, and depending also on cultural, socioeconomic, and historical factors, we must first examine, as we shall do in the next section, how law is structured and works in Canada. Since we have argued in Chapter 2 that bioethics is not a morality, we next consider the relationship of law to morality, and ask whether bioethics and law have similar or divergent relationships to the moralities in our society.

But how, then, does bioethics relate to law? We approach this central question of the chapter by first considering what law has done for bioethics, and then, what bioethics has done for law. The chapter will close with three illustrations of how law and bioethics can part ways.

HOW LAW IS STRUCTURED AND WORKS IN CANADA

What Is Law?

When we think of "the law" we tend to consider particular laws, such as that vehicles are driven on the right side of the road in Canada rather than the left, and that we must not take other people's property without their permission. We think less often about the law as a social institution that embodies certain values, although when others seem free to do what we disapprove of, we may think that "there ought to be a law to prevent that." We can begin to understand the law by considering the origin of the rules we call "law."

Law comes from two sources, namely legislation and case law, otherwise known as judge-made law.

Legislation

Legislation is made by legislatures, which in Canada means Parliament in Ottawa regarding federal legislation, and legislative assemblies in the provinces regarding provincial legislation. Legislation may be called simply that, but is also described as Acts, Bills, statutes, enactments, or, in the territories, ordinances. Legislation is passed by the politicians who sit in the federal or the provincial legislatures, and often gives legal force to the policy of the political party that has a majority of members in the legislature, and therefore forms the government.

Legislation, or an Act, will consist of a series of sections that say what people or bodies may do, must do, or must not do in defined circumstances. An Act may permit the government to perform in specified ways, empower or require public or private bodies to behave in specified ways or for specified purposes, and/or give private individuals responsibilities, or rights to require others to discharge responsibilities.

Legislatures may implement general policies through legislation, but leave minor matters of detail to be specified in *regulations* that an Act authorizes another body, such as a Minister or a provincial Lieutenant-Governor, to make. A regulation is usually not discussed in a legislature before it comes into force. The power to give a regulation the force of law must come from a particular Act, however, and a regulation is valid only if made within the limits, by the procedure, and for the purpose laid down in the Act under which the regulation states that it is made.

It is not always clear what an Act or regulation means, how it is to be applied, how it relates to other Acts or regulations or to the general background case law. Lawyers may give advice based on their opinions, and, for instance, government or police officers, prosecutors and private individuals and corporations, acting with or without lawyers, may argue that legislation or a subordinate regulation covers a particular act, or that it does not. Only a court of law can authoritatively decide, however, what legislation or a regulation permits or does not permit to be done.

Case Law or Judge-Made Law

Case law or *judge-made law* comes from decisions made by courts of law. When judges interpret legislation or regulations, their role is to find the true intention of the legislature that enacted the legislation or that, by legislation, authorized the regulation to be made, or the purpose of a valid regulation. Whether or not a regulation is valid is decided by the courts, because that is a matter of interpretation of the legislation under which the regulation was made.

Outside Québec — because the private law system of Québec is drawn mostly from the European civil tradition — much of the law is contained, not in legislation or regulations, but in case law. Some of the most important rules of behaviour are legally obligatory because judges have recognized them in case law. For instance, it is case law that requires individuals to pay their debts, and not to be negligent to others to whom they owe legal duties of care. Further, the principles by which legislation and regulations are interpreted are developed by case law. For instance, the courts presume that legislation is intended to apply compatibly with case law, unless the legislature has shown a clear intention to change it, and that it does not apply retrospectively, unless the legislation clearly so provides. Courts also presume that important legal rules are not intended to be changed simply by a regulation.

What Types of Laws Are There?

There are many different ways to classify laws. A common distinction is between criminal law and civil law.

Criminal Law

Criminal law in Canada is made by federal legislation, notably through the *Criminal Code*, but also in related Acts such as the *Narcotic Control Act*. The Canadian Constitution permits only the federal Parliament to enact crimes, because, in general, criminal law should be uniform across the country. Criminal law is designed to provide that specified acts shall not be done, under threat of punishment. The state itself is usually the party that enforces the criminal law. The state's power to punish, which means deliberately to harm or disadvantage an offender, is vast, and by case law the courts interpret criminal legislation to cover as few circumstances as necessary. Any uncertainty of fact is resolved in favour of an accused party. Every accused party is presumed innocent, and the prosecutor must prove guilty behaviour and intent beyond reasonable doubt before an accused party can be convicted and become liable to punishment.

Civil Law

Civil law is most easily understood simply as noncriminal law, although some matters, such as not taking another's property, may be governed by both civil and criminal law. The purpose of civil law is not to punish, but primarily to regulate the relationship between individual persons and to deter injurious behaviour by providing that parties whose legal interests have been harmed can recover compensation from others who are responsible. Alternatively, people who fear harms that cannot adequately be compensated can seek court orders to restrain others from committing such harmful acts.

Claims of violation of civil law are usually brought against defendants by private parties, who are described as plaintiffs or applicants. Claims may be brought against private parties, but also against public bodies and governments. Usually, plaintiffs have to prove their cases, but sometimes a defendant may bear the burden of disproving a claim. Whoever bears the burden of proof of facts in a civil action needs proof on a balance of probability, meaning that it is more likely than not that the claims that the party makes are actually true.

Civil laws may be enacted by legislation, and in some important areas, such as concern business corporations and commercial activities, sophisticated and technical Acts have been passed by provincial and federal legislatures. Much civil law remains based on case law, however, outside Québec. Québec has a codified system of private law. The *Civil Code* of Québec thus contains most of the general civil law of the province..

Constitutional and Administrative Law

Constitutional and *administrative law* are often distinguished from criminal and civil law, although the distinction is imprecise. In Canada, the *Constitution Act 1867*, originally known as the *British North America Act*, as amended notably in 1982 by introduction of the *Canadian Charter of Rights and Freedoms*, is often said to be "the Constitution." The 1867 Act, as amended, lays down powers of the federal, provincial and territorial governments. Governmental activities, including the enactment of legislation, that violate the *Constitution Act* or the *Charter*, are said to be unconstitutional.

Administrative law controls what public and quasi-public bodies do, and how they make decisions. There is no discrete body of administrative law, since its principles are drawn from such general legal rules as those of natural justice or fairness, including the right to an unbiased court or tribunal, and to know and speak to the questions at issue. Only the federal government can legislate against crime, but a province pursuing a constitutional power may penalize conduct by creating summary or quasi-criminal offences. Such offences are sometimes called public welfare or administrative offences or infractions, as opposed to true crimes, although they are tried in the courts that try and punish crimes.

The Canadian Charter of Rights and Freedoms

The *Canadian Charter of Rights and Freedoms* obliges government agencies not to violate rights considered fundamental. Such rights include life, liberty and security of the person, freedom of conscience, thought, belief and expression, democratic rights, nondiscrimination rights and, for instance, the right to be presumed innocent when charged with a criminal offence. The Charter does not bind nongovernment bodies such as public hospitals or universities, although they are bound by provincial human rights codes that contain many similar provisions. The federal and provincial legislatures are bound by the Charter, but can bypass it for five years by expressly legislating that a provision is enacted "notwithstanding" the Charter. Further, when a court finds that a legislated provision violates the Charter, the court can still uphold it under Section 1 as a reasonable limit that "can be demonstrably justified in a free and democratic society." Democratic support for legislation that violates the Charter does not compel the courts to uphold it, however, because the Charter protects fundamental freedoms and legal rights against even democratically composed majorities. In the 1988 Morgentaler case, for instance, the Supreme Court of Canada declared *Criminal Code* provisions limiting performance of abortion unconstitutional and therefore inoperative, because they violated women's rights to security of the person, notwithstanding that the provisions had been democratically enacted after full and serious debate.

What Type of Legal System Does Canada Have?

Noncriminal law in Canada is applied according to one of two legal traditions. The tradition derived from England, which applies outside Québec, is called the Common-law system, while in Québec the legal tradition is derived from France and, in another use of the term "civil," is called the Civil-law system. The Common-law system is based on judge-made law and binding precedents interpreting the law, meaning decisions of appeal courts that lower or trial courts are bound to follow. In Québec, the law is contained in the Civil Code and, while appeal courts interpret the Code persuasively, their decisions are not strictly binding on other courts. In contrast, in the Common-law system, decisions of the Supreme Court of Canada bind all other courts (but not the Supreme Court itself), and decisions of a provincial Court of Appeal are binding within the province, including on the Court of Appeal itself. Conflicting decisions of provincial Courts of Appeal may be resolved by the Supreme Court of Canada. Decisions of trial courts are not legal precedents in a strict sense, although other trial courts usually explain why they will not decide consistently with them, and do not just ignore them.

What Do Courts and Judges Do?

It follows from the discussion above that courts and judges perform two main functions. They interpret legislation, and they develop case law. Courts have significant additional functions in trials, because they hear evidence of facts in dispute in order to resolve critical disagreements. Facts are found according to the evidence presented by parties to disputes, and will be determined by juries or, when there is no jury, by the judge conducting the trial. Juries are in fact rare, being present usually only in cases charging serious crimes. Although often decisive in an individual case, facts are relatively unimportant to the development of the law. Fact findings will rarely be in issue before appeal courts, which do not hear witnesses, but consider only legal arguments relevant to the facts proved at the trial. Appeal courts' decisions on law will create precedents. The way courts approach legal issues is often referred to as their jurisprudence, meaning the prudence or judgment of, especially, the higher courts.

In interpreting legislation, courts try to find the intention of the particular legislature that enacted the law. Courts are guided by the language of an Act, but the relation between an Act and an earlier or later Act may not be clear. A subsequent Act may supersede an earlier one, but may either re-express it, perhaps with minor variations, or fundamentally change it. A later Act may, however, coexist with an earlier one but limit or expand it, or cover an issue the earlier Act did not govern. How one Act relates to an earlier Act may be implied rather than expressed in the later Act, and courts have to determine what implication the particular legislature intended from all of the relevant circumstances.

Case law is dynamic and evolutionary, in that later courts interpret the meaning and effect of earlier judgments. A later court will define the scope of an earlier precedent, and perhaps distinguish a binding precedent from the case before it, because the facts are different in some material way. On the other hand, a court may find that an earlier judgment, although given in a case in which the facts were different from those now present, was wide enough in its scope to govern the present facts, and so be applicable.

Suppose, for instance, in Case A, that a dog has suddenly run across the road outside a university, causing a car to brake, skid and crash into a lamp-post. The driver sues the dog's owner for negligence, and wins the action. The trial judge says that, in law, owners must control their animals. In Case B, a cat suddenly dashes across the same road, causing a similar crash. The judge in Case B will have to decide if Case A concerned animals, in which case driver B will recover damages from the cat owner, or only dogs, in which case driver B will not succeed. Judge B may find that dogs and cats are distinguishable, because dogs are kept on leads while cats are not expected to be, and that judge A referred only to controllable animals.

In Case C, a dog suddenly dashes across a country road, causing a car driver to skid and crash. Judge C may say that Case A is a case concerning all dog owners, even if judge B found that it was not a cat case, and award damages against dog owner C. Alternatively, however, even if driver B won because judge B found that Case A governs all animals and not just dogs, judge C may be persuaded that Cases A and B are town cases, where animal owners must guard traffic against accidents, but Case C is a country case, where animals can run free and traffic must beware. If car drivers B or C lost their actions, car driver D, injured in a crash when a cat ran across a country road, will probably not sue. Indeed, in view of that jurisprudence, driver D may be advised by an insurance company not to brake for cats in the countryside.

The Interaction of Legislation and Case Law

Judges must often determine the relation of legislation to case law. Legislation may be based on case law; for instance, legislation that requires that consent be given for a medical procedure may not define consent, but leave the definition to case law. Some legislation codifies an area of case law, filling in gaps and concretizing the *status quo* against later change. If a legislature disapproves case law, however, for instance because it politically disfavours the jurisprudence or finds that the case law has not kept up with new developments or perceptions, it may enact legislation that supersedes the case law. If legislation clearly provides that it codifies or displaces existing case law, judges will apply it accordingly, but if there is uncertainty, judges will have to find what the legislature intended through arguments of parties' lawyers. Judges may find that legislation is intended to be read compatibly with surrounding case law, and either that legislation refines a particular area of case law, or that case law offers an implied exception to the legislation.

A legislature that is dissatisfied with how the courts have interpreted an Act may reenact the legislation to reassert its purpose. The new Act will be authoritatively interpreted, however, by the courts. There is, accordingly, continuing interaction between courts and legislatures, in that legislatures react to evolving case law and judicial interpretations of legislation, and courts react to legislation that they are called on to interpret.

Through both interpretations of legislation and applications of case law, the law is in a constant state of flux. Judges often follow precedents for the purpose of keeping the law stable, but they also review and reinterpret case law to keep it contemporary. The law faces continuing tension in balancing the competing needs of predictability and updating.

Lawyers give advice on the basis of how they anticipate the courts will apply and develop case law and interpret legislation. As advocates before courts, they present evidence of facts and arguments of law that serve the goals their clients have instructed them to pursue. They do not deliberately mislead the courts, and do not conceal or ignore jurisprudence or evidence that opposes their clients' interests, but require their adversaries to discharge the burden of proof they bear under the legal rules of evidence and procedure.

THE RELATIONSHIP OF LAW TO MORALITY

There are many divergent moralities in a society as pluralistic as Canada's, and we could not possibly, in one section of a chapter, offer a detailed analysis of how law in Canada relates to each. We shall, rather, consider why four propositions on the general relationship of law to morality, propositions put forth at various times in the past and still held by some people today, do not hold true in a pluralistic society. We then consider how the relationship of law to morality is a very variable one, and conclude with the thesis that law and bioethics hold a quite similar relationship to moralities in a pluralistic society.

Law and Morality: A Generally Harmonious Relationship?

Chaim Perelman has stated that the relationship between law and morality is generally one of conformity and harmony (Perelman, 1980, 119). People may even commonly assume that law, morality, and bioethics should not issue contradictory commands and prohibitions. The law attempts to accommodate moral choices, and not to compel individuals to act against their moral conscience or religious convictions. Nevertheless, reality is often different from what we may assume it is, or should be.

We have seen conflicts between various moralities and law, for example, on the issues of abortion and use of animals in research, dramatically acted out in Canada over the last ten years. The drama included acts of violence and civil disobedience, and massive demonstrations against existing and proposed law. This challenging of law has brought people on both sides of contentious issues into contact with the police, into the courts, and even into jail.

A number of the issues we shall discuss in this book, particularly the issues raised by abortion, sterilization of mentally handicapped people, the new reproductive technologies, research with the human embryo, the transplantation of fetal tissue, and euthanasia, offer ample illustrations of the conflicts that occur when law permits what a morality prohibits, and when law prohibits what many people accept as justifiable or tolerable in particular circumstances.

Law, Morality, and the Public-Private Distinction

It is quite impossible to explain satisfactorily the relationship of law to morality by some *simple distinction of exclusive domains of operation peculiar to each*. Consider, for example, the idea that morality pertains to the sphere of *private acts*, like sexual relationships, and law to the domain of *public acts*, such as those involved in health care, in the practice of medicine, and in business. The law cannot be excluded totally from the domain of private acts, because some private acts, notably those involved in human reproduction, have public and social consequences. Accordingly, we have a need for *family law*. On the other hand, some public acts, like those involved in the practice of medicine, are too complex, and vary too much from case to case, to ever be comprehensively regulated by law. Of course, some public acts, like capital punishment and acts of discrimination, are matters of morality even when they are regulated by law. Such acts involve and provoke struggles of individual and community conscience.

There is never a legal vacuum, in that every public and private act has a status according to law, but the law regulates actions with different levels of specificity. Industrial employment, manufacture, health and safety are regulated in detail, but relations among friends enjoy wide areas of discretion. The law is frequently neutral as to moral matters, permitting rather than approving individual choices, and containing exceptions to what it generally disapproves.

The Reduction of Morality to Law

Another equally simple and erroneous idea is that *morality can be reduced to law*. Morality, on the basis of this notion, would not extend beyond the obligations, permissions, and prohibitions codified in the law. The law, then, would represent the necessary and sufficient catalogue of rationally binding constraints on human behaviour. However, there are just and unjust laws, as history amply demonstrates. If morality were just what the law contains and nothing else, where would we find the standards to distinguish between just and unjust laws? Moreover, conscience may also issue commands of reason for decisions and acts, about which the law has not yet said anything at all. And lastly, even if a majority of citizens considers a law to be just, a particular moral community in society may judge the acts the law permits to be intolerable. So, morality cannot be simply reduced to law.

A danger of law that seeks to enforce moral behaviour is that it may replace individuals' moral reflection and judgment by mere obedience to law. This may reduce the experience in society of having to exercise moral choice.

Should Law Enforce Morality?

Lord Patrick Devlin argued several years ago that if the purpose of law is to protect a community or society from disintegration, there are no theoretical limits to the state's power to legislate against immorality (Devlin, 1977, 76). Professor H.L.A. Hart adopted a quite diametrically opposed position, insisted on the distinction between law and morality, and warned that a society should not allow law to supplant morality (Hart, 1983, 54).

There are real and practical limits on the law's power to enforce morality. Even when private or public behaviour strikes gravely against the common good, it does not always follow that law should be enacted, or if it already exists, that law should be implemented to enforce morality. The law may be unenforceable, or may not be equitably enforceable, or may even provoke greater evils than those which it is supposed to prevent (St. John-Stevas, 1961, 39).

Limits on expectations that law can, or should, enforce morality also arise from the fact that positions on what is moral and immoral can be based upon little more than bias, prejudice, and the dominance of unexamined desires, fears, and repulsions. Law is likely to be discredited if it is used to enforce moralities that would eradicate the tolerance essential for the long-term good of order in pluralistic societies. Moreover, in many morally contentious areas of behaviour, it is extraordinarily difficult to claim that only one position is reasonable, and all other positions displayed in the controversy are intolerably unreasonable. Reasons put forth for and against positions in a moral controversy come from beliefs, perceptions, and assumptions. These are shaped within quite different world-views, which, when elaborated, give birth to a plurality of philosophies and moralities (Perelman, 1980, 172). The fabric of a society would shred, if law were called upon to enforce one of these moral world views against all the others.

Law and Morality: A Variable Relationship

When many moralities are contending for social acceptance, the function of the law is to create and maintain a social order, within which people can advance from moral discord to moral discourse. If we think, for example, of sexual and reproductive morality, there is perhaps great wisdom in the strong tendency of Western societies to respect the freedom of people's reproductive decisions and choices. This creates space for the so-varied ways of living love and parenthood. Legal constraints are both reasonable and necessary to prevent discrimination, the violation of fundamental rights, and a likely societal slide down a slippery slope to abuses. However, when the prevention of grave injustice is not at issue, societies are quite wise in not trying to impose legally one or another of the contending moralities in our pluralistic world.

This liberal model of law's relationship to morality does seem to reflect a dominant consensus in North America and Europe, in the scope of freedom conscience should enjoy in the area of sexual and reproductive behaviour. Even here, however, there are exceptions, as evidenced in Ireland's unusually restrictive abortion law, in the still-existing older laws of a few states of the U.S. regarding homosexuality, and in the laws of some countries prohibiting the commercial arrangement of surrogate mothering.

On the issue of euthanasia, law exhibits a more conservative relationship to morality than it does in the areas of sexuality and reproduction. Though associations have been formed, and ethical arguments have been marshalled, to promote the decriminalization of active euthanasia, there is still a strong tendency in Western societies, the Netherlands being an exception, legally to enforce the moral condemnation of this practice. The law does not, or does not yet, relate to morality in a liberal fashion on the issue of euthanasia. The law in this area is conditioned both by moral views on the sanctity of human life, and pragmatic concerns that accommodation of euthanasia would lead to abuse of vulnerable people.

The way law should relate to morality in any given society cannot be determined solely by an analysis of concepts and principles. Attention has to be given to the legal, social, economic, and health care systems within which this relationship operates. A liberal relationship on matters of reproduction may well hold its own in societies with a population size, economic order, educational tradition, and political system similar to our own. However, other societies quite different from our own, and even our own society in quite different circumstances, might, on specific issues, be constrained to adopt laws that severely restrict choice in reproductive matters. China, with its massive population and its recent policies on one child per family and coerced sterilization of intellectually deficient people, offers one current controversial example. Other societies, anxious to increase population size, have been seen to restrict access to methods of family limitation.

If enforcement of morality is seen as a continuum, law usually shifts from the weak to the strong enforcement ends of this continuum, depending on what is at stake in any particular issue. It is incorrect to place the law, even the law of any one country, at only one position on the continuum. In practice, the law may strongly enforce morality on one issue, as U.S. and Canadian law do on the issue of euthanasia. On another issue, such as abortion, the law may incorporate a minimalist ethic of fetal protection, as some think U.S. abortion law does, with the relative protection it gives the fetus in the third trimester of pregnancy. The relationship of law to morality and ethics is quite different in practice than it is often represented to be in theory. We sometimes enact laws in order to express our highest ideals, but do not enforce them strictly, in case they interfere with practices we find agreeable or appropriate to tolerate.

Law and Bioethics: A Similar Relationship to Morality

Bioethics and law share a similar relationship to the various moralities in our pluralistic society. Both bioethics and law, particularly in the area of public policy, pursue the goal of devising the compromises and the practical consensus within which people can live, while they continue to disagree on matters profound. The implication is that bioethics and law cannot, nor should they be presumed to, substitute for morality. To the extent that they do so substitute, society is suffering an impoverishment. The converse is also true. Given the extent of the divisive tension between the various moralities, a society as pluralistic as Canada's could be torn asunder, were either bioethics or law to propagate one world view against its competitors.

THE IMPACT OF LAW ON BIOETHICS IN CANADA

There is, to our knowledge, no treatise available that comprehensively examines the relationships between law and bioethics. Of course, bioethics, as indicated in the two preceding chapters, is new and still developing. A study of its relationship to law, particularly the very brief examination of that relationship that we can undertake in this section, may therefore best proceed by considering specific instances illustrating both the harmonious and the discordant intersections of law and bioethics. So we do not presume, in this section, to offer a comprehensive or theoretical analysis of the relationship, but draw attention, rather, to instances where law has exercised a positive impact on bioethics. There are also conflicts between bioethics and law, and we shall examine three instances in the closing section of this chapter, and other instances in greater detail in later chapters.

Law and Bioethics: Observations from Other Countries

The relationship of law to bioethics will vary from country to country, and we set our discussion of that relationship in Canada against the background of a summary review of key features of the relationship that observers in other countries have emphasized.

One American legal scholar, noting that the interaction between law and bioethics demonstrates both harmonies and conflicts, sees the harmony as deriving from the principles and processes that bioethics and law share in common. For example, the principle of autonomy, with its emphasis on informed consent, unites law and bioethics in opposition to a professional medical ethics that would emphasize paternalism and the principle of beneficence. As to common process, both bioethics and law have promoted interdisciplinary collaborative reasoning as the most viable approach to effective policy on controversial biomedical issues. In this view, conflicts occur between bioethics and law principally when the law is too inflexible or too general to account adequately for the complex subtleties of clinical situations (Capron, 1988).

There is a more cutting edge, however, to another observer's criticism that law in the United States has invaded medical ethics — or in the terms of this book, clinical ethics — to the point of killing it. The strongest statement of the law's negative impact on clinical ethics is that law either claims the prerogative of resolving, or is called upon to resolve, so many ethical issues that these cease to be matters of ethics and become matters of law. In this view, doctors tend to withdraw from involvement in clinical ethics. They refer uncertainties and dilemmas in clinical ethics to lawyers, and let judges decide these matters (Hyman, 1990).

A legal scholar in England has remarked that the role judges should adopt with regard to medical (or clinical) ethics is not clear. There is also uncertainty as to whether application to the courts is a satisfactory method of dealing with medico-ethical dilemmas. The fear is that the courts will be asked too frequently to resolve dilemmas that really are matters of medical or clinical ethics. English courts, it has been observed, are reluctant to pronounce definitively on the lawfulness, for example, of cessation of life-prolonging treatments, and prefer to leave these issues to debate within professional ethics groups until a trend emerges that rallies widespread professional and public approval (Dworkin, 1988).

In France, attention was focused on the relationships of bioethics to law, by a 1989 provisional draft of a law on the life sciences and human rights

(*Avant-projet de loi sur les sciences de la vie et les droits de l'homme*). Pressure had been building in France, since 1984, to move from bioethics to law. The 1989 draft proposed comprehensive and detailed regulations on a range of issues in bioethics that were, and still are, highly controversial in France and other countries throughout the world. As of 1992, this proposed law seems to have been shelved, perhaps as a result of a division of view within government circles about these controversial issues, almost certainly as a result of a governmental recognition that a law propagating one philosophy of life against others would not be quickly accepted in France. One of the leading authors in bioethics in France cautioned that current law should not be totally revamped in response to the biomedical challenge. Only those minimal legislative changes should be made that are necessary either to ban certain practices injurious to human dignity, or to regulate novel practices, for example, in the area of reproduction, so that fundamental human rights are adequately protected (Verspieren, 1991).

The Positive Impact of Law on Bioethics in Canada

What has law done for bioethics in Canada? We should be most wary of making any generalizations in answer to this question. A fair generalization should rest upon comprehensive solid data, and such data regarding the impact of law on bioethics in Canada have not yet been amassed and analysed. Nevertheless, any random selection of people familiar with law and bioethics in this country would most likely agree that we could not, in Canada, justifiably say, as some have said in the United States, that law has invaded bioethics and crippled it. Quite the contrary, law in Canada has done at least this for bioethics: it has, by and large, left bioethics alone to do its own work. That is something, but it is not all. On very important issues in the three fields of bioethics, Canadian law, particularly Canadian jurisprudence, has both guided and supported the work of bioethics. On other issues, that same jurisprudence has challenged bioethics and legal doctrine to pursue the research needed to clarify questions the court decisions have raised, but have not answered.

We shall now offer some evidence in support of this thesis affirming a remarkable complementarity between law and bioethics in Canada. Of course, any attempt to draw the lines of complementarity between the extensive legal and bioethical literatures on the multiple issues arising from the biomedical revolution would require at least one book, if not several. Consequently, we will restrict our attention here largely to Canadian case law, and to certain recommendations of the Law Reform Commission of Canada for amending the criminal law insofar as it touches upon clinical practice.

Regarding Cessation of Treatment

Clinical ethics, a field of bioethics, does not, as explained in Chapter 2, deductively apply principles to obtain conclusions about what should or should not be done in particular cases. The method of clinical ethics, rather, seeks to balance all of the elements in a clinical-ethical dilemma, to arrive at the best practical judgment about what is or is not in a patient's best interests. The full particularity of the patient, body and biography, is what should govern the practical judgments of clinical ethics. These judgments, cumulatively examined, unfold gradually, and in an always-incomplete way, the normative meaning of the principles that underline our moral and legal systems.

Cases involving cessation-of-treatment decisions, with their difficult and emotional intensity, are particularly revealing of the relationship of law to clinical ethics. We shall examine one recent case that, paradigmatically, exhibits both the synchrony of case law and clinical ethics, as well as the positive impact of jurisprudence on clinical ethics in Canada.

The case of Nancy B., a twenty-five-year-old woman affected by extensive muscular atrophy resulting from Guillain-Barré syndrome, was the focus of extensive newspaper, radio, and television commentary throughout Canada late in 1991 and during the first months of 1992. The case of Nancy B. went to the Superior Court of Québec when authorities at the Hôtel-Dieu Hospital in Québec City, where Nancy had been confined to bed for over two years, were reluctant to honour Nancy's request that the respirator, upon which she was dependent for breath and life, be disconnected. The hospital was concerned not only with violating Nancy B.'s rights, but also with violation of the *Criminal Code* regarding homicide.

Nancy was a young person, healthy and active prior to the Guillain-Barré attack on her muscular system. She would, according to expert medical opinion, never improve or recover from the extensive muscular atrophy that destroyed the muscles necessary for breathing and made her dependent on a respirator for life. She was lucid and not pathologically depressed, and she demanded cessation of life-prolonging treatment. The court was called upon to decide whether Nancy B.'s request should be honoured.

Judge Jacques Dufour, in his decision rendered on January 6, 1992, clarified two important points of law in support of his judgment that Nancy B.'s refusal of respirator treatment should be honoured. First, a doctor's act of disconnecting a respirator, in response to her patient's informed and free request that this be done, cannot be said to be either an unreasonable act or an act of criminal negligence. Secondly, disconnection of a respirator, in the circumstances of Nancy B.'s case, in no way amounts to either homicide or to aiding suicide.

This decision of Judge Dufour implicitly endorses two of the recommendations made by the Law Reform Commission of Canada early in the 1980s, as to how the *Criminal Code* of Canada should be changed in sections dealing with a physician's obligations to provide or continue life-prolonging treatment. The *Criminal Code*, drawn up long before the development of modern life-prolonging technology, is ambiguous and unclear about the legal status of withholding or discontinuing life-prolonging treatment. The Law Reform Commission recommended that these ambiguous sections of the Code be changed, so that the criminal law of Canada could not be interpreted as obliging physicians either to treat patients against their informed and free refusal, or to initiate or continue treatments that are therapeutically useless and not in the patients' best interests (Law Reform Commission, 1983, 32).

The decision of Judge Dufour on how the *Criminal Code* is to be interpreted and applied, and the two recommendations of the Law Reform Commission of Canada, confirm and reflect the direction of numerous practical judgments of clinical ethics in Canada, on issues involving life-prolongation decisions. This trend is away from a rigid "prolong-life-at-all-costs" ethic, towards an ethic based primarily upon the dignity and quality of life rather than on the duration of life taken as an absolute value.

This trend of clinical ethics, in the case of Nancy B., would emphasize that human dignity is strongly linked to the power to command respect for one's considered and cherished intentions. That trend would also accept the claim implicit in Nancy's request, the claim that, for some people, to be a human being, and to be bearably alive, requires more than being just a functioning brain. The bottom line is that there is no law that can justifiably command a patient like Nancy to be enslaved to a life-support machine. The judgment of Judge Dufour recognized that extension of life at all costs, particularly at personal costs of suffering the patient cannot bear, is not the right thing to do.

The decision of Judge Dufour in this case has a particular importance for clinical ethics, for two reasons. First, the eminently reasonable recommendations of the Law Reform Commission of Canada have been largely ignored by the legislature. They have never been passed into law. The ambiguity of the *Criminal Code* remains, and it is threatening both to doctors and hospitals. This judgment, then, offers some legal security for those who struggle with cessation-of-treatment decisions in clinical ethics. Second, members of a clinical team, with extensive experience in deciding about cessation of life-prolongation measures for unconscious patients, may well experience a strong visceral response against stopping such treatment for a conscious, lucid patient. The "executioner syndrome" should not be taken lightly. Physicians and others, though realizing the justification of a patient's request to disconnect respirator support, may find it most difficult to shake off the perception that they are executing the patient in so doing. The Dufour judgment may not dispel that personal perception, but it at least clarifies that withdrawal of life-prolongation treatment in cases similar to Nancy B.'s is neither an act of homicide, nor an act of aiding suicide in the eyes of the law. It is difficult to overestimate the powerful impact this decision is likely to have on clinical ethics in Canada.

Regarding Palliative Care

Physicians have a professional and a moral mandate to use every *proportionate* means available, to afford dying people the release from suffering that they desire — and for which they so often have to beg — so that they can die in tranquillity, and not in knots of agony. Relief from suffering is the moral act of respect for humanity and for human dignity.

Constant, wracking, and mind-twisting pain separates a person from himself and from loved ones. It shatters human integrity. Adequate control of pain is, then, an essential part of living an integrated life. Induction of the neuronal tranquillity that is prerequisite for an integrated human life, and for dying as an integrated human being, is the goal that should govern both the choice and combination of analgesics and the route, dosage, and frequency of administration. It is indeed foolish to deny patients relief from suffering, because of foolish fears or uncertain concerns that analgesics may shorten life.

However, physicians are far from foolish in fearing the consequences of the law, if they follow the pain-relief dictate of clinical ethics. Given the ambiguity of Canada's *Criminal Code*, some, perhaps many, physicians believe they have to be courageous and daring to go far enough with their use of drugs to relieve suffering effectively.

On this sensitive issue, the Law Reform Commission of Canada has done a great service to the clinical ethics of palliative care, in proposing to amend the *Criminal Code* so that it cannot be interpreted as obliging doctors to curtail the use of pain-killing drugs because of a fear that such drugs will shorten an incurable patient's life. This recommendation supports the view that the possible effect of analgesics on a dying person's length of life is no basis whatsoever for holding physicians criminally liable when they administer palliative medicine proportionate to the patient's need for relief from suffering (Law Reform Commission, 1983, 35). Indeed, the English judge, Lord Patrick Devlin, who claimed that law should uphold morality (see above), so instructed a jury in 1957, in the celebrated trial and acquittal of Dr. John Bodkin Adams.

Regarding Consent

Chapter 2, in its section on clinical ethics, emphasized that the patient, in his or her full particularity, is the norm that should govern practical judgments in the resolution of ethical dilemmas in clinical care. In Chapter 5, we shall emphasize the four ethical characteristics of a doctor-patient and professional-patient relationship. The second of these characteristics, lucidity, dictates that communication with patients should be open, honest, and impart to the patients all the information that could influence their decisions on treatment options.

The particularity of the patient's situation was a central issue in the Supreme Court of Canada case of *Reibl v. Hughes*. This case will be discussed in greater detail in Chapter 5, but we refer to it here to support the thesis of this chapter that law has had a positive impact on bioethics in Canada. This legally and ethically important judicial decision, finding a doctor civilly liable for negligence, illustrates the essential ethical difference between "obtaining" informed consent as a ritual kind of act, performed primarily to get treatment or research moving, and "educating" a patient or research subject in an open, searching conversation. The goal of such an exchange is to ensure that the patient knows everything that he or she requires to make a free and reasonable decision; and to ensure that the doctor knows enough about the patient's life, his or her story and life plans to inform the patient adequately about available choices of care.

The Supreme Court emphasized that merely because medical evidence establishes the reasonableness of a recommended operation does not mean that a reasonable person in the patient's personal and social situation would undoubtedly agree to the operation. Because Mr. Reibl was only eighteen months away from receiving full disability insurance benefits if he continued at his job, he would have preferred to postpone the risk of a stroke linked to the operation itself, by not agreeing to the operation Dr. Hughes was recommending until he had full financial protection if he were to become disabled. Had Dr. Hughes discussed this latter risk, the risk of stroke directly linked to the operation, adequately with Mr. Reibl, the conversation would very likely have brought out into the open the great importance Mr. Reibl attached to continuing in his work. Dr. Hughes asked if Mr. Reibl's house mortgage was paid, but did not alert him to the implications the operation had on his income, and that it might reduce his income to the level of his disability insurance benefits. The risk was very low that Mr. Reibl would have been disabled within eighteen months, had he decided to postpone the operation for that time, and his informed choice to run that risk would have protected Dr. Hughes against liability, had it resulted in disability.

The discussion of risk in consent negotiations is a very difficult and complex matter. Physicians and clinical investigators may have a tendency to downplay discussion of, or not even to mention, risks that are known in the medical literature to occur only rarely. However, patients may place greater emphasis on the severity of risk than on its frequency. They may, given their particular circumstances, quite reasonably refuse an operation, or prefer to delay an operation, or refuse to participate in research if these procedures carry even a remote risk of serious complications, such as paralysis or cardiac arrest or death. On the other hand, courts have held that very remote possibilities, such as of contracting hepatitis B from a blood transfusion, need not be disclosed to patients for whom a blood transfusion is indicated, because reasonable patients would not decline therapy on the basis of such low risk.

Regarding Abortion

Nearly ten years ago, one of the co-authors of this book was invited to speak to Catholics, Protestants, and Jews gathered for a meeting of the National Tripartite Liaison Committee, to discuss the subject of abortion. In a long open letter sent to the Committee members as a substitute for an academic text on the issue, the observation was made that those holding absolutely to the position that abortion merits no moral tolerance whatsoever, whatever the circumstances, would find it odd, maybe even obscene, to bother about whether Canadian law assures equitable access to abortion. The letter proceeded to warn that those who were, at the time, happy that Canadian law reduced the number of abortions and made them more difficult to obtain should not remain overly sanguine. The warning was that a law harbouring or causing basic inequities, as interpreted within the moral framework of a society, was destined to be overturned (Roy, 1983, 21).

Bioethics, in its field of public ethics, works with at least the three following criteria for justifiable legislation: the criteria of feasibility, justice, and minimization of greater evils. The first and third of these criteria would require ethical opposition to any law that would attempt a total ban on abortion. The second criterion, the criterion of justice, offered solid grounds to question the ethical justifiability of Canada's criminal abortion law, as it stood until rendered inoperative by the Supreme Court of Canada's 1988 decision in the case of *R. v. Morgentaler*.

This book will offer a more extensive discussion of abortion in Chapter 8, so mention of abortion here is restricted to an indication of the harmony that exists between law and bioethics on this most contentious and socially divisive of issues.

Regarding Limited Resources

The Canadian health care system, as we shall examine in greater detail in Chapter 4, expresses the strong commitment of Canadians to the principle that the provision of care and the pattern of health care funding should be the same for everyone. This is one of the central characteristics by which Canadians define ourselves. As Canadian health care economist, Robert G. Evans, has expressed it: "We are all equal when faced with disease or death, and our institutions reflect that sense of equality." (Evans, 1988, 169) This is the Canadian ideal upon which the *Canada Health Act* is based. The purpose of the Act is to dismantle economic barriers that limit reasonable access to high-quality medical care. Such care is supposed to be available to meet the medical needs of everyone in Canada.

However, maintenance of universal access to the best available care is not possible, when the volume of the best available care is constantly expanding and the costs for universal access are consuming increasing amounts of available resources. Hard choices have to be made, and they are hard, in part, because they challenge the legally buttressed ethical ideal that is the basis for the Canadian health care system.

These challenges may grow in number over the coming years, but one such challenge is already evident in the question about whether all Canadians should have governmentally paid access to a new contrast medium used in radiological (X-ray) examinations. Contrast media are iodine containing substances injected into the bloodstream to block the passage of X-rays. Use of these media gives a clearer diagnostic image, for example, of the heart, blood vessels, and kidney system. The new contrast media lessen unpleasant severe and minor reactions, as compared with the still widely used older contrast media, but the new media are much more costly.

If cost were not important, everyone would receive the new media. However, the Québec Council for the Evaluation of Health Care Technologies estimated that universal access to the new media would cost the province $15 million dollars a year more than the cost of the older media. So, cost cannot be ignored and raises the question of whether limiting access to the newer media, for example limiting access only to patients who can be identified to be at high risk for severe reactions, can be justified.

This question poses a challenge to the Canadian ideal of equal access. The challenge involves both legal and ethical issues, and a recent study exhibits additional evidence of harmony between law and bioethics in Canada. The study argues that there is neither a legal nor an ethical obligation to use the new costly media for everyone needing contrast media for diagnostic examinations (Roy, 1992).

THE IMPACT OF BIOETHICS ON LAW

Legislation

Because bioethics, as now understood, has evolved in relatively recent times, instances of its impact on case law are relatively few in Canada. Many bioethical perceptions have so influenced the political process of law-making, however, as to result in legislation. Most provinces have human-tissue gift laws, for instance, that recognize the principle of beneficence, and give effect to individuals' intentions to donate organs to others when alive, and particularly to their willingness, after they die, that their bodies be used for organ donation, scientific research or medical education. The ethical duty to protect the vulnerable is recognized, however, in that legal minors or those under sixteen years of age cannot be donors of solid organs. This prevents parents from giving legally effective consent. However, the province of Québec allows minors capable of discernment to do so, subject to certain conditions. When the minor will personally benefit from donating renewable tissues, however, such as blood or bone marrow, for instance to a brother or sister whose survival the minor will appreciate, parental consent may justify the minor serving as a donor if the minor does not object or resist. Ethical perceptions on human dignity and non-exploitation have also shaped the provision prohibiting commerce in human body materials, except blood and blood constituents.

Recognition of the bioethical value of the autonomy of competent adults in determining their medical care has resulted in several legislatures implementing, or considering recognition of, midwifery as a health profession for attending planned home births, without acting under the orders of doctors or nurses. Medical professional associations and licensing authorities have condemned home births, because babies and mothers may require care during or immediately after delivery that only hospitals have available. Legislatures have been persuaded, however, that the balance of benefits and disadvantages for both mother and child of home birth, attended by a midwife, over hospital birth should be struck by mothers individually, and not by the medical profession, because, of the available decision-makers, mothers are most affected by such decisions.

Courts' Interpretations of Legislation

The courts presume that legislatures intend their enactments to operate consistently with, rather than in violation of, bioethical principles. This is evident in cases considered above, such as the Nancy B. case. Here, the *Criminal Code* provisions regarding duties of maintaining life were considered subordinate to provisions of the Québec Civil Code on competent patients' rights to decline unwanted treatments. The trial judge invoked the *Reibl v. Hughes* judgment of the Supreme Court of Canada, which originated in Ontario, to tie the Québec jurisprudence to that of other Canadian provinces. The courts' presumption of consistency with bioethical principles is rebutted by clear provisions in legislation. The *Canadian Charter of Rights and Freedoms* may be violated, however, by legislation that endangers individuals' physical or mental health.

The Supreme Court of Canada, in the 1988 Morgentaler case, found the criminal abortion law to violate the Charter, for instance, because the law permitted abortion only to preserve a woman's life or health, but the procedure was made legally available in facilities that no one was legally obliged to set up and that, in fact, one province did not provide at all. The Chief Justice of Canada reflected bioethical principles of non-maleficence in observing that forcing an endangered woman, by threat of criminal sanction, to carry a fetus to term, unless she meets certain criteria unrelated to her own priorities and aspirations, is a profound violation of her bodily integrity because of its physical and emotional impact on her. The Charter protection of security of the person was interpreted to render the *Criminal Code* abortion provisions inoperative.

Case Law Developments

Canadian courts have been persuaded to adopt decisions of courts in other countries that give effect to bioethical principles. Several Canadian courts have expressed sympathy, for instance, with the New Jersey decision in the celebrated case of Karen Ann Quinlan, in which a court accepted a caring parent's right to speak the words his persistently vegetative daughter would have wanted spoken, to discontinue mechanical life support. The court accepted the authority of decisions jointly reached by patients' health attendants, representatives such as parents, and hospital ethics committees. Combining principles of autonomy and justice that incompetent persons not suffer discrimination, courts have concluded that incompetent individuals do not lose the autonomy they once possessed when others may reliably express it on their behalf.

Similarly, in the Wren case, the Alberta Court of Appeal adopted the reasoning of the highest court in England, the House of Lords, in the Gillick case. This gave effect to mature legal minors' rights of autonomy to consent to beneficial and protective medical treatments without their parents' consent and, because of patients' confidentiality, without their parents' knowledge. The case law has a broad application, because it concerned such sensitive and emotional issues as adolescent contraception and abortion.

A leading instance of bioethics influencing case law occurred in the 1991 Ontario Court of Appeal decision in *Malette v. Shulman*. A Jehovah's Witness was taken to hospital unconscious and bleeding after a terrible vehicle accident. The physician attending her was informed that she was carrying a signed card refusing blood products, but he undertook transfusion in order to prevent her death from heavy loss of blood. Mrs. Malette sued him for the civil wrong of battery, meaning unauthorized touching, and was awarded a favourable judgment that the Ontario Court of Appeal upheld. The trial judge observed that transfusion may have saved her life, but he and the unanimous appeal judges agreed that, in this case, the bioethical principle of respect for autonomous persons prevailed over principles of beneficence and non-maleficence. The patient was entitled to the priority of her own values, not her physician's, in determining what medical care she received, even when her choice endangered her survival. She was ethically and legally entitled to place her religious convictions over her need to survive. Society may not share her priorities of interests but, in a pluralistic country, can tolerate her freedom of preference.

CONFLICT BETWEEN LAW AND BIOETHICS

Law and bioethics have already entered into conflict in Canada for a number of quite different reasons, and they may continue to do so. If we have drawn attention, in previous sections, to instances where law intersects harmoniously with bioethics, we must now identify certain instances of conflict in the relationship.

When the Law Is Out of Date

We have already alluded several times to the judgment shared by the Law Reform Commission of Canada and by persons active in clinical ethics that the *Criminal Code* of Canada, in certain of its sections, is both ambiguous and out of date with respect to important areas of clinical practice.

Certain sections of the Code, as they now still stand ten years after the Law Reform Commission's suggested amendments, definitely do place physicians in the following dilemma: *either* to hope that the law as written does not actually mean what it seems to say, and to practice medicine in the patient's best interests; *or* to assume that the law as written intends to say what it seems to say, and then to practice defensive medicine. This would mean practicing medicine so as to minimize the likelihood of legal problems, even if this means jeopardizing the patient's best interests (Law Reform Commission, 1983, 10).

When the law is out of date with clinical practice and, for this reason, is creating harmful tensions and uncertainties, the law should be changed.

When the Law Should Be Maintained Despite Conflict with Ethics

The *Criminal Code* prohibits active euthanasia and assistance to suicide, and the Law Reform Commission steadfastly refused to recommend the legalization (or decriminalization) of either. This refusal is based, in part, on fear of likely abuse.

There are, indeed, many good reasons, some of which will be discussed in Chapter 17, to oppose the legalization of euthanasia and assistance to suicide. We should realize, however, that there is no law, not even a law interdicting euthanasia, that can match up to the infinite variety of human and, at times, tragic situations. This is the reason, in part, for the difference between statutory law and jurisprudence, and also for the difference between law and bioethics.

In medicine, as in war, situations occur that fall outside all existing rules. What should one do when a husband and adult son ask, in front of a wife and mother dying from throat cancer, and with her nodding agreement, that the doctor put her "to sleep" Saturday or Sunday, the days when everyone expects her to die? Her pain was bearable, but the periodic choking episodes were terrifying to this woman. She wanted to die in peace and tranquillity, not during a choking episode. What should one do when a young man, in the terminal stages of AIDS, asks for enough drugs, and for instructions about how to use them, so that he can take an overdose at a time of his choice. He does not want to die, but knows he will, and he then wants to die before he wastes away and loses his mental competence.

In these and other, similar situations, advancing a death that is inevitable may well be ethically justifiable. It is not, however, inconsistent to judge certain acts of hastening death to be ethically justifiable, and yet, simultaneously, to hold that the law should not be changed to grant doctors, or anyone else, legal authorization in advance to carry out these acts.

Chaim Perelman has considered this situation. He draws attention to the fictions that juries and judges use in exceptional circumstances, to avoid applying the law against persons who have committed acts against the law, but acts that are seen as ethically understandable and justifiable in the particular circumstances. The fiction in question consists in a jury qualifying facts in a way contrary to reality, by rationalizing that the accused has not committed murder, in that his or her intention, however misguided, was to relieve pain but not to risk death, and it does this to avoid applying the law punitively. In Perelman's view, this recourse to fiction is better than providing expressly, in law, for the fact that euthanasia is a case for justification or excuse. He believes that we would risk grave abuse in promulgating indulgent legislation in this matter of life or death (Perelman, 1980, 118).

This use of legal fiction to protect doctors who would administer ethically justifiable euthanasia is not an ideal solution. This conflict between ethics and law illustrates the point that the values we cherish cannot always fit into a single system, without one having to be compromised or sacrificed to preserve another. Actions that are lawful are legally justified, but actions that are unlawful may nevertheless be legally excused in individual cases, when they are undertaken to serve an ethical principle. When abortion was criminal, for instance, it might be excusable because of the facts of an individual instance.

Should the Supreme Court Be Challenged?

Since 1977, numerous symposia, workshops and position papers, involving a cross-section of professionals and professional associations, have concluded that contraceptive sterilization can be ethically justified as truly beneficial for some mentally retarded persons. The benefit would consist in their being freed from parental burdens they could never carry, while not being barred from loving sexual relationships in which they could find personal fulfilment. The controversy centred on the decision-making process: who should be involved, and what conditions have to be fulfilled, to protect mentally retarded persons from being sterilized for someone else's benefit?

This ethical consensus resulted from the grass-roots initiative of many people, in solving a pressing problem in the absence of legal guidelines. However, a decision of the Supreme Court of Canada, delivered in the autumn of 1986 in the Eve case, has now clarified the law in this matter. The Supreme Court of Canada declared categorically that sterilization should never be authorized for nontherapeutic purposes. In the absence of the affected person's consent, the Court believed that it can never be safely determined that such sterilization is for the benefit of that person. The Court even found it difficult to imagine a case in which nontherapeutic sterilization could possibly be to the benefit of a mentally retarded person (see Chapter 9).

This decision will prove to be a millstone for clinicians, parents, those carrying institutional responsibility for the care of mentally retarded persons, and, perhaps, for mentally retarded persons themselves, whose social lives and privacy in relations with members of the other sex may be restricted for fear of pregnancy. Of course, the latter may never fully comprehend why they are being restrained from being with the persons to whom they are attracted, and whom they would want to love. The decision will also serve as a lodestone for continuing discussions in Canada about what should be done, when what is judged by many to be ethically justifiable has been declared to be illegal. The Supreme Court of Canada can change its own decisions. Should it be challenged to do so?

CONCLUSION

We now differ greatly, in pluralistic societies, about the content and extent of moral obligations and ethical imperatives. Some of these differences derive from the very divergent philosophies of life people espouse; other differences reflect the peculiarities of the social, economic, and health care systems within which people live. So long as these differences endure, it would be illusory to expect law to exhibit a relationship of complete harmony with morality and ethics.

Much is achieved, though, if law can assure the conditions essential for tolerance in today's pluralistic societies.

The question about the relationship between law, bioethics, and the moralities in a pluralistic society has not yet found a definitive general answer, and probably never will. Any general theory in this relationship will be tested over and over again, on one particular issue after another, as societies themselves change and propose new solutions to new problems of right and wrong.

REFERENCES

Capron A.M. "Harmonies and Conflicts in Law and Biomedical Ethics." In: D. Callahan and G.R. Dunstan, eds. "Biomedical Ethics: An Anglo-American Dialogue." *Annals of the New York Academy of Sciences.* Vol. 530. New York: The New York Academy of Sciences, 1988, 37-45.

Devlin Lord P. "Morals and the Criminal Law." In: R.M. Dworkin, ed. *The Philosophy of Law.* Oxford: Oxford University Press, 1977, 66-72.

Dworkin R.M. "The Delicate Balance: Ethics, Law and Medicine." In: D. Callahan and G.R. Dunstan, eds. "Biomedical Ethics: An Anglo-American Dialogue." *Annals of the New York Academy of Sciences.* Vol. 530. New York: The New York Academy of Sciences, 1988, 24-36.

Evans R.G. "'We'll Take Care of It for You.' Health Care in the Canadian Community." *Daedalus* 1988;117:155-189.

Hart H.L.A. *Essays in Jurisprudence and Philosophy.* Oxford: Clarendon Press, 1983.

Hyman D.A. "How Law Killed Ethics." *Perspectives in Biology and Medicine* 1990;34/1:134-151.

Law Reform Commission of Canada *Euthanasia, Aiding Suicide and Cessation of Treatment.* Report #20. Ottawa: Minister of Supply and Services, 1983.

Perelman C. *Justice, Law, and Argument.* Dordrecht, Boston, London: D. Reidel, 1980.

Roy D.J. An Open Letter to Members of the National Tripartite Liaison Committee. Unpublished manuscript, 1983.

Roy D.J., Dickens B.M. and **McGregor M.** "Editorial. The Choice of Contrast Media: Medical, Ethical and Legal Considerations." *Canadian Medical Association Journal* 1992;147/9:1321-1324.

St. John-Stevas N. *Life, Death and the Law.* Bloomington: Indiana University Press, 1961.

Verspieren P. "De la bioéthique à la loi." *Études* Avril 1991:481-482.

4

THE CANADIAN HEALTH CARE SYSTEM

There are at least three reasons justifying our inclusion of a chapter on the Canadian health care system at the beginning of this book. First, that system strongly influences the way the issues of bioethics are formulated and resolved in Canada. Second, the way access to health care is organized in a country is not only the context, it is also the source, of some of the most difficult questions we discuss throughout this book, and particularly in Chapter 14. Third, some of the most intense controversy in public ethics in the 1990s centres on the large and comprehensive issue of what kind of health care system a country can, in fact, and should, in justice, adopt and protect against political change. The Canadian health care system, then, is a context, a source, and a focus of discussion in bioethics.

In this chapter, we first examine, in general terms, why health care systems are both a framework and an issue of bioethics. Then we concentrate on the history and structure of the Canadian health care system, followed by a comparison and contrast of the Canadian system with those of several other countries. We close the chapter with a consideration of current uncertainty and controversy about whether maintenance of the Canadian health care system, as it now stands, will be possible over the coming years.

THE HEALTH CARE SYSTEM: A FRAMEWORK OF BIOETHICS

In the preceding chapter, we cited the issue of whether all Canadians should have access to the safer, but much more costly, new contrast media for radiological examinations. The question, though centring on only one health care technology, goes to the heart of what we should understand distributive justice to require of us in Canada. Other questions of a similar kind arise on a daily basis in health care institutions in Canada, and in countries throughout the world. For example, if a hospital's budget for liver transplantation is depleted at some point in a given year, may patients on the waiting list be allowed to have a transplant if they are able and willing to pay? What about the others on the waiting list, equally in danger of dying, who cannot pay? When hemodialysis resources are limited, should they be used for elderly persons suffering from kidney failure? For patients with AIDS? Waiting lists or queues, a common feature of many health care systems that have a national health insurance programme, are generally thought to be a fair way of organizing access to costly and scarce kinds of care. Yet, at what point does length of wait, for example for heart surgery, become an intolerable injustice?

These difficult and emotionally trying questions, some of which we consider in Chapter 14, where we discuss limited resources and tragic choices, are answered quite differently in various countries of the Western world. The different answers derive, in part, from significant differences between the health care systems within which these questions, questions of both clinical ethics and public ethics, are posed and have to be resolved.

Bioethics, as emphasized in Chapter 2, is not armchair applied philosophy. The methods of bioethics in each of its fields demands close attention to the contexts of the issues it is attempting to analyze and resolve. These contexts are many and often intermeshed, but they are always influenced, sometimes explicitly, at other times more subtly, by the way health care, including medical and hospital care, is delivered in a country. Two examples, one from Canada, the other from the U.K., illustrate this point.

For the Canadian example, we return to the issue of contrast media, cited in Chapter 3 and mentioned again above. There is, as of this writing, continuing discussion, not only in the province of Québec, of limiting access to the safer, but much more costly, new low osmolality contrast media. The general idea is that only patients who can be identified as being at high risk for severe reactions to the older contrast media would receive the costly newer media for their X-ray exams. Were a policy of limited access to be adopted as a way of justly distributing scare resources in the Québec health care system, how would the relationship of doctors to patients be affected? What would the principle of honesty then require doctors to tell patients, when seeking their informed consent for these examinations?

A doctor normally should inform patients about all significant risks and benefits of a treatment, and of existing alternative treatments. But if doctors were to do this, how many patients would agree to having the older contrast media, which are less safe and more likely to cause discomfort, injected into their veins? One could argue, and some have so argued, that if a policy of limited access is justified, then the newer contrast media are not, in fact, available as an alternative treatment for patients who are not at high risk for severe reactions to the older media. Therefore, doctors do not have to discuss the pros and cons of each contrast medium in informed consent negotiations. Such a discussion would amount to a patient-by-patient referendum on the health care policy, and to its likely collapse.

Without going into an analysis and critique of the various arguments involved in this issue, the issue itself of limited access to safer and much more costly newer contrast media does illustrate how a particular policy of a health care system could influence the relationship of doctors to patients, and shape the way information is given to or withheld from patients when their consent to treatment is sought.

In the U.K., the Sidaway case illustrates how the health care system can influence the relationship between law and ethics in the matter of informed consent.

Mrs. Amy Sidaway was left partially paralyzed after an operation, called a laminectomy, to remove one or more thin layers from her vertebrae. Because of this paralysis, she could no longer work or carry out her cherished leisure activities. In a malpractice action she launched against the estate of her since-deceased doctor and the hospital where the surgery was done, Mrs. Sidaway did not accuse the doctor of negligence in the performance of the surgery. She rather claimed that he failed to inform her of the risks of injury and subsequent paralysis that were a possibility with this particular operation. Mrs. Sidaway said she would not have agreed to the surgery, had she known about the operation's inherent risks of paralyzing injury.

The Sidaway case went through three courts in England. Mrs. Sidaway's claim was rejected each time, and the courts also rejected what was described as the transatlantic standard for informed consent, which, in fact, also operates in such countries as France and Germany. According to that standard, as we shall discuss in Chapter 5, a doctor's legal duty to disclose information should be determined by reference to what a reasonable person in the patient's position would want to know, to make a decision about accepting treatment.

The English courts rejected this standard, in part because of the traditional commitment in England to the professional standard. According to that standard, what doctors are legally bound to tell patients is determined by reference to what reasonable physicians normally do disclose to patients. However, commentators on the Sidaway case find that the U.K. health care system is itself an important factor in explaining the decisions of the English courts.

In the U.K., the amount of money to be used for health care is determined by a central planning authority and, after that amount is set, doctors are the ones generally responsible for deciding how, and for whom, that money will be spent. This system simply could not work if doctors were to follow the North American standards of wide and open disclosure in informed consent negotiations. According to one interpretation of the courts' decisions in the Sidaway case, the U.K. health care system could not tolerate the North American doctrine of informed consent, because the system could not bear up under the financial effects of all possible reasonable patient decisions. Pressure of the health care system on the doctor-patient relationship leads, then, to a split between a doctor's ethical and legal duties regarding consent. Though disclosure of all risks a particular patient would reasonably want to know about might be a doctor's ethical duty, such disclosure is not a doctor's legal duty (Schwartz, 1985).

THE HEALTH CARE SYSTEM: A CONTEMPORARY ISSUE OF PUBLIC ETHICS

Ideal access to medical and health care would mean that people could obtain whatever they need and wish, whenever they could benefit, wherever they are. Universal access to ideal care never has been, and never will be, possible. A somewhat less utopian prospect did, for a time, seem achievable in countries of the Western world, around the middle of this century. Before the end of World War II, Winston Churchill proclaimed that disease must be attacked in the poorest or in the richest, in the same way that a fire brigade will devote no less complete assistance to a humble cottage than it would to a mansion (Gemmill, 1960, 20).

The policy of the National Health Service (NHS), adopted in 1948 in the U.K., was to assure that everyone would have equal opportunity to benefit from the best and most up-to-date medical and allied services available. Medical treatment and cure, according to Aneurin Bevan, the then-Minister responsible for introducing the NHS, was to be made available to rich and poor alike, in accordance with medical need and by no other criterion (Abel-Smith, 1978).

This admirable ideal rested upon an illusion of abundance, an illusion from which the U.K. had to retreat shortly after institution of the NHS. One year after promising unlimited free medical care of the best possible standard to the entire population, the U.K., in 1949, had to set an annual ceiling for NHS spending (Macrae, 1984). Rationing by queue became essential.

Countries throughout the Western world are now having to free themselves, more and more each year, from the illusion that resources can ever match needs. The key problem is that supply creates its own demand. Needs are constantly reinterpreted, and expand in response to available new health care services and technologies.

Any attempt to apportion equal access to available technologies and services is doomed to frustration, when research activity is continually creating costly innovative procedures. It is impossible to escape the conclusion that some kinds of medical care within national health insurance systems must always be unevenly available, if they are not simply to be unavailable altogether (Office, 1979, 283).

We must distinguish two related, but quite different, questions. How limited resources are to be justly distributed within a health care system, when innovation is limitless, is one matter. Every health care system has to face this question, and we shall discuss some of the related ethical issues in Chapter 14. The larger issue of public ethics centres on how the health care system as a whole is organized. The issue is one of public ethics, not just an issue of economics and administration, because it is deeply rooted in a clash between powerful interest groups and the requirements of justice.

This central issue of the 1990s is different in each country. In the United States, where over thirty million people have no private or public health care insurance, the movement is growing to institute some kind of system of universal access to health care. Though the American Medical Association and the Health Insurance Association of America are mounting campaigns against national health insurance plans such as Canada's, others, including the leaders of the American College of Physicians, claim that universal access to health care is a moral and medical imperative (Greenberg, 1990). The issue in Canada is whether the provincial and territorial health insurance plans, based on the principle of universal access to care with equal terms and conditions for all, can be maintained. The Canadian system necessarily depends upon a viable economy and, of equal importance, on sensible interaction between the federal and provincial governments. One observer from outside Canada has warned that, without more meaningful dialogue than currently exists between the federal and provincial governments, Canadians place at risk the future of their health insurance plans, a health care arrangement that is admired throughout the Western world (Iglehart, 1990).

Current uncertainties and controversies about the Canadian health care system will come up for discussion again at the end of this chapter. However, some of the current tensions between the federal and provincial governments, and between the professions and provincial governments, were visible and prominent at the origin of the Canadian system, and at key turning points in its evolution.

THE CANADIAN HEALTH CARE SYSTEM: A SUMMARY HISTORY

Up to now, we have been speaking of a single Canadian health care system. In reality, there is no such thing. Rather, there are ten distinct provincial and two territorial health systems in this country. Despite this multiplicity, the systems share several basic features. The source of this coherence was a series of federal-provincial accords, whereby the federal government provides a considerable part of the funds to the provinces and territories for health care, and in return, the latter governments agree to incorporate the basic features of the programme into their systems.

Medicare, the national health insurance programme, is scarcely twenty-five years old (Taylor, 1990). A proposal for a comparable programme, made by the federal government shortly after World War II, failed to win approval by the provinces. Instead, medical insurance plans were developed by non-profit organizations such as Blue Cross and provincial physician organizations, and various commercial insurance companies also offered health coverage.

First, Insurance for Hospital Services

Rather than wait for a national programme to materialize, several provinces decided to go ahead with their own public health insurance plans. The first to do so was Saskatchewan, which launched its Hospital Services Plan on January 1, 1947. The programme was universal and compulsory, it paid for all essential hospital services, and it was financed by an annual premium (initially $5 per person, with a limit of $30 per family). British Columbia inaugurated its programme in 1949. This was similar to Saskatchewan's, although B.C. encountered great difficulties in collecting premiums. In 1951, a per diem charge for hospital stays was introduced, in addition to the insurance payment. In 1954, premiums were abolished, and the hospital system was funded by an increase in the provincial sales tax. Alberta was the third province to venture into public health insurance. On July 1, 1950, the Alberta Municipal Hospital Plan was established. It did not provide universal coverage, but rather, subsidized existing municipal hospital insurance plans. Premiums were $10 per year for an individual or family, and there was an additional per diem charge of $1. When Newfoundland entered Canada in 1949, it had a system of provincial hospitals with salaried physicians, who provided services to those who paid an annual premium. This programme covered approximately 47% of the population.

Even though no other provinces established public health insurance plans during the 1950s, there developed a strong consensus in favour of a national plan. On April 10, 1957, Parliament adopted, by a unanimous vote, the *Hospital Insurance and Diagnostic Services Act*, which provided for federal grants to provinces for making hospital services available to all residents on uniform terms and conditions. Payments began in 1958 to the provinces with plans in place, and by 1961 all ten provinces and the two territories were included.

Next, Insurance for Medical Services

Once hospital insurance was in place, the next step was to insure the other major component of health care costs, physicians' services. Here again, Saskatchewan led the way. In 1959, Premier Tommy Douglas announced the government's intention to institute a comprehensive medical care programme for all the residents of the province. The main opponents of the proposed programme were doctors, who did not want to lose their control over the provision of medical services. Despite their fierce opposition, the Saskatchewan *Medical Care Insurance Act* was passed in November 1961. It provided for universal, compulsory participation in the insurance plan, which was to be financed by premiums. All physician and surgeon services were covered, whether in hospitals, offices, or the patient's home.

Saskatchewan doctors did not take kindly to this legislation. At a meeting of their professional association, the College of Physicians and Surgeons, on May 3-4, 1962, which was attended by two-thirds of the membership, they resolved to go on strike on July 1, if the government did not withdraw the legislation. In anticipation of this action, the Medical Care Insurance Commission, the body that administered Medicare, began to recruit doctors in other countries, especially Great Britain. The strike went ahead as resolved, with approximately 40% of the doctors providing only emergency services, almost 50% going on vacation, and a small minority continuing regular practice. Some 110 doctors were recruited from other countries, and began to provide regular services. After twenty-three days, an agreement was reached with the help of an informal mediator, Lord Stephen Taylor from England. The doctors accepted the basic principles of Medicare, and the government allowed the doctors several options for billing their patients.

Once the Saskatchewan plan was in place, three other provinces — B.C., Alberta and Ontario — inaugurated their own Medicare plans. Meanwhile, the federal government had established, in 1961, a Royal Commission on Health Services under the leadership of Emmett Hall, chief justice of Saskatchewan and later a member of the Supreme Court of Canada. The Commission released its report on June 19, 1964. First among its two hundred recommendations was that the federal government enter into agreements with the provinces, to provide grants to assist the provinces to introduce and operate comprehensive, universal provincial programmes of personal health services. The federal government accepted this recommendation and, on July 19, 1965, it hosted a meeting of the provincial premiers to determine how the programme might be implemented.

Although the provinces were not all in favour of universal Medicare, the federal government went ahead and introduced the *Medical Care Insurance Bill* in July 1966. It was passed on December 8, with only two members of Parliament opposed, and came into effect July 1, 1968. At that time only two provinces met the qualifications of the Act, Saskatchewan and B.C. Five others — Newfoundland, Nova Scotia, Manitoba, Alberta and Ontario — joined the following year. By April 1, 1972, all provinces and territories were in the plan.

Then, Consolidation of the System

Both the 1957 *Hospital Insurance Act* and the 1966 *Medical Care Insurance Act* were essentially financial in nature. They specified the conditions under which the federal government would transfer sums of money to the provinces and territories for hospital and medical services. Every five years, such arrangements are renegotiated by the two levels of government. The passage of the *Federal-Provincial Fiscal Arrangements and Established Programs Financing (E.P.F.) Act* for the 1977-1982 period allowed the provinces more flexibility in how they spent the federal transfer payments, but it also gave rise to accusations that the provinces were spending funds destined for health care and higher education on other things. In order to investigate this charge, and to determine whether extra-billing by doctors (by which doctors could bill patients for charges exceeding what the health insurance plan paid doctors for a medical service) and hospital user fees were violating the principle of universal access to health care, the federal government, in 1979, appointed a Health Services Review Commission with Emmett Hall as the sole member.

In his report, which appeared in 1980, Justice Hall refuted the charge that the provinces were misusing federal health care funding. On the issue of extra-billing, he issued a strong condemnation: *"The practice of extra-billing is inequitable. Not only does it deny access by the poor but it also taxes sick persons who, besides paying premiums, are already paying the major cost of the system through their taxes."*(Hall, 1980, 26). In order to protect the right of physicians to be adequately compensated for their services, Hall proposed a system of binding arbitration to resolve disputes between physicians and provincial health authorities.

In 1983, the federal government decided to implement the recommendations of the Hall Commission on extra-billing and user fees. The *Canada Health Act* was introduced in December 1983, and received unanimous approval the following year. It consolidated the *Hospital Insurance Act* of 1957 and the *Medical Care Insurance Act* of 1966, and specified with greater precision the conditions for the transfer of funds to the provinces and territories. These included the elimination of extra-billing and user fees. Provinces could be penalized if they did not comply, notably by the federal government making deductions from its transfer payment to a provincial or territorial government that violated its agreement to comply with the *Canada Health Act*. By 1987, all the provinces and territories had passed legislation in accordance with these provisions.

Now, Is the System in Peril?

Since the passage of the *Canada Health Act*, the federal government has introduced a series of measures designed to reduce its contributions to the funding of health care. For example, in the February 1990 budget it announced that it would freeze E.P.F. contributions for health care at the 1989-90 level for two years, following which E.P.F. per capita entitlements would grow at a rate of G.N.P. minus 3%. In the February 1991 budget, this freeze was extended for three more years, to 1994-95. If this policy were to continue, the federal contribution to health financing would eventually reach zero. Without the threat of withheld transfer payments, many observers feel that the federal government will have no means of enforcing the national Medicare standards on the provinces and territories. We shall return to this issue at the end of the chapter.

PRINCIPLES AND PRINCIPAL FEATURES OF THE CANADIAN SYSTEM

The ethical significance of the heated controversies over extra-billing and hospital user fees, after passage of the *Canada Health Act* in 1984, stems from the fact that the Canadian system has been founded upon a principle of public ethics to which the Canadian people fiercely adhere. Equality before the health care system, as R. Evans has phrased it, is as strong a principle in Canada as equality before the law (Evans, 1988, 165). The governing idea of this principle is that all Canadians should have access to a similar level of care, regardless of their ability to pay for it (Iglehart, 1986, 778). The *Canada Health Act* is designed to ensure that all Canadians have access to services that are "medically necessary for the purpose of maintaining health, preventing disease or diagnosing or treating an injury, illness or disability."

The principal features of Canadian Medicare, as originally included in the *Hospital Insurance Act* and reaffirmed in the *Canada Health Act*, derive from the health care system's fundamental principle of equality. These features are five in number:

- comprehensiveness: coverage extends to all hospital and all physician and surgeon services; some provinces add other health care benefits, such as dental services for children, drugs for the elderly, chiropractic, optometry and physiotherapy treatments.

- universality: these services are available to all Canadians, regardless of income or other considerations; nor do poor people have to undergo a means test to establish their eligibility for coverage.

- accessibility: Canadians must have reasonable access to medically necessary services.

- portability: a resident of one province or territory is covered while travelling in other parts of Canada and, at least partially, in other countries.

- public administration: either by an independent commission or by the health department.

Medicare is, it should be remembered, a system of health care *insurance* and the Canadian health care system is one of socialized insurance, not of socialized medicine (Evans, 1988, 170). Like other forms of insurance — personal accident, automobile, house, etc. — one pays for it regardless of whether one has the opportunity to collect. Despite the intricacies of federal-provincial/territorial fiscal arrangements, the ultimate source of payment for health insurance is the taxpayer. There is no one single health tax in Canada; rather, the health system is financed from general government revenues. We pay for it through income, sales and business taxes and through other schemes devised by governments to raise revenues.

Unlike some forms of insurance, such as automobile collision coverage, Medicare does not charge different premiums to different individuals according to the likelihood of their claiming benefits. Even though some illnesses are obviously self-inflicted, such as lung cancer in heavy smokers or broken bones in reckless motorcycle drivers, hospital and medical services are provided to everyone on the same basis. Good health habits are encouraged, but there is no penalty for neglecting them.

Another feature of Medicare is its relative open-endedness, with regard to reimbursement of service costs. There is no individual limit on such reimbursement. No matter how often persons become ill and how expensive the treatment, they will not be refused needed medical services. Determination of need is generally in the hands of physicians, whose only constraints are their own time and their access to hospital facilities. Patients may have to wait, sometimes many months, for an appointment with a specialist or a hospital bed for elective surgery, but they will not be denied these services just because they have already consumed more than their fair share of health care dollars. There is no such thing as one's fair share in Medicare.

As noted above, Medicare does not pay for all health care. Indeed, government funding accounts for only 75% of Canadian health expenditures. The remaining 25% must be borne by individuals, either directly or through supplementary insurance plans. Many employers provide group plans to cover such expenses as prescription drugs, eyeglasses, medical devices and dental care, all of which are excluded from most provincial and territorial health insurance plans.

The Canadian health care system, then, involves a triangular relationship between members of the general public, professional providers of care, and the provincial and federal governments (Evans, 1988, 160).

Though a majority of Canadians have regularly expressed general satisfaction with Canadian Medicare, the system is far from ideal. There are many shortages, which result in waiting lines and suboptimal conditions, especially in institutions. Nevertheless, high-quality care is readily available to most Canadians most of the time, and patients do not directly pay for that care when it is delivered. Payment is indirect, and the burdens of cost are distributed across the income spectrum through general taxation.

The Canadian health care system is largely funded by governments, who wish to exercise control over how this money is spent. Payments to health professionals constitute the major category of expenditures on health, and are therefore subject to special controls. When doctors are paid on a fee-for-service basis, as most are, those who deliver many services, and may decide how many services they deliver, are highly paid. Governments often prefer that doctors be on fixed salaries. Professionals encounter the heavy hand of government in various ways: limited rates for specific services, income caps for self-employed physicians, and negotiated or legislated salaries for unionized hospital employees.

Like the Canadian public, health professionals in this country report general overall satisfaction with the health care system. Government control of licensure and remuneration may be resented, but they also provide security of income to the vast majority of health workers. A small majority feel so constrained by these controls that they depart for what they consider to be greener pastures, usually in the United States. However, the majority remain loyal to the Canadian system, and hope that the constraints will not get any worse.

Government has two principal concerns in regard to health: the general improvement of the health status of the population, and the cost of the system. These concerns are usually in conflict, since most measures to improve health cost money. In recent years, the first priority of all Canadian governments has been cost containment. In order to control large budget deficits, strict limits have been set on public expenditures such as health care. Governments officials usually deny that such restrictions have a negative impact on health. They claim, instead, that with greater efficiency the same results can be achieved with less funds. Nevertheless, it is clear that, at the very least, Canadians are being inconvenienced by these budget cuts, as is evidenced by longer waiting lines for elective procedures, slow acquisition of new medical technologies, and an increasing shortage of chronic care facilities.

Many commentators have stated that the Canadian health care system is in a state of crisis, because of these funding issues. If this is true, it would not be the first such crisis. Indeed, the basic features of the Canadian system were the result of government responses to several earlier crises. However, the crisis of the 1990s may well be quite different from those of the past. The health care system does not run, sovereignly independent, on its own financial energy. As Jake Epp, former federal Minister of Health and Welfare, emphasized several years ago: "Our entire health care system and our social safety net are based on one condition — economic growth." (MacDonald, 1986). What depth and duration of economic recession can the Canadian health care system endure? The future of that system, as we shall discuss below, is not certain.

INTERNATIONAL COMPARISONS AND CONTRASTS

In one respect, at least, medicine is the same the world over. Thanks to modern methods of communication, new discoveries in medical research and practice are instantly transmitted from country to country and continent to continent. Moreover, physicians and other health care professionals often travel abroad for education, training and conferences. As a result of these interactions, there is a remarkable similarity in the treatments available to patients, at least the wealthy ones, in all the major cities of the world.

Closer inspection will reveal that this similarity is limited to a very small segment of national health care systems, namely, well-funded urban hospitals. At all other levels of these systems, the differences from one country to another are likely to be much greater than their common features. In what follows, we will limit our comparison of several national systems to those aspects that we dealt with in the Canadian context, namely health care delivery and financing.

U.S.A.

Like their Canadian counterparts, Americans who get sick or are injured usually seek out a physician or a hospital. Whereas all Canadians can expect reasonably equal access to these providers of health care, Americans fall into several very unequal categories. Those who are wealthy or who participate in a good private or group insurance plan can receive the very best of care. Many hospitals compete with each other, through expensive advertising campaigns, and are only too happy to see a patient coming through their doors. Waiting lines are often nonexistent, and patients are treated with the most modern technologies and can order whatever type of service they desire.

A second group of patients, senior citizens and welfare recipients, are entitled to a limited range of free medical benefits through two national health insurance plans, Medicare for the elderly and Medicaid for people with low income. Since the fee schedules of these plans have been progressively reduced during the past decade, many physicians and private hospitals will not accept patients from this group. Instead, they are sent to inner-city clinics and public or charity hospitals, where they receive a minimal level of treatment, greatly inferior to what is experienced by the first group.

The third group of patients is made up of 15% to 20% of the American population. They have no health insurance, either private or public. Many of them are the working poor, too well off to qualify for welfare (and Medicaid), but with no employer plan either. They must pay for their own medical care, but often cannot afford to. As a result, they simply go without or, if they are lucky, they may obtain free treatment as charity cases. Even then, they will be at the very end of the line. A similar plight affects many millions of additional people who have insurance, but are underinsured for the services they need.

Why does this three-tier system of health care exist in the richest nation of the world? The U.S. is one of the very few countries in the world to embrace wholeheartedly the entrepreneurial/market approach to health care (Sutherland, 1990, 48). Health services are regarded as commodities to be bought and sold like any others, such as food, clothing, and housing. It is believed that the terms of exchange of such goods should be left to free market forces; government intervention is at best a nuisance, and at worst extremely destructive, resulting in either shortages or oversupply of services. A large number of American hospitals are privately owned and operated as for-profit businesses, unlike Canada, where almost all hospitals are either publicly owned or charitable institutions.

According to this free-market ideology, the provision of compulsory health insurance programmes by governments in countries such as Canada represents a serious attack on individual human freedom. It forces people to spend money on one thing (health insurance), rather than on other items that they might have chosen (such as stocks or a new house). Moreover, it interferes in the relationship between providers and clients (patients) by unilaterally imposing conditions, such as a specific fee for a service, on the providers, thereby taking away their freedom to negotiate the terms of the relationship. Proponents of this view argue that governments do not regulate other sectors of the economy in this way, so to single out health is arbitrary and unfair.

An additional argument against national health insurance that holds sway in the U.S.A. is that to provide something for free is to devalue it. Individuals are likely to abuse the system if there is no deterrent, such as a charge for each service. Furthermore, no other commodity is provided for free, including such necessities of life as food and shelter. Thus, it is reasoned, there is no cause for exempting health care from the market.

Underlying this approach to health care financing is a very strong individualism, and a correlative antipathy to Canadian-style collectivism, especially government action on behalf of the entire population (Tuohy, 1989). Such action is regarded by many Americans as a manifestation of socialism, or even communism, and is summarily rejected without an examination of its possible advantages.

Despite this deeply ingrained suspicion of government intervention in health care, the U.S. has, over the years, instituted several national health funding programmes. In 1986, federal, state and local governments paid approximately 42% of national health costs (compared to 75% in Canada). The largest programme is Medicare, which was established in 1965 to provide health insurance for senior citizens. Another programme, Medicaid, is a federal-state partnership that pays for health care for low-income people, primarily women and children. Benefits vary from state to state. Both of these programmes experienced severe cutbacks during the 1980s. The federal government also pays the cost of kidney dialysis for all patients with end-stage renal disease.

One of the results of this melange of free-market ideology and limited government intervention is that, for many years, Americans have paid far more for health care than any other country. Moreover, these expenditures have risen more rapidly than elsewhere. One commonly used measure of a nation's health care expenditures is the percentage of the gross domestic product (G.D.P.) that is devoted to health care. By that standard, the American figure rose from 9.3% to 11.8% of G.D.P between 1980 and 1989 (the Canadian increase was from 7.4% to 8.7%).

This combination of high spending and lack of health care for a great many citizens has given rise to numerous proposals for reform of the U.S. health system. Many Americans are looking to Canada as a model in this respect. Others, such as the American Medical Association, strongly reject the prospect of a Canadian- or European-style system, and have launched well-funded campaigns to convince Americans to avoid this path. At the same time, the American approach, despite its faults, has some defenders in Canada, especially among wealthy business groups who want to see government spending reduced. All this is to say that Robert Evans's description of the Canadian health care system as "one of the most convincing forms of evidence, perhaps *the* most convincing, that we are not Americans after all," (Evans, 1988, 157) may be less true in the future than at present, because of changes in both countries.

Great Britain

In contrast to the U.S.A., with its entrepreneurial/market health care system, and to Canada, with its national insurance model, in some countries government oversees not just health care financing, but delivery as well. One example of this approach is Great Britain. Since 1948, most health care has been provided through the National Health Service (NHS), a government-run system of hospitals, salaried physicians and auxiliary health services, financed out of general tax revenues and available to all citizens at no extra charge.

When the British are in need of health care, the first point of contact with the system is their family physician. Every citizen is registered with a physician. The latter will decide what treatment is needed, and whether or not the patient should be seen by a consultant specialist and/or admitted to hospital. The quality of health services is comparable to that of Canada, but for many years in Great Britain, the availability of hospital beds for non-emergency treatments has been severely limited, even more than in Canada. As a result, one may have to wait two years or more for a hip replacement, cataract operation or other elective procedure.

The main reason for these restrictions is that the British have traditionally spent less on health care than Canadians or Americans. In 1987, they devoted only 6.1% of G.D.P. to health, compared to Canada's 8.6% and the U.S.'s 11.2%. This represented a very small increase from their 5.8% in 1980. The British government has claimed that the NHS is more efficient in providing services to the entire population than, for instance, the American system, and so they do not need to increase spending to North American levels. Nevertheless, the long waiting lines and relatively low salaries for health care professionals are signs that health care in Great Britain could benefit from greater funding.

One of the ways that recent British governments have dealt with demands for better health services has been to encourage the growth of a private health care industry. During the 1980s, private hospitals doubled in size, and NHS salaried physicians were permitted to take on private, fee-paying patients. The private hospitals provided rapid access to services for which there were long waiting lists at the NHS hospitals. In order to pay for these services, many individuals took out private health insurance; during this period the number of those covered by such insurance rose from 5% to 10% of the population (Day, 1989, 14).

The mixture of a publicly funded health care system, available to all citizens, and another, private system for a well-to-do minority of the population reflects the deeply rooted class consciousness of British culture. In the words of Robert Evans, "In the United Kingdom most citizens find it right and proper that the 'better' class of people should receive their care under more genteel surroundings and pay for the privilege." (Evans, 1988, 167) He contrasts this attitude with the more egalitarian approach found in Canada, where every citizen is supposed to have equal access to health care, regardless of their "social worth" or ability to pay.

Other Countries

The health care systems of other capitalist industrialized countries, especially the wealthier ones such as Japan, Australia, New Zealand and the nations of Western Europe, are more similar to that of Canada than to either the U.S.'s or Great Britain's. All of these countries have national health insurance but, with the exception of Sweden and Finland, none of them has a health care delivery system comparable to Great Britain's NHS.

Outside of the major industrialized countries, one finds a great variety of health systems. The one common characteristic of most of these countries, apart from a few oil-rich ones, is that they have very little money to devote to health care. The way in which these limited funds are spent differs greatly from one country to another, even between neighbours with similar income levels. For example, China has developed a comprehensive, though low-cost, system of health services for most of its population. India, on the other hand, has no such system, but rather a tangled array of private and public hospitals and health professions, whose services are beyond the reach, financial and often geographical, of a large proportion of Indians. As a result, by one rough measure of health status, namely life expectancy, China far exceeds India (69 vs. 58 years).

As Canadians face mounting financial pressures on our health system, we may be able to learn a great deal from those countries that have always had to make do with much less. Many of them have been able to achieve better results, in terms of life expectancy and care of the chronically ill, than we have, in spite of spending a considerably lower proportion of their G.D.P. on health. In our search for ways to improve our system, we should not limit ourselves to sources in Canada, the U.S.A and Europe. Despite our different histories and cultures, we should learn what the so-called underdeveloped countries have done with regard to the financing and delivery of health services, and see to what extent their experience can be applied to the improvement of our own system.

THE CANADIAN SYSTEM: AN UNCERTAIN FUTURE

The policy of the federal government to limit progressively its financial contributions to health care has resulted in severe pressures on the provincial and territorial health systems. The poorer provinces, such as Newfoundland, Nova Scotia, Prince Edward Island and New Brunswick, have no alternative sources of revenue to replace the federal shortfall, and have been forced to reduce health care services by closing hospital beds, freezing salaries, and other equally drastic measures. Even the wealthiest provinces, Ontario, Alberta and British Columbia, find themselves able to maintain health services at their present level only by reducing expenditures in other areas, such as education and social services, or by running higher deficits.

In the late 1980s and early 1990s, most provinces and territories launched extensive reexaminations of their health systems, in order to determine how the goals of health care can be achieved with greater efficiency and, hopefully, at less cost. Some of these studies, for example the Québec Commission of Inquiry into Health and Social Services (1988) and the B.C Royal Commission on Health Care and Costs (1991), issued massive reports with many detailed recommendations. Even when governments agree with such recommendations, it can take years before they are formulated as legislation, debated by the provincial legislature, adopted as law, and implemented as policy. Many of the recommendations of the Québec Commission were eventually incorporated into Bill 120, *Loi sur les services de santé et les services sociaux*, which was given first reading in December 1990, and finally passed, after much opposition and many amendments, in August 1991. Its various provisions were to be phased in over the next several years.

Depending on their financial capabilities and the attitudes of their governments towards health care, the Canadian provinces and territories may adopt significantly difference responses to the current financial crisis. Québec has already opted for a user-fee of five dollars for unnecessary visits to hospital emergency departments, a policy that is in clear contradiction to the *Canada Health Act*. Other provinces are considering measures, such as the revival of premiums, which can lawfully be charged, in order to generate additional funds for health care. More positively, Québec has also created a provincial council for the evaluation of health technology, with the goal of determining which technologies, old and new, are really beneficial and cost-effective. This initiative has generated considerable interest in other provinces and territories, which realize that they can no longer afford to spend considerable sums on unproven technologies while neglecting other, clearly effective, ones.

It is clear that the first half of the 1990s is destined to be a period of instability in the Canadian health care field. Although the financial crunch is the principal catalyst for much of the rethinking and eventual reorganization of provincial and territorial systems, many other factors are influencing this process. Provinces may adopt a more restricted view of what services are "medically necessary," and of the levels of service to which citizens are entitled to have "reasonable access," according to the *Canada Health Act*. These include constitutional issues, especially the division of responsibility for health between the federal government and the provinces and territories; the changing roles and relationships of the various health professions; an increasing concern with the *quality* of health care; and continued attention to the *ethical* aspects of health care practice and organization. The remaining chapters of this book will concentrate on this last topic, and the final chapter will provide a summary of this discussion and suggest the overall impact of ethics on the future of health care in Canada.

CONCLUSION

Although the organization and funding of health care raises many ethical issues, it has not been the purpose of this chapter to discuss, or even identify, these issues. (Chapter 14 will be devoted to this topic.) What we have done here is to provide an outline of the basic elements of the Canadian health care system, to serve as background for the discussion of specific bioethical issues in the rest of this book.

Our contention that the organizational context of health care is an essential factor in bioethical analysis has the following consequence: we must question the pertinence of non-Canadian authors to the Canadian discussion of bioethical issues. To question in this sense does not mean to reject; it means simply not to accept without question. Much of what has been written in the U.S.A., Great Britain or France is extremely useful for understanding the ethical status of abortion, care of the elderly or organ transplants in Canada. Conversely, other books and articles on these same topics are either useless or positively misleading when applied to the Canadian scene, because they presuppose laws or attitudes that are not valid here.

In the following chapters, we will examine specific bioethical issues in a Canadian perspective. In addition to the *organizational* context, as described in this chapter, we will situate each issue within the Canadian *legal* framework, as discussed in the previous chapter. And we will build wherever possible on the *ethical* status of the question, as developed by Canadian ethicists. We will not neglect the writings of non-Canadians; on the contrary, we will make considerable use of their insights, as long as they help us achieve the goal of this book: to understand bioethical issues as they arise in the Canadian context.

REFERENCES

Abel-Smith B. *The National Health Service: The First Thirty Years.* HMSO, 1978.

Day P. and **Klein R.** "The Politics of Modernization: Britain's National Health Service in the 1980s." *The Milbank Quarterly* 1989;67/1:1-34.

Evans R.G. "'We'll Take Care of It for You': Health Care in the Canadian Community." *Daedalus* 1988;117:155-189.

Gemmill P.F. *Britain's Search for Health.* Philadelphia: University of Pennsylvania Press, 1960.

Greenberg N.J. et al. "Universal Access to Health Care in America: A Moral and Medical Imperative." *Annals of Internal Medicine* 1990;112:637-639.

Hall E.M. *Canada's National-Provincial Health Programs for the 1980s: A Commitment for Renewal.* Ottawa: Department of National Health and Welfare, 1980.

Iglehart J.K. "Canada's Health Care System" (Second of three parts). *The New England Journal of Medicine* 1986;315:778-784.

Iglehart J.K. "Canada's Health Care System Faces its Problems." *The New England Journal of Medicine* 1990;322:562-568.

MacDonald N. "Health Care Linked to Economy: Epp." *Ottawa Citizen* February 20, 1986.

Macrae N. "Health Care International. NHS, Born 1948, Died 1949." *Economist* April 28, 1984:18.

Office of Health Economics (London) "Scarce Resources in Health Care." *Milbank Memorial Fund Quarterly 1979*;57:265-287.

Schwartz R. and **Grubb A.** "Why Britain Can't Afford Informed Consent." *Hastings Center Report 1985*;15:22, 24-25.

Sutherland R.W. and **Fulton M.J.** *Health Care in Canada: A Description and Analysis of Canadian Health Services.* Ottawa: The Health Group, 1990.

Taylor M.G. *Insuring National Health Care: The Canadian Experience.* Chapel Hill and London: The University of North Carolina Press, 1990.

Tuohy C. "Conflict and Accommodation in the Canadian Health Care System." In: R.G. Evans and G.L. Stoddart, eds. *Medicare at Maturity: Achievements, Lessons & Challenges.* Calgary: The University of Calgary Press, 1989, 393-434.

5

THE RELATIONSHIP BETWEEN DOCTORS, NURSES, AND PATIENTS

The first five chapters of this book are designed to offer a framework for our discussion of specific issues in bioethics in the remaining chapters. The relationship between doctors, nurses, and patients, the focus of reflection in this chapter, is particularly relevant for clinical ethics and research ethics, two of the fields of bioethics discussed in Chapter 2. This chapter is a brief exercise in professional ethics, with which clinical ethics and research ethics necessarily maintains interdisciplinary collaboration.

This chapter has two purposes. The first is to describe some important themes of professional ethics in the health care professions. Each of these professions has its own distinctive ethical principles, rules, and guidelines to regulate the behaviour of its members and their relationships with other health professionals, patients, and society. The codes of ethics of these professions are summary statements of behaviour that is expected or required. In this chapter we will focus on two aspects of professional ethics in the health care setting: relationships among members of different health care professions, and the relationship between health care workers and patients.

The second purpose of the chapter is to clarify and analyse two bioethical topics that are factors in all of the issues to be discussed in subsequent chapters. These topics are informed consent and confidentiality. Although their application to particular types of patients (e.g., infants, elderly persons, mentally ill persons) will be discussed in detail in other sections of the book, the general ethical principles that support these concepts will be treated here.

The plan of this chapter is as follows: we begin with an analysis of the key concept in the relationship of health care professionals among themselves and with patients, namely, *authority*. We will see how the traditional hierarchy among these professions, with doctors at the top, is under revision as nurses, administrators, social workers, and other groups call for a more collegial relationship within the health care team. We will also examine various models of the professional-patient relationship, with particular emphasis on physician-patient interaction. Next, we will deal with two key aspects of these relationships, informed consent and confidentiality. The chapter will conclude with a summary of the key points on this topic that will recur throughout the remainder of the book.

THE RELATIONSHIP BETWEEN HEALTH CARE PROFESSIONALS AND PATIENTS

The identification, analysis, and resolution of many of the ethical issues we are considering depend upon the understanding we currently have about the way doctors, nurses, other health professionals, sick people, and families should behave towards each other. The behaviours involved are complex, and involve publicly accredited knowledge and skills, services, expectations, responsibilities, rights, and basic human needs. We use the term *relationship* to encompass all the interactions brought into play when sick people turn to professionals for cure, care, comfort, and counsel. Unlike the relationship of parent to child, wife to husband, or friend to friend, the relationship of doctors, nurses, and other such groups to sick people and their families is *professional* in character. This professional relationship is also *normative*, because it serves to determine what is mandatory, permissible, tolerable, or to be prohibited in the specific words and deeds that link people in achieving the goals of health, prevention of disease, rehabilitation and cure, comfort, and, when all else fails, in achieving the goals of a peaceful and dignified death. In this sense, the professional-patient relationship is *a foundation* of professional ethics: it is upon our concept of this relationship that we, in part, base our decisions about right and wrong, about rights, obligations, and responsibilities in the care of sick and dying people.

Our concepts of the relationships involving health care professionals, especially the relationships between doctors and patients, doctors and nurses, and nurses and patients, have evolved and changed over the past several decades, and that evolution is still underway. Attention to some of these shifts in understanding will clarify some of the significant developments in professional ethics that have occurred over the past twenty-five years.

RELATIONSHIPS AMONG HEALTH CARE PROFESSIONALS

Relationships among the health care professions have changed dramatically in North America over the past twenty-five years, and change is still underway. The basic *shift* has been from a *hierarchical* to a *collaboration model* of relationship. We focus your attention here on the nature of this change, rather than on all the factors that have brought the change about. For the purposes of discussion, we will concentrate on the relationship between nurses and doctors, although other health care professions are going through similar redefinitions of their roles in relation to one another.

Until quite recently, nurses (nearly always thought of stereotypically as female) were expected to be handmaidens, who executed the orders of doctors (nearly always thought of stereotypically as male). Court cases in England and the United States supported these images and the hierarchical model of the doctor-nurse relationship. Nurses were to "follow the directions of the patient's doctor." The doctor was seen as "supreme." If a nurse obeyed the express orders of a doctor, even when she was convinced that it would be harmful to the patient, she was not guilty of negligence, for to obey these orders was seen as the duty of a nurse (Langslow, 1987).

There is a trend in court decisions, though, to adopt a quite different view of the way nurses should now relate to doctors and patients. There is increasing recognition that nurses have a *therapeutic relationship with patients that is distinct* from the relationship between doctors and patients. A United States court in a case in 1977 supported this concept of the nurse's distinct therapeutic relationship: "Nurses are specialists in hospital care who, in the final analysis, hold the well-being, in fact in some instances the very lives, of patients in their hands."(Langslow, 1987, 65) This fact has already been recognized in a number of provinces. Québec, for instance, allows nurses to perform a number of medical acts as professionals, independent from physicians.

Nurses are now increasingly recognized for what they have become: specially-trained and certified advanced practitioners, with independent duties and responsibilities to their patients. The hierarchical model has increasingly given way to a collaborative model of the doctor-nurse relationship. Within this model, doctors and nurses work closely together, not only on purely technical questions of optimal care, but also in clinical ethics, as we shall discuss later in this text.

This collaborative model is reflected in the Code of Ethics of the Canadian Nurses Association (revised 1991), where it is stated: "The nurse should participate in the assessment, planning, implementation and evaluation of comprehensive programmes of care for individual clients and client groups" (p. 13). Of course, not all physicians are likely to agree with nurses about when and how such collaboration should take place. Whereas under the hierarchical model of authority, there was never any doubt about who was in charge and who should prevail when conflict occurred, the collaborative model can give rise to disputes about appropriate patient care, which often have to be solved by a third party such as the hospital administration or ethics committee.

THE HEALTH PROFESSIONAL-PATIENT RELATIONSHIP: IN TRANSITION

The exercise of authority can be a problem, not only in the relationships among health care professionals, but also in those between professionals and patients. Here it is necessary to describe briefly the notion of a profession. Professions are established in a society to achieve a reasonable division of labour and, especially, to minimize the harm, anarchy, and chaos caused by undisciplined charlatanism and quackery. Professionalization brings responsibility out into the open, and assures a measure of public control over what people claim to be able to do for others. It sets up a framework within which reasonable expectations are likely to be reasonably fulfilled. Of professionals, we expect knowledge, skill, experience, and high standards of performance in those areas of expertise for which they have acquired social recognition and accreditation. With public accreditation and responsibility comes authority.

The Doctor's Aesculapian Authority: A Traditional View

Professions vary with respect to their credentials of competence, and also with respect to the authority they carry in our society. Physicians, in particular, have enjoyed and exercised a very special and powerful kind of authority in their care of sick and dying people. The term *Aesculapian authority* has been given to the peculiar power physicians have possessed, to command the attention, respect, and compliance of patients, families, and support staff to their diagnostic and treatment decisions. Aesculapius, the deified healer of ancient Greece, was believed to have ministered to the Greek army at the siege of Troy. The term *Aesculapian authority* has served to synthesize several other types of authority that doctors have traditionally enjoyed.

Sapiential authority (from *sapientia*, the Latin word for wisdom) is based on knowledge and expertise. Doctors have exercised such authority because of their presumed ability and competence to read and interpret symptoms, to diagnose disease, and to select effective means of treatment and cure. Who has not heard the expression, "I am under doctor's orders"? We are more conscious now than people used to be that doctors' sapiential authority does not really give them the power "to order." Sapiential authority is not structural authority, is not the authority, for instance, of elected office. However submissive patients may be, and however pretentious doctors may be, a doctor, on the basis of sapiential authority, "may advise, inform, instruct, and direct, but he may not order." (Siegler, 1973, 42)

Doctors have been presumed to know what is good for patients, what is good and necessary for their health, and, in limited cases, for their survival. *Moral authority* is based not only on technical knowledge and expertise, but on a knowledge of what is good and right. As Paterson has observed: "What the doctor is doing is socially right as well as individually good. This is an unbeatable combination. There is no other profession which matches this." (Paterson, 1973)

People are quite sensitive today to the limits of a doctor's moral authority to direct their decisions about how they should live, and even about treatment decisions when they are sick. Decisions about alternative treatments for various disease conditions, and about aggressive life-prolonging treatment versus palliative care for patients threatened by death, are rarely reducible to their strictly medical components. In matters of life's goals and of value choices, a doctor's moral authority is no greater than anyone else's authority.

A doctor's *charismatic authority,* though a real component of Aesculapian authority, is more difficult to define. Charismatic authority is not based specifically upon scientific knowledge and technical skills, nor does it specifically rest upon the ability to interpret what is right and good for health and life in normal circumstances. Charismatic authority rests upon the ability of knowing what to do when all known rules fail to apply, when available knowledge leaves a concrete situation clouded by uncertainty. This authority is expressed in people who know how to prescribe the original, perhaps ordinarily unthinkable, solution or course of action in a situation marked by uncertainty, danger, and threat to life. This authority is not bestowed automatically with a medical degree, nor do doctors necessarily grow to such authority with years of practice.

A Shift Away From Aesculapian Authority

At least in North American and European societies, people are realizing more and more that it is no longer possible to resolve the multiple and complex ethical issues of contemporary medicine by direct and simple appeal to the doctor-patient relationship. This is particularly true if that relationship is conceived exclusively, or even primarily, in terms of the patient's trust and the physician's conscience. The shift today is away from this paternalistic model, however tolerable it may have been in simpler times, towards basing medical ethics on the physician-patient or physician-family partnership in shared decision-making.

However, this dialogical model is not the whole story either. Physicians are not alone when they treat and care for patients. Particularly in cases of complex and grave illness, an individual physician works with many consultants, and always needs to collaborate closely with nurses, social workers, therapists, psychologists, and other health care professionals. These groups have increasingly developed their own particular areas of experience, knowledge, and technical expertise. They no longer see themselves, and are increasingly no longer seen in society, as the simple servants of the doctor. The courts and others more generally in society have come to recognize that these groups now carry professional responsibilities commensurate with their knowledge and expertise.

In a broad and real sense, society as a whole is at the bedside when individual health care professionals, patients, and families take decisions and make choices that nudge the foundations of community among human beings. Indeed, a society's ethos and values are today more frequently at stake in the decisions and practice of health care professionals than ever before in the history of the healing sciences and crafts. The many discussions and models of the doctor-patient relationship proposed over the past twenty-five years reflect attempts to understand a profession, a societally central profession, in transition.

MODELS OF THE DOCTOR-PATIENT RELATIONSHIP

Although each health care profession has established particular standards of care for the interactions of its members with their patients, almost all of the attention of ethicists has been directed towards the physician-patient relationship. Descriptions of this relationship range from the development, in the photographic sense, of images implicit in everyday clinical practice, to the construction of explicit and theoretical models. Generally, these images and models are not totally true or false, nor are they mutually exclusive, nor do they individually account adequately for the interactions between doctors and sick people, interactions that vary enormously across the many human diseases in quite different cultures and historical periods. We draw your attention to the aspects of the doctor-patient relationship that have particular significance regarding both the causation and the resolution of ethical issues, and dilemmas occurring in the care of sick and dying people.

The Biomedical Engineering Model

For many years, the basic science model of disease has dominated clinical practice. Although the central reality of clinical practice is the individual patient in his or her full human, physiological, psychic, and personal particularity, clinicians often see patients through "scientific spectacles" that penetrate right through the person of the patient, to focus physician attention on disorders in the patient's organs, tissues, cells, and molecules. No informed person, of course, will doubt that scientific competence and objectivity are absolutely essential for effective medical care of sick people. The difficulties appear when the physicians are so totally and exclusively focused on organs and cells that they cannot notice or relate to all the "soft" information — the information about patients' personal distress, suffering, and life goals — that differentiates people from simple organic, cellular, and molecular systems. The exclusive scientific focus and image of the doctor also favours the untrue and unrealistic idea that doctors really should have nothing to do with ethics. They should intervene, act, and correct what is wrong with the body — period.

Though it covers an important part of what doctors should do for sick people, this perspective alone fails to do two critically important things. First, the model does not illuminate what doctors should do and be for patients, when intervention to cure and control symptoms has reached its limits. Second, the model has little to suggest about who is to decide what is to be done or what is to be stopped, when the decisions cannot be reached on the basis of scientific and medical data alone. Many of the uncertainties, battles at the bedside, and court cases of recent years in the area of life-prolongation decisions have centred on this question.

The Authoritarian Model

Michael Balint has used the expression "apostolic function" to summarize the observation or opinion that every doctor "has a vague, but almost unshakably firm ideal of how a patient ought to behave when ill."(Balint, 1964, 216) For many years, patients were seen as incapable or unwilling to share responsibility for their treatment and care; either because the knowledge required for treatment decisions was thought to be beyond their understanding, or because the physical and emotional disturbance caused by illness was assumed to have rendered them untrustworthy judges of their own best interests. The role of the physician, within this "priestly" image of the doctor, included the responsibility to make decisions about what was in patients' best interests and to act accordingly, without the expectation that patients, or their families, if they were unconscious or incompetent, should participate in the decision-making.

This image or model of the physician is the primary focus of critiques of medical *paternalism*. Basically, paternalism means treating adults as a father treats his young children. How far may we go in "preventing" adults from harming themselves by their own actions, or by their likely failure to act? How far may we go in "protecting" adults from truth about a diagnosis or prognosis we think they will be unable to bear? These questions occur frequently in the care of the sick and dying.

Prevention of harm and protection of adults may, at times, be necessary and ethically justifiable. However, the burden of proof should always rest with those who believe they are right in interfering with another person's life and restricting another person's liberty, when this interference and restriction are for the "person's own good." The shift today is away from the preconceived idea that doctors generally know better than patients themselves what is truly in the patients' best interests.

Human dignity does not reside in the power for thought and knowledge alone. Dignity comes to mature expression in the power to act knowledgeably and sensibly, and to command respect for one's considered and cherished intentions. Patients are not always able to act in accordance with their considered and cherished intentions. They often need help so to act, and they often cannot command attention, understanding, and respect from doctors and nurses for a choice or decision that seems to contradict a sacred purpose of medicine: to save life. These persons may wonder about their own worth, when they come to feel inferior to a life-support machine because of their inability to command if, when, and for how long it will be used.

The main criticism of paternalism is that it simply assumes that people are untrustworthy guardians of their own lives. This is an affront to human dignity, and often occurs at patients' moments of great vulnerability, moments, when they need all possible help to be, and to stay, in control.

The Contract Model

There is something fundamentally wrong, Robert Veatch has argued, with taking the doctor-patient relationship as the basis for medical ethics, if the medical profession is exclusively in charge of determining what this relationship requires of doctors. If professional obligation is nothing more than what the profession says it is, then, so Veatch believes, ethical positivism has run amok in professional conceit (Veatch, 1981, 108-138). Why should only doctors be involved in determining the ethics of a relationship that intimately involves and affects the lives and liberties of patients?

Veatch proposes a triple-contract theory to counteract the limitations of an exclusively professional ethic of the doctor-patient relationship. The *basic social contract* determines the fundamental principles, such as contract-keeping, autonomy, honesty, respect for life, and justice, that are essential for maintaining a society. These principles are the basis for a *second contract* between society and a profession, the contract that specifies the duties of a professional role. The *third contract*, between individual physicians and lay persons, is based on the first two, and clarifies the specific responsibilities inherent in each doctor-patient relation.

Whatever one may think of this triple-contract theory as such, Veatch has at least emphasized that medical ethics cannot find its adequate foundation solely in a professional code. On the basis of this theory, medical ethics "can no longer be seen as a set of principles or commitments generated from within a profession."(Veatch, 1981, 6)

The Healing Model

Edmund Pellegrino and David Thomasma view medicine as belonging primarily to the category of relationships. Medicine is rooted in the special relationship of healing. They attempt to base medical ethics on values and goals that are intrinsic to this relationship of healing. The ultimate test of clinical judgment in this relationship is whether it is in conformity with the "living body, the lived body, and the lived self" of the patient. Prior to contracts and social-legal arrangements between society and the medical profession are the facts of disease and illness. The doctor-patient relationship, and the range of physicians' duties, are primarily based on the primordial event of the "intrinsic need of a living body for help in restoring itself to health." This theory of medical ethics roots medicine, the doctor-patient relationship, and medical ethics in the event of "the living organism in need." The goal of the theory is to derive medical ethics from the nature of medicine and the nature of medical acts, the latter epitomized in the central act of healing (Pellegrino 1981).

The Covenant Model

In William F. May's analysis, there is no one, simple, all-inclusive model of the doctor-patient relationship that can serve as an adequate basis for medical ethics. The model has to be as complex as that relationship is. The relationship is that of a professional to a human being in need. It has to offer not only personal presence and concern to a patient, but proficiency, skill, and highly specialized services. Professional competence is an essential characteristic, but not an exhaustive characterization of the relationship. It is also true that elements of a contractual relationship — particularly information exchange and informed consent rather than blind trust, legal enforcement of terms of agreement, and mutual advantage of partners rather than philanthropy of one human being towards others — are indeed additional essential characteristics of the relationship between patients and physicians.

Nevertheless, May cannot accept a reduction of the physician-patient relationship to a contractual relationship, in which "two partners calculate their own best interests and agree upon some joint project in which both derive roughly equivalent benefits for goods contributed by each."(May, 1975, 33) This reduction would amount to a commercialization of the doctor-patient relationship. A commercial relationship is not marked by a personal and professional commitment to confront the realities of disease, pain, suffering, loss, and death with competence and, when that fails, with a personal presence to suffering persons. Covenantal ethics implies a readiness to serve that reaches beyond the borders of calculated self-interest, a readiness also to confront one's own vulnerability in facing the incurability, the suffering, and the impending death of patients. This is a commitment not to abandon patients, especially when professional skill and the terms of a contract have reached their limits.

THE PROFESSIONAL-PATIENT RELATIONSHIP: PERSONALIZED CARE

The professional-patient relationship is an authentic human relationship, when it manifests four fundamental characteristics. Charles Fried has identified these with the terms: *lucidity, autonomy, fidelity,* and *humanity*. These characteristics are essential qualifications of how health care professionals and patients should behave towards each other (Fried, 1974, 101-104).

In a human relationship, a person is not treated simply as one of a class. The characteristic, *humanity,* stresses that each person is a unique individual with a correspondingly unique biology, as well as individualized needs, weaknesses, strengths, and life plans. Humanity means attention to, and respect for, this "full human particularity." *Autonomy,* or self-determination, implies the need and the capacity to deliberate about personal goals, and the liberty to act accordingly. A relationship that fosters autonomy is notable for the absence of fraud, force, and the tendency to use another human being as a disposable resource.

Lucidity qualifies communication as honest, candid, and open to imparting all known information that is material to another's self-determination, deliberation, and choice of alternatives to realize individual life plans. This means sensitivity to another person's total life interests, and, as well, to a person's capacities for comprehension. Lucidity is ill-served if clinicians look upon "obtaining informed consent" as some kind of legally imposed ritual. Clinicians and clinical investigators sometimes speak as though consent is something *they* need for *their* work. They then fail to grasp that adequate information is primarily a need of the patient, and a moral requirement of integrity in a human relationship.

Fidelity means faithfulness in responding to justified expectations that are integral components of a relationship. These expectations will vary from one kind of relationship to another. Patients enter into relationships with doctors justifiably expecting, however implicitly, that their doctors are suitably qualified, are up-to-date with current standards of good medicine and skillful surgery, are committed to restoring their patients to good health, and are not using access to them to advance an undisclosed interest or purpose of their own.

A relationship involving such intense scrutiny of a person's body and of the intimate details of a person's life can only be lived within the framework of an ethic of personal care. It is a right, not just an interest or preference, of patients to be treated by doctors and nurses according to the norms of autonomy, lucidity, fidelity, and humanity. If the normative relationship of doctors and nurses to patients is one of personal care, then "these rights must not be compromised, because candor and faithfulness are the very conditions of any significant personal relations at all. To stand ready to compromise them is not to be a little bit impersonal, a little bit unfaithful, somewhat fraudulent and violent. It is to deny the integrity of personal relationships altogether; personal relationships and the recognition of the rights in them are correlative concepts." (Fried, 1974, 99)

CONSENT, CHOICE, CONTROL, AND SHARED DECISION-MAKING

The term *informed consent*, and multiple discussions of its meaning, have dominated the literature on medical ethics and medical law since 1980. However, these years of discussion have not totally cleared away confusion, misunderstanding, and simple lack of comprehension of "informed consent," one of the most important norms of professionals' relationship to patients. We cannot cover the many aspects of consent exhaustively in this chapter, but you should attend closely to the following points.

The Foundation of the Norm: Informed Consent

One of the most succinct and frequently quoted expressions of the *norm* of informed consent is Justice Benjamin Cardozo's statement in the United States 1914 case of *Schloendorff v. Society of New York Hospitals*: "Every human being of adult years and sound mind has a right to determine what shall be done with his own body." (Faden, 1986, 123) That norm serves to support the broader and more primary principle of *respect for persons*, and also to specify what respect for persons requires of doctors and nurses in their care and treatment of sick people. Persons are *inviolable* and *autonomous*, so the norm of informed consent to medical and surgical treatment serves, first of all, to protect sick people from unacceptable intrusions of professionals into their bodies and their lives. The equally important purpose of the norm is to foster a sick person's control over his or her own life.

This understanding has ancient roots in Plato's concept of the ideal relationship of a physician to a sick person. In *The Laws*, Plato distinguished the slaves' doctor from the doctor of free men. The slave doctor would hurry from one patient to another, prescribing treatment quickly and dictatorially, without giving reasons for the treatment, and without any effort to help sick people to understand their condition. The free doctor behaved very differently. He would speak to patients as though they were students, and would teach them, helping patients to acquire a conscious understanding of their sickness and its treatment (Jacquer, 1944, 215).

The ideal image of the physician-patient relationship is a basis and a measure of the norm of informed consent. Consent may be interpreted as acquiescence, compliance, permission, agreement, approval, or collaboration. These terms *are not* synonyms. They express different grades of intellectual and voluntary assent to the treatments and alternatives doctors and nurses propose and administer. The degree of assent sought from patients will vary with physicians' and nurses' commitment to the above-mentioned four characteristics of a relationship in which they see themselves as servants, not of life in the abstract, but of the life plans of this particular patient.

Informed Consent: Misconceptions

There are still doctors around today who believe patients are generally unable to understand either the nature and course of their illness, or the reasons for and against treatment options. An extreme expression of this misconception is found in the paternalistic view put forth by a physician in 1976:

> Informed consent is a legalistic fiction that destroys good patient care and paralyses the conscientious physician. ... It is not applicable, even by definition, to a large segment of the population. The term has no place in the lexicon of medicine. The integrity of the physician continues to represent the most effective guarantee of the rights of the patient and of the experimental subject. (Laforet, 1976)

Some physicians treat informed consent as a kind of legal password they need from the patient, so they can get on with their work of treatment without fear of legal harassment. They seem to be unaware that the norm of informed consent is meant to help patients stay in control of their own lives. The goal is to foster real dialogue between professionals and patients, so that patients will share in the decisions that affect their bodies and their biographies.

This new and contemporary emphasis on *shared decision-making* has motivated a plea to abandon use of the *expression* "informed consent." The expression is so encrusted with years of accumulated misleading ideas that the *reality* behind the expression is often overlooked. The expression may suggest that patients are not informed if they decline to consent; that the purpose of information is to gain consent; and that only patients need to be informed (Dickens, 1985). This last idea loses sight of the fact that physicians and nurses also need information from patients. The responsibility and right of patients is not exhausted with the giving or refusing of consent or permission for treatment. They also need the time for, and the environment favourable to, sufficient disclosure about themselves that physicians and nurses can come to understand what patients' life plans really are, and how treatment decisions should honour patients' goals, values, and plans.

Informed Consent: The Standard of Disclosure

Though each of the four characteristics of a genuine human relationship between professionals and patients shapes the process of consent, the characteristic, *humanity*, is the most difficult to respect and exercises the greatest effect on *lucidity* of communication between doctors, nurses, and patients. *Humanity* means that a patient "has a right to have his full human particularity taken into account by those who do enter into relationship with him." (Fried, 1974, 103)

The particularity of the patient's situation was a central issue in the 1980 Canadian Supreme Court decision involving John Reibl, a patient, and Robert A. Hughes, a surgeon. After surgery to remove a blockage in the left carotid artery, Mr. Reibl suffered a massive stroke, which left him paralyzed in the right side of his body and sexually impotent. Though Mr. Reibl had formally consented to the operation, and it had been conducted without apparent negligence, Dr. Hughes had failed adequately to inform him of the irreducible risks of stroke during, or as an immediate result of, surgery. Dr. Hughes had, rather, emphasized the risks of stroke due to the artery blockage if Mr. Reibl did not have the operation. Mr. Reibl was forty-four years old at the time of his operation, and only a year and a half away from fulfilling the employment time-eligibility condition for a lifetime retirement pension and extended disability benefits from the Ford Motor Company where he worked.

The operation Dr. Hughes proposed was reasonable and indicated for Mr. Reibl's condition. However, Mr. Reibl was not in an emergency situation.

He claims that he would have postponed the surgery, had he really understood the comparative risks of surgery versus postponed surgery. He would have preferred to live a shorter normal life than to live crippled, as a result of surgery designed to prevent the very paralysis from stroke that it caused. More importantly, Mr. Reibl would have postponed this surgery at least until the time he reached eligibility for his company's full pension benefits.

Bora Laskin, the Chief Justice of the Supreme Court of Canada, concluded that a reasonable person in Mr. Reibl's position would, on a balance of probabilities, have opted against the surgery rather than undergoing it at that particular time. Moreover, the Chief Justice also emphasized how critically important it is for physicians to consider the particularity of a patient's situation when informing patients about the risks of both a proposed treatment and its alternatives:

> Merely because medical evidence established the reasonableness of a recommended operation did not mean that a reasonable person in the patient's position would necessarily agree to it, if proper disclosure had been made of the risks attendant upon it, balanced by those against it. The patient's particular situation, and the degree to which the risk of surgery or no surgery were balanced, would reduce the force, on objective appraisal, of the surgeon's recommendation. In deciding what decision a reasonable person in the patient's position would have made, the patient's particular position should be considered objectively, and not subjectively. *(Reibl v. Hughes,* 1980, 882)

This decision in the *Reibl v. Hughes* case indicates that of three possible standards to measure the scope of information physicians and patients should impart to each other — the professional standard, the subjective patient standard, and the objective patient standard — the latter is to be followed. The *professional standard* would give the medical profession the power to set the standard of disclosure of information at a lower level than would serve the public interest and protection. On the other hand, the *subjective patient standard* would place physicians at the mercy of the patient's bitter hindsight. The *objective patient standard* requires that physicians take account of a patient's particular position, a position, obviously, that will vary with each patient. This standard, however, is not completely relative to each patient. The standard across the varying situations of many patients is *reasonableness.* The patient's particular concerns that a physician must know about and honour in consent discussions are those that are reasonably based. Since these reasonable particular concerns of patients cannot be determined without physicians coming to know their patients, the real ethical imperative of informed consent is: know thy patient!

The Institutional and Social Context of Consent

Few would deny that doctors and nurses need better education and training about how to communicate with very different kinds of patients. However, perfecting communication between professionals and patients depends on more than education alone.

Several years ago, Bernard Barber warned about the individualistic error of conceiving informed consent as the outcome of a transaction that occurs between two, and only two, individuals — the physician and patient or subject. Barber advised that we shall not understand informed consent until we look beyond the doctor and patient as two isolated and insulated individuals. We have to examine the actual structure of the social system that exercises a determining influence on the behaviours of both professionals and patients involved in the consent process (Barber, 1980, 6-7).

The way medical and nursing care is organized and delivered to patients is one aspect of the social system that can, today, easily distort communication between professionals and the sick people they serve. Achieving informed consent as shared decision-making is hardly possible when care is provided "by teams of highly specialized professionals whose individual responsibilities may be defined less by the overall needs of the patient than by particular diseases or organ systems. When this occurs there may be no single professional in effective command of the entire care of the patient, no one who knows the patient well and to whom the patient may turn for information, advice, and comfort." (The President's Commission, 1982, 96)

Shared decision-making will remain largely an illusion, and consent will continue to pose problems, until we succeed in fashioning structures of care that favour a genuinely human professional-patient relationship.

RESPECTING PATIENTS' WILL WHEN EXPLICIT CONSENT IS IMPOSSIBLE

There are situations, notably emergency situations, when physicians may be unable to inform patients about, and obtain their consent for, treatments or operations that have to be undertaken to preserve health or life. The legal doctrines of apparent, implied, or presumed consent have evolved to qualify the need for a patient's *explicit* consent. These doctrines and their ethical foundation, however, do not justify a physician or nurse in going ahead with treatments "where there is knowledge or reason to believe that the particular patient would *not* consent to a procedure." (Fried, 1974, 41)

This was the issue in the Supreme Court of Ontario case involving Georgette Malette, victim of multiple injuries in an auto accident, and Dr.

D.L. Shulman, the physician who treated Mrs. Malette in the Kirkland and District Hospital Emergency Department in Kirkland Lake, Ontario. Mrs. Malette, a Jehovah's Witness, was unable to give or refuse consent to blood transfusions administered to her during emergency treatment. However, her purse did contain a card, signed by her but without date of signature, indicating her request that blood or blood products not be administered to her under any circumstance. The judge in this case concluded that this card was a valid restriction of Dr. Shulman's liberty to treat this patient with blood transfusions, even though they may appear necessary to save her life. The case went to appeal, and the Appeal Court supported this conclusion. This case illustrates the principle that the presumption of consent, justified in certain circumstances, must give way to reliable evidence of a patient's prior refusal of a treatment, when that patient can no longer directly express his or her intentions.

There are many other situations in which informed consent is impossible to obtain from patients. Some of these will be treated in subsequent chapters, those dealing with newborns (Chapter 16), intellectually disabled persons (Chapter 9), mentally ill individuals (Chapter 11), dementia patients (Chapter 12), and patients who are comatose (Chapter 16). Others arise as a result of linguistic and cultural factors, for example when trained interpreters are not available. In these situations decisions about medical treatment for patients must be made by others, who are known as substitute, or proxy, decision-makers. Who should serve in this capacity, and what criteria they should use to make their decisions, present major ethical and legal difficulties. These problems, and the tentative resolutions that have been suggested to date, will be considered in later chapters.

TELLING THE TRUTH AND THE THERAPEUTIC PRIVILEGE

The term *therapeutic privilege* refers to the legal doctrine, buttressed to a certain extent by common sense, that physicians may justifiably withhold information from patients or their proxies, if they reasonably believe this information would not be in the patients' best interest, or would interfere with treatment and cure. Of course, legal doctrine, ethical teaching, and even common-sense notions change with time. Few today would extend this therapeutic qualification of the doctor's duty to inform patients to the point of justifying withholding of information simply because the physician fears adequate information would provoke patient refusal of treatment the physician thinks is necessary.

Therapeutic deception is the other side of the coin of the therapeutic privilege. A consensus has been in the building for many years now that patients should generally be told the truth about their diagnosis and prognosis. The burden of justification should be on those who claim that telling patients the truth will do them more harm than the paternalistic deception that would shield them from the truth.

People did not always think this way about cancer in the past. There was a trend in North America, still detectable even several years ago, to shield patients from a cancer diagnosis, and from a prognosis of the disease's course. In answer to the question, "Should the cancer victim be told the truth?" one physician in 1943 responded: "I not only feel certain that, as a general rule, the patient should not be told he has a malignant tumor but, also, I am no less certain as to why he should not be told." (Seelig, 1943, 34) The reason for not telling was to protect the patient from living in the shadow of doubt as to when death would strike, or as to when the disease would strike again if treatment succeeded in bringing about a temporary remission.

There still exists, in this respect, a difference between North America and Continental Europe — more particularly France and Italy — where for cultural reasons, and perhaps because of a more authoritarian model of physician-patient relationship, truth is often withheld from the patient.

This practice of shielding cancer patients from the truth about their condition was brought into serious question more than thirty years ago. A study of patients' own views about what they want to be told, published in the *British Medical Journal* in 1959, concluded that most people *do* want to know the truth about their condition (Aitken-Swan, 1959). The study also discovered that patients are not really shielded from the truth, when doctors try to deceive them about their cancer condition. They generally perceive the truth is being withheld from them. Patients are then isolated, not reassured. And that isolation can be devastating: devastating for the patients themselves, and devastating to their relationships with their families, their doctors, and their nurses.

These insights are now widely accepted, and increasingly shape the attitudes of health care professionals and the ways they communicate with people who face incurable and terminal disease. The hospice and palliative-care movements have exercised great influence on these changes of attitude. Hospice and palliative care, conceived in the crucible of the neglect of dying cancer patients, arose in opposition to separations of *cure* from *care*, of *patient* from *family*, and of *clinical objectivity* from *human compassion*.

The real moment of truth and of the greatest challenge occurs when patients face the threat of disintegration and death. Health care professionals are then challenged to do more than minister to the needs of a patient's body. They may be invited to enter the innermost sanctum of another human being's personal history. The trust and identification with another, required to face another person's suffering, also open windows on to the communication of hope. The challenge is to touch, awaken, and release the saving power of a suffering person's latent beliefs. Communication that starts with truth can end with hope.

CONFIDENTIALITY

Informed consent and truth-telling are two essential aspects of the relationship between health care professionals and patients. Another key feature of this relationship is *confidentiality*. This has been an integral element of medical ethics since Hippocrates, who admonished his physician associates to "guard the patient's secrets." A similar rule is found in virtually every health care profession's Code of Ethics. For example:

- An ethical physician will keep in confidence information derived from a patient, and divulge it only with the permission of the patient except when otherwise required by law. (Canadian Medical Association)

- The nurse respects the client's right to confidentiality within the nurse-client relationship. (College of Nurses of Ontario)

- The health service executive shall respect the confidentiality of information, unless it is in the public interest or required by law to divulge information. (Canadian College of Health Services Executives)

Confidentiality of health information is also protected by laws in most, if not all, Canadian provinces and territories.

The high value that is placed on confidentiality has several sources. We will deal with each in turn.

Autonomy
As we saw when dealing with the notion of informed consent, Canadians consider personal autonomy to be a fundamental value of our society. Autonomy relates to confidentiality, in that personal information about an individual belongs to him or her and should not be divulged to others without his or her consent. When an individual reveals personal information to another, a physician or nurse for example, or when information comes to light through a medical test, those in the know are bound to keep it confidential unless authorized to divulge it by the individual concerned.

Respect for Others
Confidentiality is considered to be important, not just because of adherence to the abstract principle of autonomy, but also because human beings deserve respect. One important way of showing them respect is by preserving their privacy. In the medical setting, privacy is often greatly compromised, but this is all the more reason to prevent further unnecessary intrusions into a person's private life. Since individuals differ regarding their desire for privacy, we cannot assume that everyone wants to be treated as we would want to be. Discretion is an important virtue for determining which personal information a patient wants to keep secret, and which he or she is willing to have revealed to others.

Trust

Whereas respect for others (in this case, patients) is the principal foundation for the duty of health care professionals to preserve confidentiality, the primary basis of the patient's relationship to his or her caregivers is *trust*. In order to receive medical care, patients have to reveal personal information to doctors and others who may be total strangers to them — information that they would not want anyone else to know. They must have good reason to trust their caregivers not to divulge this information. The basis of this trust is the ethical and legal standards of confidentiality that health care professionals are expected to uphold.

Despite the importance of confidentiality, it is neither possible nor desirable to guarantee it absolutely. The nature of our health care system and institutions is such that many individuals — doctors, nurses, laboratory technicians, students, etc. — require access to a patient's health records, in order to provide adequate care to that person and, for the students, to learn how to practise their profession. In the increasing number of cases where patients speak a different language than their caregivers, there is a need for interpreters to facilitate communication. In small linguistic and cultural communities, it may be very difficult for these interpreters to maintain confidentiality. In cases of patients who are not competent to make their own medical decisions — children, intellectually handicapped persons, those who are unconscious or senile — other individuals have to be given information, in order to make decisions on their behalf. Some medical conditions, such as sexually transmitted diseases and genetic abnormalities, affect other persons, who may have a right to this information. Each of these potential limitations on confidentiality will be discussed in later chapters of this book.

Although confidentiality is not absolute, it is still a primary obligation for health care professionals, and exceptions have to be justified. Along with informed consent, it is an essential element of the relationship between patients and health care professionals, and of contemporary bioethics.

CONCLUSION

The five preceding chapters have established a framework for dealing with specific bioethical issues. Our discussion of these issues in the remaining chapters will presuppose a knowledge of the matters treated above. Some of them will figure more prominently in one of the chapters than in others; for example, the nature of the Canadian health care system is crucial for the problem of resource allocation (Chapter 14), informed consent raises particular problems in the research setting (Chapter 13), and confidentiality has been severely questioned in relation to AIDS (Chapter 10). Nevertheless, the themes of each of the preceding chapters recur throughout the book, and readers are encouraged to refer to these sections as you encounter these themes in later chapters.

REFERENCES

Aitken-Swan J. and **Easson E.C.** "Reactions of Cancer Patients on Being Told their Diagnosis." *British Medical Journal* 1959;1:779-783.

Balint M. *The Doctor, his Patient, and the Illness.* New York: International Universities Press, 1964.

Barber B. *Informed Consent in Medical Therapy and Research.* New Brunswick, New Jersey: Rutgers University Press, 1980.

Dickens B.M. "Informed Choice in Medical Care." In: R.S. Abella and M.L. Rothman, eds. *Justice Beyond Orwell.* Montréal: Les Éditions Yvon Blais, 1985, 244-245.

Faden R., **Beauchamp T.L.** and **King N.M.P.** *A History and Theory of Informed Consent.* New York, Oxford: Oxford University Press, 1986.

Fried C. *Medical Experimentation, Personal Integrity and Social Policy.* Amsterdam, Oxford: North-Holland Publishing Company, 1974.

Jacquer W. *Paidera: The Ideals of Greek Culture.* Vol. III. *The Conflict of Cultural Ideals in the Age of Plato.* New York: Oxford University Press, 1944.

Laforet E.G. "The Fiction of Informed Consent." *Journal of the American Medical Association* 1976;235:1579-1585.

Langslow A. "Legal Issues and the Role of the Nurse." In: Monash University Centre for Human Bioethics. *The Role of the Nurse: Doctor's Handmaiden, Patient's Advocate or What?* Australia: Monash University Centre for Human Bioethics, 1987, 61-72.

May W.F. "Code, Covenant, Contract, or Philanthropy." *Hastings Center Report* 1975;5:29-38.

Paterson T.T. Notes on Aesculapian Authority. Unpublished Manuscript. Cited in M. Siegler and H. Osmond. "Aesculapian Authority." *Hastings Center Report* 1973;1:42, note 3.

Pellegrino E.D. and **Thomasma D.C.** *A Philosophical Basis of Medical Practice.* New York, Oxford: Oxford University Press, 1981.

Reibl v. Hughes (1980), 2 Supreme Court Reports 880.

Seelig M.G. "Should the Cancer Victim Be Told the Truth?" *Journal of the Missouri Medical Association* 1943;40:33-35.

Siegler M. and **Osmond H.** "Aesculapian Authority." *Hastings Center Report* 1973;1:41-52.

The President's Commission for the Study of Ethical Problems in Medicine and Biomedical and Behavioral Research *Making Health Care Decisions*. Vol. I: Report. Washington, DC: U.S. Government Printing Office, 1982.

Veatch R.M. *A Theory of Medical Ethics*. New York: Basic Books, 1981.

P A R T 2

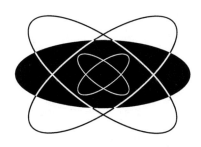

AT THE
BEGINNING
OF LIFE

6

WHEN PEOPLE CANNOT CONCEIVE A CHILD: THE REPRODUCTIVE TECHNOLOGIES

For thousands of years an aura of mystery enveloped the entire phenomenon of human reproduction, from the event of conception, through pregnancy, and up to the blissful or, at times, tragic moment of birth. Mystery meant at least this: invisibility and technical inaccessibility. The ovum, zygote, embryo, and fetus were hidden within the woman's body. The need for sexual intercourse to unite spermatozoon and ovum, and the hiddenness of fertilization within the fallopian tube served as a shield against imaginative, reproductive experiments; served as a barrier also to the development of innovative treatments of infertility (Combined Ethics Committee, 1990, 1).

All this has changed radically. Properly trained people with the required technical equipment and expertise can now observe and experiment with the basic elements of human life — the ovum and spermatozoon and the chromosomes and genes they carry — and they can also intervene in the human reproductive process along its entire course.

Applications of techniques and technologies, to be discussed in this and the following chapter, that were developed in tandem with scientific advances in reproductive biology, as well as in molecular biology and genetics, permit powerful control over the origins and early development of human life. Bentley Glass, a biologist, said over fifteen years ago that this growing power to control human reproduction had influenced the lives of men and women, and he could have added, of children, more than any other advance in biological technology in this century (Glass, 1974).

THE CONTEXT AND OBJECTIVES OF THIS CHAPTER

The reproductive technologies were originally developed to assist infertile couples to conceive and have children. However, various applications of the techniques of artificial insemination and in vitro fertilization in the treatment of infertility have led to novel, complex, and controversial reproductive arrangements. Moreover, these same techniques can be, and have been, used by quite fertile people who, for various reasons, want to have children without sexual intercourse, or without the personal burdens of pregnancy, or who want to found a nontraditional family, for example, a family consisting of children, a lesbian mother, and her lesbian companion. So ethical issues related to the uses of assisted reproduction in circumventing infertility will be a prime, though not exclusive, focus of discussion in this chapter.

The Context: The Separation of Reproductive Functions Leads to Novel Reproductive Relationships and Research

A variant of the principle, *divide and conquer*, namely, *separate and control*, generates much of the power people can now exercise over various dimensions of the reproductive process. The development of relatively safe and effective methods of contraception has allowed people *to separate sexual intercourse from reproduction*, and that separation has increased people's *control over fertility*. Methods of assisted reproduction, such as artificial insemination and in vitro fertilization — to be discussed at length later in this chapter — allow people *to separate reproduction from sexual intercourse*, and this separation has delivered increased *control over infertility*. When these methods of assisted reproduction, enlisted to circumvent infertility, use the sperm and ova of a married couple — as they do in artificial insemination with a husband's sperm (AIH), and in in vitro fertilization (IVF) when the wife's ova are fertilized with her husband's sperm — reproduction, indeed, takes places in separation from sexual intercourse of the married couple, but little else marks these forms of reproduction and the resultant relationships of parenthood and family, as being any different from the relationships of parenthood and family constituted when fertile couples reproduce by sexual intercourse.

However, the basic techniques of artificial insemination and in vitro fertilization may be used to set up *socially novel and controversial reproductive arrange-*

ments. Artificial insemination with donor sperm (AID), increasingly called therapeutic donor insemination (TDI), used when a husband's sperm cannot fertilize his wife's ova, sets up a reproductive arrangement in which the child has two fathers: a genetic or biological father, the sperm donor, and a social father, the man who will raise the child and is usually recognized as the child's father. This reproduction arrangement, though not unique to the use of artificial insemination with donor sperm, used to circumvent infertility, in effect *separates genetic from social fatherhood* in human reproduction.

When single or lesbian women seek artificial insemination with donor sperm, or when they perform such insemination on themselves, the child is isolated from its genetic father and usually has no social father. The converse can happen if a homosexual man or couple commissions a woman to be artificially inseminated and serve as a surrogate mother. The woman, in this case, is both genetic and gestational mother, and the child will be isolated from its genetic-gestational mother and will usually have no social mother. When a woman, after the death of her husband, is artificially inseminated with her father-in-law's sperm, the child's social grandfather is also its genetic father.

The use of both donated sperm and donated ova, or the use of donated embryos, in combination with IVF, can lead to even more complex reproductive arrangements and relationships. When, to cite a relatively rare event, a child is conceived from the sperm of one man (the genetic father) and the ovum of one woman (the genetic mother), is carried through pregnancy to birth by a second woman (the gestational mother), only to be reared by a third woman and a second man (the social, and often adoptive, parents), the parental and familial relationships thereby established are so new and so different from traditional family ties that we even lack a suitable language for them. This particular arrangement *separates three functions of motherhood* — genetic, gestational, and social motherhood — and assigns them to three different women. How many grandparents, half-brothers and sisters, uncles, aunts, and cousins does this child really have?

The techniques for the retrieval of ova from the ovaries, and the methods of in vitro fertilization also *separate the early human embryo from the niches* (the fallopian tube and the uterus) *where it was always previously hidden*. This new and relatively recent separation of the early human embryo from the woman's body permits novel kinds of basic, as well as clinically oriented, research on the human embryo.

The Objectives: Towards a New Reproductive Order?

Human reproduction is a profoundly interpersonal act with eminently social consequences. The human values clustering around reproduction, its relationships, and its institutions have emerged slowly and, indeed, not without pain, peril, and tragedy over long periods of history. It has also taken a long time to work out the customs, ethics, and laws of reproduction, however culturally and socially variable these may be from country to country and across different historical periods.

Today's innovations in reproductive biology and medicine introduce — some would say, invite — rapid and radical moves away from traditional ways of building a family. The separations, mentioned above, of genetic, gestational, and social motherhood, and of genetic and social fatherhood as well, inevitably complexify — some would say, confuse — a child's genetic and social identity. The transformation of traditional reproductive behaviour and reproductive values, rendered possible by various applications of the reproductive technologies, jostles the biological and social foundations of personal identity, of parenthood, marriage, and family.

When ancient wisdom, past experience, and the long-standing ethics, law, and politics of reproduction no longer deliver clear and unambiguous social guidance for novel reproductive experiments, people inevitably enter a period of normative transition, perhaps even a period of normative crisis. Simply put, people no longer know what is right or wrong, what can be tolerated, or where lines have to be drawn. In such periods, fears, emotions, and passions are aroused, uncertainties abound, and controversy dominates the forums of public discourse.

In the face of deep divisions among people on important matters — and there is little to rival human reproduction either in importance or in the depth of ethical divisions it elicits — there is hardly a substitute in open societies for the long process of careful monitoring of innovations, and of civilized discourse about them. For over two decades now, people in countries around the world have mobilized commissions and working groups of the most varied sorts, to deliberate about whether and how today's innovative reproductive practices can be housed within the reproductive ethics and law that were framed when people had little control over the reproductive process. That prolonged deliberation, reflected in hundreds of reports from national, regional, and local governments, from the professions and from religions, is a search for a possibly new, or a possibly reconfirmed older, reproductive order.

The numerous and varied applications of the reproductive technologies raise a host of issues in clinical ethics, research ethics, and public policy ethics. They also exemplify fundamental conflicts on the levels of ethos and morality, as discussed in Chapter 2. It is impossible, in one chapter, to cover the entire spectrum of clinical ethics, research ethics, and public policy ethics and law as these relate to the reproductive technologies. So we need a strategy for this chapter, and this is the one we shall follow.

A great deal depends upon whether people accept these technologies in principle. Some do, others do not; and, in both cases, for quite different reasons. So, after presenting a scientific, medical, and historical overview of the reproductive technologies, we shall concentrate *first* on the ways of thinking, on the reasons and rationales put forth to support acceptance, rejection, or measures of reserve regarding social implementation of innovations in reproductive biology and medicine. The focus is primarily on public policy ethics. Moreover, many who accept the use of the reproductive technologies do so only under specific conditions. We shall, then, *secondly* examine how this "conditional ethics" works for certain of the reproductive technologies. In this connection, we will *thirdly* consider the status of the reproductive technologies within Canadian law. *Fourthly*, we shall then identify, without extensively analyzing, some of the currently most controversial ethical issues raised by use of the reproductive technologies. One focus of our discussion will be on research on the human embryo.

THE REPRODUCTIVE TECHNOLOGIES: A SCIENTIFIC, MEDICAL, AND HISTORICAL OVERVIEW

The title of this chapter links the reproductive technologies to people who cannot have children at all, or who have been unable to have children despite their efforts to do so for some period of time. The reproductive technologies have been developed and primarily used as treatments for infertility, as techniques for assisting reproduction. So, before describing the various procedures encompassed by the general terms *reproductive technologies* or *methods of assisted reproduction*, we direct attention first of all to infertility, a medically and socially complex phenomenon.

Infertility

People are fertile when they produce children, and infertile when they do not. Both fertility and infertility, then, are couple-related achievements or failures, since a man and a woman are needed for fertilization and the initiation of a pregnancy. The inability of a couple to conceive and produce children may be due to the combined deficits of both the man and the woman, or to deficits that affect only the male or the female partner in a couple.

If *fertility* and *infertility* refer to the facts of having or not having children, the terms *fecundity* and *infecundity* refer to the male and female capacities to achieve fertilization, conception, and successful pregnancy, where success in pregnancy refers to the birth of a living child. Whereas *sterility* refers to the total or absolute incapacity to fulfil either the male or the female functions in reproduction, fecundity is subject to degrees. A man who can produce no sperm whatsoever, a condition called azoospermia, is sterile. A man who can produce sperm, but only in quantities that are below the minimal standards of adequacy to achieve fertilization, a condition called oligospermia, offers an example of *reduced fecundity*. A woman who cannot produce fertilizable ova and who has no uterus is sterile. A woman who produces fertilizable ova only irregularly or rarely, or whose uterus is irregular in its capacity to sustain a pregnancy, offers an example of reduced fecundity.

Infertility may be *chosen*, as when men freely undergo a sterilization procedure such as vasectomy, or women request sterilization procedures such as hysterectomy or tubal ligation. Infertility, however, may result from a wide range of injuries or damages to the reproductive organs and the reproductive systems of men and women. Such injury or damage may be congenital, accidental, or the consequence of treatments needed for life-threatening conditions such as cancer. Surgical removal of the ovaries or of the uterus may be required in the treatment of cancer in women. Chemotherapy or radiotherapy in the treatment of cancers in men may result in irreparable damage to their capacity to produce sperm. Sexually transmitted diseases may lead to pelvic inflammatory disease (PID) in women and cause scarring, blockage, and permanent damage to the fallopian tubes, the channels required for passage of ova from the ovaries to the uterus, and the site also where fertilization normally occurs.

While some conditions leading both to female and male infertility, particularly those resulting from sexually transmitted diseases and infections, are *preventable*, other conditions causing infertility may be *treated* either surgically or with medications, though the rates of success vary. Drugs, such as clomiphene citrate, can help women who are not producing ova to return to normal cycles of ovulation. Both medication and surgery can help to reverse infertility in women affected by a condition called endometriosis, where endometrial tissue from inside the uterus grows outside the uterus onto the fallopian tubes, ovaries, or other organs in the pelvis. The growth of endometrial tissue on the reproductive organs can cause infertility. Surgery may help to improve the quality of sperm in men affected by varicocele, a condition in which excessive blood flows around the testis, due to defects in valves in the testicular veins. The sperm of some men with this condition are low in count and poor in motility, the capacity of sperm to move being of critical importance for its ability to fertilize the ovum. When all available diagnostic methods can find no cause, either in the man or the woman, of a couple's infertility, the infertility is said to be *idiopathic* or *unexplained*.

The reproductive technologies, to be described below, are increasingly used to assist people in achieving reproduction when infertility is resistant to other methods of treatment. There is some controversy over the timing and extent of use of the reproductive technologies, particularly of those methods of assisted reproduction that have modest success rates, are costly, and are physically and emotionally stressful for a couple, particularly for the woman.

A frequently used definition of infertility has been criticized in this context. People are often diagnosed as having fertility problems on the basis of the one-year test: a couple is judged to have fertility problems or to be infertile if they have been unable to produce a child after one year, or twelve menstrual cycles, of sexual intercourse without use of contraceptives. This criterion quite surely does confound sterility, or the inability ever to conceive, with slow fecundity, or the inability to conceive quickly (Menken, 1986, 1391). Use of this criterion can lead to an excess diagnosis of infertility, and to a premature diagnosis of infertility as well.

Premature, as well as inadequate, diagnosis of infertility can lead to premature and even unnecessary treatment. Dr. John Collins, in a study published in Canada ten years ago, found that pregnancy independent of treatment occurs frequently in couples who have been diagnosed as infertile. *Treatment-independent* pregnancies include these pregnancies that occurred spontaneously in couples diagnosed as infertile but who received no treatment, and those pregnancies that treated couples had long after treatment was completed. Nearly a fourth (23%) of 1,145 couples diagnosed as infertile had spontaneous or treatment-independent pregnancies (Collins, 1983). However, when a woman is in her mid-thirties, approaching so-called "advanced maternal age," she may be impatient about pregnancy, and unwilling to wait to see if her marriage is infertile, as diagnosed by more than a twelve-month test.

Use of the reproductive technologies has undoubtedly enabled couples, who otherwise would have remained infertile, to have children, children of their own or partially of their own. Though some people have cited world overpopulation, limited resources, and the numbers of parentless children needing adoption as reasons militating against the treatment of infertility, there seems to be a quite general consensus, as the Warnock Committee emphasized, that infertility is a condition meriting treatment (Warnock, 1984, 10). The desire to have children has deep wellsprings in the human spirit, and infertility can cause profound distress and suffering (Seibel, 1982; McEwan, 1987; Wright, 1989). For this reason, if for no other — and wise use of limited resources is another reason — infertility merits treatment. Untreated and unremedied infertility can cause emotional and marital disturbance, requiring a greater outlay of health care resources than the treatment of infertility itself. Infertility merits prevention, and prevention of infertility merits a larger investment of research and education resources than societies have generally made, to date.

The reproductive technologies that have been the object of hundreds, if not thousands, of reports, studies, and scientific publications, and the focus of high controversy as well, are used primarily to treat infertility. They may also be used to enable couples to have children without some kinds of congenital abnormalities they would pass on to their children, were these to be conceived by sexual intercourse. The same technologies can enable people to found nontraditional families. We shall now describe the most frequently used and discussed procedures referred to as the reproductive technologies.

Artificial or Therapeutic Insemination

The oldest technique of assisted reproduction, artificial insemination, now more generally called therapeutic insemination with husband's sperm (TIH) or with donor sperm (TID), is the placement of sperm by means of a small plastic catheter or a syringe into a woman's upper vagina or into the cervical canal. Therapeutic insemination has been known for two centuries, but has been widely practised in North America and Europe only since the Second World War. The first recorded pregnancy and birth of a child conceived by TIH, which took place in England in 1790, is credited to assistance from Dr. John Hunter. Several sources mention 1884 as the date of the first successful TID pregnancy (Rubin, 1965; Fuller Torrey, 1963).

Though therapeutic insemination is now widely practised in many countries, accurate and up-to-date statistics on the number of children born after use of either TIH or TID are not always available. In the United States, a 1988 survey conducted by the Office of Technology Assessment estimated that 172,000 women received therapeutic insemination from 1986 to 1987, with 35,000 births due to TIH and 30,000 births resulting from use of donor sperm (TID) (Office of Technology Assessment, 1988). The Centre d'étude et de conservation du sperme humain (CECOS), the centre of a network of sperm banks and therapeutic insemination services in France, reported 7,160 TID requests accepted and 1,825 TID pregnancies, for the period 1973-1978 (David, 1980, 18). A more recent report (1987) states that 15,000 children have been born in France, since TID with use of frozen donor sperm began in 1972 (Clément, 1987, 2388). Canadian practitioners calculated that at least 1,500 births had occurred in Canada as a result of TID over the ten-year period 1968-1978 (Advisory Committee, 1982, x and 72). More recent statistics for Canada are not available to us, as of this writing.

Therapeutic insemination with a husband's sperm (TIH), quite widely practised in the United States as noted above, may be considered in a number of circumstances; for example, when the husband, due to impotence, cannot achieve ejaculation into the vagina or cannot penetrate the vagina, due to vaginal abnormalities. TIH is also considered when the husband has to undergo surgery, chemotherapy, or radiotherapy that would destroy or reduce his capacity to produce viable sperm. His sperm can be obtained before these treatments, then be frozen and stored for future thawing and insemination of his wife. Scientists demonstrated, in the 1950s, that the use of frozen, then thawed, sperm in therapeutic insemination can result in conception and birth of a normal child.

Therapeutic insemination with donor sperm (TID) is usually considered when the husband is affected by azoospermia, severe oligospermia, or when the husband's sperm have very low motility or other abnormalities that prevent his sperm from fertilizing an ovum. A husband may also carry a genetic defect that would lead to severe congenital malformation of the child, or to transmission of serious genetic diseases. TID, where donors are suitably screened to rule out transmission of known genetic defects, would enable a couple to have a child and avoid passing on the husband's genetic defect. Some men, who are carriers of the gene defect for Huntington's disease, which usually appears in middle age and leads, over several years, to loss of motor control, dementia, and death, have opted with their wives to have children by TID.

The pregnancies of therapeutic insemination, properly conducted, approach those of natural insemination by sexual intercourse. Estimates are that over 90% of couples coming for therapeutic insemination should be expected to conceive within a year. Findings differ regarding the superior pregnancy rates obtained by use of fresh, as opposed to frozen-thawed (cryopreserved), sperm in therapeutic insemination (Hummel, 1989, 926). If there is a reduction in conception rates due to the use of frozen sperm, this may be due to a decrease in the number of motile sperm that results from the cryopreservation process. Scientists estimate that 30 to 50 million motile, frozen-thawed sperm are probably needed to achieve pregnancy rates similar to those resulting from the use of fresh (unfrozen) sperm (CECOS Federation, 1989, 757).

Since the outbreak of the epidemic of HIV infection and AIDS, authorities and professional societies in the United States and Canada, and in other countries as well, have strongly recommended that only frozen sperm be used in therapeutic insemination. Cryopreservation of sperm intended for use in therapeutic insemination allows time to test the sperm donors for presence of the human immunodeficiency virus in their bodies. The American Fertility Society's 1990 *Guidelines* for the use of donor insemination require that donor semen be kept frozen for 180 days, to allow sperm donors to be retested for the human immunodeficiency virus (HIV) and for the hepatitis B virus (Moghissi, 1990, 400). This is a reasonable and mandatory precaution, since there are reports that women have become HIV-infected from sperm donated for insemination.

In Vitro Fertilization (IVF) and Embryo Transfer (ET)

In October 1937, an unsigned editorial in *The New England Journal of Medicine* speculated about possible future "conception in a watch glass," and proclaimed what a boon successful extracorporeal fertilization of ova and reimplantation of embryos would be for infertile women (Editorial, 1937). The birth of Louise Brown in England in 1978, the first successful pregnancy leading to birth of a normal baby as a result of in vitro fertilization (IVF) and embryo transfer (ET), turned the 1937 *New England Journal* speculation into reality. Many babies, surely numbering now in the thousands, have been born after use of these methods of assisted reproduction pioneered by Doctors R.G. Edwards and Patrick Steptoe. Hundreds of clinics are now using these methods as a remedy for certain kinds of female, and even male, infertility.

The *process* of in vitro fertilization and embryo transfer is conceptually rather easy to grasp, but technically much more difficult to perform than is generally appreciated. There are basically five steps to the process: (1) stimulation of the woman's body with hormones and drugs, to assure ovulation or production of several ova or eggs, called oocytes at this stage, that are mature enough for fertilization; (2) properly timed retrieval of ova (oocytes) from the ovaries, now generally done with a small suction needle guided by ultrasound; (3) placement of the ova (oocytes) in a petri dish containing a proper nutrient fluid to sustain the ova; (4) addition of suitably prepared active sperm to the nutrient fluid containing the ova, to achieve fertilization; (5) sustenance of the fertilized ova until they have divided into the optimal number of cells (usually six to ten cells, reached about three days after petri-dish insemination) for embryo transfer and implantation within the uterus; (6) embryo transfer to the uterus.

There is disagreement about the number of early embryos that should be transferred to the uterus after IVF. Embryo transfer frequently does not lead to a pregnancy, even when a woman's ova are successfully fertilized with her husband's sperm in the laboratory. Many complex biochemical factors, even when conception is achieved by sexual intercourse, have to be properly balanced in a woman's body if an embryo is to successfully implant in the uterus. In the early 1980s, practitioners of IVF and ET noted that multiple embryo transfers increased the probability of achieving a pregnancy after IVF. In one study, John Kerin and others observed a steady increase in overall pregnancy rates as two, three, and four embryos were simultaneously transferred after IVF (Kerin, 1983, 538).

Multiple embryo transfers also increase the chances of multiple pregnancies and of twin, triplet, or quadruplet births. Sometimes, such an event turns out happily, as in the case of the Collier five, Canada's first quintuplets born after in vitro fertilization, to Wayne and Mac Collier in Toronto in 1988 (Swainson, 1993). However, multiple pregnancies, particularly three and higher, are risk-laden both for the mother and for the fetuses. It is for this reason that some have proposed freezing a woman's extra embryos, so that they can be thawed and transferred to her uterus, one at a time, in her next reproduction cycles, if a first or second attempt at embryo transfer does not result in pregnancy. The cryopreservation (freezing) of early human embryos will be discussed below.

Women whose fallopian tubes (the channels through which eggs pass from ovary to uterus) have been severely damaged or surgically removed are those who will likely benefit most from in vitro fertilization. If IVF works in these situations, it will permit a couple to have their own child. IVF, however, is now used in a number of other situations where blocked or absent fallopian tubes are not the cause of a couple's infertility. IVF is also used in some cases when a couple's inability to have a child by sexual intercourse is due to the husband's infertility.

The proliferation of IVF programmes has led to controversy about the efficacy, safety, costs, and benefits of this method of assisted reproduction (Wagner, 1989). The mandate of Canada's Royal Commission on Reproductive Technologies, chaired by Dr. Patricia Baird, covers these and other issues related to assisted reproduction. The Commission's delayed report is now said to be due in the summer of 1993.

There is still considerable uncertainty and controversy about the success rates of IVF and ET. The controversy, in part, deals with the choice of nominators and denominators used by various programmes in reporting their success with IVF. To obtain fair and realistic, as opposed to inflated and misleading, quotes of success rates of IVF, one proposal recommends using the number of maternities achieved as the nominator, and the number of women who received at least one cycle of IVF-ET treatment as the denominator, to express rates of success (Page, 1989, 338). Though live birth of normal babies is the real "bottom-line" measure of success of IVF and ET, use of the number of live births as the nominator could, because of multiple pregnancies, produce inflated and misleading quotes of success.

The bottom-line measure of success with IVF and ET varies from clinic to clinic. The most experienced clinics now have live birth success rates for IVF and ET that are not far from the estimated chance of live birth when conception is achieved through sexual intercourse (Tan, 1992). Clinics, though, have to go through a learning curve, and increasing success rates depend upon accumulated experiences, as well as upon advances in research. This variance in success rates is an important part of the information couples need to receive, if they are to consent meaningfully and freely to start the laborious, emotionally straining, and often financially costly process of in vitro fertilization and embryo transfer.

Gamete Intrafallopian Transfer (GIFT)

Gamete intrafallopian transfer, or GIFT, has been used as a treatment for certain kinds of infertility since 1984. GIFT differs from IVF and ET in the following ways. As in IVF, a woman is treated with hormones to produce superovulation (to produce several ova mature enough for fertilization) and the ova are retrieved, usually by needle aspiration under ultrasound guidance. However, unlike IVF, the retrieved ova are not fertilized with the husband's sperm *in the laboratory*. Rather, both the woman's ova and her husband's sperm are transferred to the end of the fallopian tubes, to allow fertilization of the ova to take place within the woman's body, with subsequent migration of the fertilized ovum to her uterus for implantation.

An *International Cooperative Study*, set up to use a common protocol, or set of procedures, for GIFT in ten centres in the world, reported in 1988 on the results of the first 800 cases of women who had been treated with GIFT. 499 of the women who received the GIFT procedure were from couples affected by unexplained or idiopathic infertility. Of the 800 women treated with GIFT, 201 delivered babies and 69 of these were multiple deliveries, though data were not given to indicate how many of these were twin, triplet, or quadruplet births (Asch, 1988, 724).

GIFT has also been used to treat women whose fertility has been reduced due to a previous ectopic pregnancy, a pregnancy in which the embryo implants outside the uterus, usually in the fallopian tube. One report offers data on 87 women who received 111 gamete intrafallopian transfers, as treatment for infertility due to previous ectopic pregnancy: 28 pregnancies were achieved, with 23 live births, 4 spontaneous abortions, and 1 ectopic pregnancy (Guirgis, 1992, 586). The 1990 *IVF-ET Registry* has reported a U.S. live-born delivery rate of 14% for IVF-ET and 22% for GIFT (Medical Research International, 1992, 15).

Ovum and Embryo Donation

Ovum donation is now practised fairly commonly in the treatment of infertility when a woman's ovaries are absent, either congenitally or due to surgery — for example, in cases of ovarian cancer; or when a woman is affected by ovarian failure, an inability to produce ova; or when a woman fears passing on a genetic defect to her child. Ovarian failure can occur prematurely, or naturally with the onset of menopause. Many women are menopausal, or nearly so, in the early forties. Ovum donation to enable older women to have babies has been attempted a number of times, but experience with this practice in older women is limited, and the risks for both the woman and child are not negligible (Sauer et al., 1990). The practice raises both the medical and ethical question: "How old is too old?"(Sauer et al., 1992, 1279)

In these circumstances, ova donated by another woman are fertilized with the sperm of the infertile woman's husband by the methods of IVF, and the resulting embryos are transferred to the infertile woman's uterus.

Some infertility treatment clinics favour anonymity in ovum donation, and use extra ova (oocytes) donated by couples undergoing IVF treatment. There are reports that the sisters of infertile women are often used as ovum donors in other programmes (Sauer and Paulson, 1990, 1422; Sauer et al., 1988).

One of the earliest reports of ovum donation, leading to pregnancy and birth of a healthy child, goes back to 1984 (Lutgen, 1984). In the U.S. in 1990, 498 women received 547 transfers of donated ova, from which 122 live deliveries resulted. Among these there were 36 sets of twins, 3 sets of triplets, and 1 set of quadruplets (Medical Research International, 1992, 21).

Embryo donation is contemplated in situations, less frequent than those in which ovum donation is used, when both the wife and the husband are infertile, or when the husband cannot produce sperm and the wife cannot produce ova. As we shall discuss below, couples now quite frequently request the freezing and storage (cryopreservation) of their extra embryos resulting from IVF. Donated embryos, at times, come from this cryopreserved supply; for instance, when a couple treated with IVF achieves pregnancy and live birth, and no longer needs their cryopreserved embryos. A donated embryo may also result from laboratory fertilization of a donated ovum with donated sperm. If the donated embryo is transferred to the infertile woman's uterus, the resulting child has two fathers (one biological, the other social) and two mothers (one genetic, the other being the gestational-social mother).

Both ovum and embryo donation, as we shall discuss below, raise particular kinds of ethical and legal issues (Robertson, 1988-1989).

Surrogate Mothering

The term *surrogate mothering* or *motherhood* has several meanings relating to quite different reproductive and parental relationships. These meanings and relationships need to be distinguished, to understand adequately both the procedure of surrogacy and the ethical, legal, and social issues it raises.

Some women are able to produce fertilizable ova, but they have disorders of the uterus or heart disease so severe that they could never become pregnant or carry a child to birth. When a woman is infertile due to uterine disorders, her ova can be retrieved and fertilized with her husband's sperm by IVF methods, and the resultant embryo can be transferred to the uterus of a woman willing to carry the embryo through pregnancy to birth, and then, by prior agreement, to give the baby over to the couple whose ova and sperm were united in the laboratory. In this arrangement, the woman with uterine infertility is both the *genetic* (she furnishes the ovum) and the *social* mother. *Surrogacy* is limited to *gestational surrogacy*: the "surrogate" mother is the woman who becomes pregnant and carries the baby to birth. The apparently first case of IVF gestational surrogacy was reported in 1989 (Utian, 1989).

In ovum donation, as described above, some women are quite capable of becoming pregnant and carrying a fetus to live birth, but they cannot produce normal ova or they cannot produce ova at all. When ovum donation is used in these circumstances, the woman, who is infertile due to ovarian problems, becomes pregnant after transfer of a donated ovum fertilized in the laboratory with her husband's sperm. She is the gestational and social mother. *Surrogacy* is limited to *genetic surrogacy*: the "surrogate" mother is the woman who donates the ovum.

However, the kind of "surrogate mothering" that has led to a number of court cases and to intense controversy over the last decade involves a quite different reproductive arrangement. In this arrangement, a woman, married or not, previously a mother herself or not, agrees to conceive a child by artificial insemination with sperm from a husband whose wife is infertile, to carry the embryo through pregnancy to birth, and then, in keeping with a prior agreement, to give the child over to the infertile couple after birth. In this situation, the infertile wife is only the social mother of the child. *Surrogacy* here includes both *genetic* and *gestational surrogacy*: the "surrogate" mother is the woman whose own ovum is fertilized and who carries the embryo, resulting from artificial insemination, through pregnancy to birth.

"Surrogacy" in these situations means that one woman, the surrogate, stands in for another woman with respect to one or another or at least two of a woman's reproductive or mothering functions. Is it really meaningful, however, to call a woman a "surrogate" mother when, as in the third, typical situation just described, she is, in fact, both the child's genetic and gestational mother? Is not the child biologically her very own child, and is not she biologically the child's very own mother?

It is difficult to obtain accurate, up-to-date statistics on how widely "surrogate mothering," in the third sense described above, is practised. A 1990 report on obstetrical aspects of these surrogate pregnancies mentioned that 17 surrogate-parenting programmes, many run by physician-attorney private firms, had arranged for 600 births in the U.S. as of 1987 (Reame, 1990, 1220). The Royal Commission on the Reproductive Technologies will most likely offer an update on Canadian data in its report. Countries, and provinces and states within countries, differ considerably on how surrogate mothering should be regulated, understandably so, since the practice challenges and changes the very concepts and language traditionally used in ethical and legal discussions of parenting (Macklin, 1991).

The Frozen Storage, or Cryopreservation, of Human Embryos

In 1983, Alan O. Trounson and Linda Mohr reported from Australia that a pregnancy had been achieved, after thawing and transfer of an embryo that had been frozen at the eight-cell stage and preserved in liquid nitrogen for four months. They reported that there appeared to be no abnormality of the fetus at week 24 that could be associated with the freezing, storing, and thawing procedure (Trounson, 1983, 709). This particular pregnancy, however, ended in spontaneous abortion at twenty-four weeks, due to infection. The use of cryopreserved embryos in the treatment of infertility has increased considerably over the last decade. The *IVF-ET Registry*, for example, reports that there were 3,290 frozen-embryo transfers performed in 129 clinics in the U.S. in 1990. These transfers of frozen-thawed embryos resulted in 382 clinically verifiable pregnancies and in the delivery of 291 babies, including 45 sets of twins and 5 sets of triplets (Medical Research International, 1992, 21).

There are three main reasons proposed in favour of the frozen storage of human embryos. First, this offers a way to save excess embryos created by the in vitro fertilization process. Second, use of frozen and thawed human embryos would enable a woman to have a second or third try at pregnancy without undergoing the ova retrieval process, if her first embryo transfer after IVF did not lead to pregnancy. Third, frozen storage of embryos would render possible pretransfer genetic diagnosis of embryos, when couples carry a risk of transmitting genetic defects to their children. Embryos found, after genetic diagnosis, to be free of defective genes could then be thawed and transferred for pregnancy.

Though clinics around the world are now keeping a considerable number of human embryos in frozen storage and are frequently using frozen-thawed embryos to initiate pregnancies, there is still much to learn to perfect the freezing-thawing process. Moreover, as we shall discuss later in this chapter, the status of the frozen-stored human embryo poses major legal, social, and ethical issues.

Sex Selection

In 1974, an editorial in the *Lancet*, a British medical journal, referred to two techniques indicating that predetermination of sex of offspring, through artificial insemination with a sample of sperm containing only, or primarily, X- or Y-chromosome-bearing sperm, might be possible in the near future (Editorial, 1974). Methods have not yet been devised that can reliably and consistently separate X- from Y-chromosome-bearing sperm, so that use of artificial insemination with such sperm could be used to guarantee a couple a boy or girl.

However, a different approach to preimplantation determination of sex, announced in the spring of 1990, is now being used in connection with in vitro fertilization. A team of doctors at Hammersmith Hospital in London determined the future sex of an embryo by analyzing just one cell from the cluster of cells that form the three-day old embryo after in vitro fertilization (Handyside, 1990). One of the women undergoing embryo transfer of embryos selected for female sex was doing this to avoid having boys with Duchenne's muscular dystrophy, a crippling, genetically based disease that is fatal early in a boy's life. This woman had already suffered through the deaths of three of her brothers who had been affected by this disorder. We shall discuss preimplantation diagnosis in greater detail in the following chapter.

ETHICAL EVALUATION OF THE REPRODUCTIVE TECHNOLOGIES

Innovations in reproductive biology and medicine, the methods of assisted reproduction deriving from these advances, and the novel reproductive arrangements that the new reproductive technologies render possible set the stage for change in traditional reproductive behaviour. Some of these changes are, in nearly everyone's opinion, *ethically quite prosaic* when use of a particular technology buttresses, without transforming, the long-standing values and patterns of reproduction, marriage, and family. Such would seem to be the case when a wife is therapeutically (or artificially) inseminated with her husband's sperm. Other applications of the reproductive technologies introduce quite *dramatic* changes into reproductive behaviour, *ethically dramatic*, in the sense that the changes are really quite profound transformations of the relationships and roles traditionally played by people in the drama of reproduction; *ethically dramatic*, also, because these changes illustrate radical shifts in people's judgments about what is really important in reproduction.

How, then, are the reproductive technologies, and the various uses made of them, to be ethically evaluated? We centre attention in this section and in this chapter on the quite different approaches people have taken to support the positions they have adopted on these technologies, or on specific applications made of them. People will arrive at quite different, and even contradictory, conclusions, depending on what assumptions, perceptions, beliefs, values, and principles they are considering and emphasizing; depending also on the methods they use to demonstrate or verify that the values and principles they are defending are, in fact, protected and honoured, or threatened and violated by innovations in human reproduction.

Because a detailed discussion of the myriad issues of clinical and research ethics in human reproduction, as related to each of the technologies, would require a book, we organize our consideration here around the ways people have evaluated the reproductive technologies, in their responses to *questions* centring on how these technologies relate to: the integrity of the human person; the development and welfare of children; the institutions of parenthood, marriage, and family; the freedom and respect of women; and the just distribution of power and control over human reproduction.

The Integrity of the Human Person

Do the reproductive technologies preserve and promote, or do they threaten and diminish, the integrity of the human person?

The report, *Artificial Human Insemination* (1948), of a commission appointed by the Archbishop of Canterbury in 1945, and cited in a Canadian publication in 1977, considered therapeutic artificial insemination with donor semen to be a high point in the depersonalization of human sexuality. Why? Because this technique achieved procreation, conception of a child, outside the context of human relationships (Creighton, 1977, 8). A Roman Catholic textbook, written about the same time as the Canadian Anglican study, emphasizes the same reasoning in its moral rejection of therapeutic insemination with donor sperm: the technique completely dissociates procreation from conjugal love, from a wife's and a husband's expression of mutual love in sexual intercourse (Lobo, 1975, 149).

If therapeutic donor insemination, in fact, depersonalized and dehumanized sexuality, it would constitute a serious affront to the integrity of the human person and to the true and integral good of human beings. This criterion of integrity is central in two influential reports on the reproductive technologies, published in the 1980s. Both The American Fertility Society's *Ethical Considerations* and the Roman Catholic Congregation for the Doctrine of the Faith's *Instruction* refer, on somewhat different terms, to the integrity of the human person as the fundamental criterion for ethically evaluating the reproductive technologies. The American Fertility Society states that "the human person integrally and adequately considered" is the criterion of evaluation. That criterion includes the sum of the dimensions of the person that constitute human well-being, such as bodily health, intellectual and spiritual well-being, the freedom to form one's own convictions on moral and religious matters, and social well-being in all its forms (Ethics Committee, 1990, 1S). The Roman Catholic Congregation proposes that science and technology "must be at the service of the human person, of his inalienable rights and his true and integral good according to the design and will of God." This is a matter of unconditional respect for the fundamental criteria of the moral law (Congregation, 1987, 12).

The American Fertility Society and the Roman Catholic Congregation apparently agree on the fundamental criterion, "the integrity of the human person and the human good," according to which the reproductive technologies should be evaluated, yet each arrives at radically different and opposed ethical evaluations. The Roman Catholic Congregation rejects therapeutic insemination with a husband's sperm, and in vitro fertilization even when a husband's sperm and a wife's ova are used. The American Fertility Society found both TIH and IVF utilizing a husband's sperm and a wife's ova to be ethically acceptable.

How could these two groups differ so radically on what are generally considered to be the ethically most simple and uncontroversial applications of the reproductive technologies, as they will be seen to differ also on other applications of these technologies? This difference is due, in great part, to their profound difference regarding *how to judge whether the reproductive technologies respect or measure up to the criterion* of integrity.

The American Fertility Society's method is *inductive* and *experiential*. The *Ethical Considerations* report explicitly states that verification of whether the reproductive technologies match up to the fundamental criterion requires:

- an inductive approach based on experience and reflection;

- recognition that some things so offend an inner sense of what is proper and sacred that no experience is necessary to reveal their moral character;

- experience of the comprehensive impact on persons as essential to judge the morality of many human actions;

- openness, caution, and a willingness to revise evaluations; the basic willingness to say "no" where we have said "yes," and "yes" where we have said "no." (Ethics Committee, 1990, 1S).

The Roman Catholic Congregation's method is *deductive* and *authoritative*. The *Instruction*'s method is one of "rational reflection on the fundamental values of life and of human procreation." (Congregation, 1987, 15) Rational reflection, here, is not on experience, but on Church interpretations of what the design of God and the natural moral law have shown the integral human good to be. The *Instruction*'s *assumption* is that what constitutes integrity of the human person and of human reproduction is *already known*. That knowledge is expressed in official Church teaching, so that, in comparing the reproductive technologies to that teaching, one can deduce whether or not they match up to the fundamental criterion.

The *Instruction* finds that TIH and IVF do not match up to the demands of personal integrity and of reproductive integrity, because these techniques separate conception of a child from a couple's expression of married love in sexual intercourse. Procreation, separated from the sexual expression of married or conjugal love, violates an integrity that the *Instruction*, basing itself on Church teaching, sees as consisting of an inseparable connection between two meanings of the conjugal act: the unitive meaning (furthering union of wife and husband) and the procreative meaning (Congregation, 1987, 35-36).

No other major commission or working group in the world has been able ethically to reject TIH and IVF on this basis. If TIH and IVF, in the *Instruction*'s terms, deprive procreation of its proper perfection because of the above-mentioned separation, the *Ethical Considerations* report failed to see why an act "deprived of its proper perfection" is for that very reason immoral, particularly when the "deprivation of perfection" is no fault of the spouses involved. Most people would affirm, along with the *Instruction*, that a child should be conceived as a fruit of parental love. But the American Fertility Society, and many other groups and individuals, fail to understand why "conceived as a fruit of parental love" has to mean conceived as a result of the parents' act of sexual intercourse.

The Good of the Child?

Do the reproductive technologies promote, or do they endanger, the good of children and their healthy development?

In the past, the focus of concern on this question was on artificial or therapeutic insemination with donor semen, but the concern now centres on the use of donated ova and embryos, and especially on surrogate mothering. Will the separation of genetic, gestational, and social mothering, and the fulfilment of these by two or three different women, necessarily or generally endanger the harmonious development of a child? There seems to be no evidence that couples who turn to therapeutic insemination with donor semen offer any less a congenial family environment for the healthy development of a child than do couples who have conceived their children through sexual intercourse. But will this also hold true for ovum and embryo donation, for surrogate mothering, for uses of the reproductive technologies to found nontraditional families? Is it possible, prior to acquiring the evidence of real experience, reliably to predict that children conceived by these applications of the reproductive technologies, and born into these multiple-parent arrangements, will generally suffer, and suffer serious harm to their normal development?

Some have asked: if an infertile couple wants a child so desperately that they turn to such "bizarre" methods as ovum or embryo donation or surrogate mothering, are they not too desperate about their own desires and needs, are they not too selfish ever to exercise genuine concern and care for the child? The question may be fair, but it is only fair to admit that the same question applies equally well to couples who become parents in the traditional ways. Would this not suggest that responsible parenting and the harmonious development of a child depend more on the characters of the parents involved than on the ways parenthood is achieved? Parenthood also has a history. Couples may be initially very dominated by their *desire* for a child, but they usually grow, when changed, comforted, and challenged by the presence of a new human being, to serve genuinely the desires and needs of their children. One need not and should not demand a higher degree of pure altruism of an infertile couple using nontraditional reproductive methods than one would of couples conceiving by sexual intercourse.

The relationship of parents to a child is said to be *symmetrical* when each parent has both a genetic and social relationship to the child. Otherwise, the relationship is said to be *asymmetrical*. Asymmetry of relationship to the child, in TID, in ovum and embryo donation, and in surrogate mothering could adversely affect parenting and the harmonious development of the children, if the social fathers in TID, or the social mothers in the cases of gestational surrogacy or genetic-gestational surrogacy, find it impossible to come to terms with their infertility, if they fail also in their ability lovingly to embrace a child who is not biologically their very own.

Western societies have had a considerable length of experience with TID. That experience has failed to deliver evidence to support suspicions expressed, from time to time, that infertile fathers generally find it most difficult to consider, treat, and love as their own, children who have genetically come from the wife and the sperm donor. It is probably reasonable to expect that the experience of infertile women will be similar, when infertile couples turn to ovum or embryo donation, or to surrogate mothering. However, some experiences with surrogate mothering, as we shall note below, do justify concern about the good of children conceived and born in surrogate arrangements, and direct attention to other risks, as well.

This way of looking at the reproductive technologies does not imply that the use of donor gametes (sperm or ova) or surrogate arrangements is for everyone. The key idea is that it is impossible, prior to the accumulation of actual experience, to generalize one way or the other about what the experience of an infertile couple, and what the impact of that experience on the child's development, will be. Asymmetry of the husband-wife or the social mother-father relationship to the child is not a sufficiently solid and general basis for ethical rejection of therapeutic donor insemination, ovum and embryo donation, or various forms of surrogate mothering. These techniques do separate a child's genetic and social identities. Both the Roman Catholic *Instruction* and the American Fertility Society *Ethical Considerations*, the latter particularly with regard to surrogate mothering, identify this separation as a significant concern. Will children be seriously or permanently harmed, psychologically and socially, and will their own future parenthood be harmed by the truth, however long it is kept secret, that one or both of their parents are not their "real," or genetic, or biological parents?

This question should not be brushed aside as mirroring little more than the fears peculiar to primitive thinking. Twenty years ago, in a symposium on artificial insemination and embryo transfer, Dr. Massimo Piatelli-Palmarini emphasized the need to be concerned about "the collapsing of the historical and biological web which constitutes the human person."(Piatelli-Palmarini, 1973, 24) He emphasized, in the sex-specific language of that time, a very important consideration that may, in the general excitement, euphoria, or controversy about the reproductive technologies, be easily forgotten, namely: "The whole concept of a person and his existential 'feeling-in-the-world' depend as much on the history of how he came into being and on awareness of all the bonds linking him with nature and his fellow men as it does on his having a healthy body and a well-balanced mind."(Piatelli-Palmarini, 1973, 21)

These bonds linking a child with nature and history are not insignificant. One's genetic history links one to a network of persons. Grandparents, great-grandparents, and the collateral relationships of uncles, aunts, cousins, are integral strands in the pattern of human connections essential to one's sense of personal identity. One may experience a very shallow sense of identity, if one's social identity rests upon no identifiable underlying grid or network of connections to one's genetic ancestors and relations. Some adopted children, it would appear, are deeply marked by the separation of their social from their genetic identities. Children born from reproductive arrangements using donated gametes, or in surrogacy arrangements, may be similarly marked. However, one may justifiably ask whether these children will, in the future, suffer more, as some have suffered in the past, from being deceived about their origins than from the separation of their genetic and social identities.

In some countries, through not in Canada, single and lesbian women can now obtain donor sperm from commercial sperm banks, to artificially inseminate themselves without medical assistance. Women are now challenging, as we shall discuss below, the medicalization of the reproductive technologies and, in particular, of artificial therapeutic insemination. There are sperm banks, at least in the United States, that are controlled by women. One such institution, the Northern California Sperm Bank in Oakland, provides semen to single, as well as married, women, and does not have sexual orientation or sexual preference restrictions. There seems to be considerable evidence that self-insemination is quite widely used by single women and by lesbian women to have children (Wikler, 1991).

The rise of nontraditional families — of families consisting of gay men with children or of lesbian women with children, and in particular of families that are designed to be either fatherless or motherless — challenges ethical evaluation of the reproductive technologies, perhaps more intensely than do other applications of assisted reproduction, to strike a balance between the good of children and the rights of persons to be protected against unjust discrimination in matters of parenthood and the founding of a family. This evaluation is still in evolution (Case Conference, 1978; Hanscombe, 1983; St. Clair Stephenson, 1991).

The Good of Women?

Ethical evaluations of the reproductive technologies have tended to focus on a wide range of front-line, first-order issues, dealing with the many possible combinations of sperm and ova from different sources that can be attempted to conceive a child. There are concerns with the novel ethical, legal, and social complexities that occur when the various biological and social functions of parenthood are separated and assumed by several people, and with the conditions under which untraditional reproductive arrangements and innovative research on the embryo can be accepted within existing or modified frameworks of policy and law. These issues have been grouped into twenty-five categories, and one study has tabulated the varying responses of ten major commissions or working groups to each (Walters, 1988).

In this section we take a different direction, and return to this chapter's opening statements about power and control over reproduction. Evidently, that power has increased enormously, and has had a major impact on the lives of men, women, and children in this century. Moreover, women are absolutely at the centre of every social experiment undertaken with the reproductive technologies. But are they there as subjects, or as objects of control? How do *women* interpret and evaluate the impact of the reproductive technologies on their lives, on the lives of children, and on the institutions of parenthood and family? Answers to these questions are essential in any ethical evaluation that would pretend to be objective, fair, and comprehensive.

Feminist thinkers have not been alone, though many have been prime leaders, in directing ethical reflection to the issue of power, and in adopting an ethically critical perspective on the reproductive technologies (Overall, 1987; Overall, 1989; Sherwin, 1992). While few feminist evaluations would reject assisted reproduction outright, the leaders in feminist analysis exercise the critical ethical task of directing people to reflect on the hidden, subtle, and unexamined assumptions that dominate sexuality and reproduction, and that shape the goals of the reproductive technologies and the ways in which these are being used. That reflection challenges any ethical evaluation of the reproductive technologies to consider the presence of male dominance, of oppression, of exploitation, of discrimination, and of racism that can be detected when reproduction, the activity upon which the entire future of society depends, has to be medically and technologically managed and controlled (Sherwin, 1992).

Have women been unfairly, unknowingly, and unnecessarily experimented upon during the preceding twenty years or so of pressured, if not feverish, attempts to push to the frontiers, to explore the entire space of possibilities, of technology in assisted reproduction? A balanced answer would require research far exceeding this chapter and book, but there are good reasons to raise the question, if only to stimulate the conduct of such research.

Research on women to develop treatments for infertility due to fallopian-tube defects reaches back to the last century, as do the first attempts to fertilize the ova of rabbits and guinea pigs in the laboratory. Work on fertilizing human ova in the laboratory intensified in the late 1960s and 1970s and, as already noted, the first baby conceived by IVF methods was born in 1978. A great deal of experimentation has been conducted on women, prior to that birth and since then. Is there any substance to the charge that much of this experimentation was undertaken on women without prior research, for example, on primates?(Sherwin, 1992, 128). Have women been used as guinea pigs in the development of the reproductive technologies?

In considering these questions, one may be given pause for thought in reading a report on the use of IVF and ET in nonhuman primates. It was only recently that the first rhesus monkey twins were born, following IVF and ET. The report announces that *now* (early 1990s), primate models are available for studies that cannot be conducted on women for ethical and practical reasons (Wolf, 1990, 261). Has the ethical order of experimentation been reversed, with experimentation on women preceding that on primates, in perfecting the reproductive technologies? Whether women have been used as guinea pigs, and whether their consent to the reproductive research under-taken upon them over the last two decades has been informed, comprehend-ing, and voluntary are two necessary and justifiable questions (Testart, 1990; Pfeffer, 1991).

Have women been subjects, or primarily objects, of control, and of manip-ulation, in the development and use of the reproductive technologies? Physicians, it has been charged, have tended to treat women as passive bodies to be subjected to medical manipulations: professional attention has focused on the technology, rather than on women (Sherwin, 1992, 128). It is difficult to escape the impression that physicians have attended very little to the good of women when they have implanted multiple embryos, at times as many as eight to ten, in their single-minded commitment to achieve pregnancies and births. The risks and rigours of carrying multiple pregnancies, and the pressures of rais-ing triplets, quadruplets, or quintuplets have been just too much for some women, both physically and psychologically. Some women, after suffering through the years of infertility, and after undergoing all the stressful IVF and ET procedures, have then been forced to face the tearing choice of fetal reduction, of aborting one, two, or three of the fetuses they conceived with technology's assistance (Gemmette, 1991).

Do efforts to extend pregnancy beyond the age of 50 really serve the good of women or, rather, the drive by all means available to surpass the limits of nature? Three (male) physicians have recently shown that the uteri of women between 50 and 54 years of age can be suitably prepared, with a regimen of steroids, to achieve implantation of embryos resulting from in vitro fertilization of donated ova, and to sustain pregnancy up to birth of a child. A recent report gives data on 9 pregnancies established in 14 women over 50 years of age. At the time of publication of the report, 2 of 3 deliveries had been by caesarean section; 4 pregnancies were continuing. Though admitting that the psycholo-gical effect of giving birth beyond age 50 is unknown, the physicians involved believe that this new technology will be unlikely to "have a serious influence on the fabric of society, other than to open new doors and possibilities to some people." (Sauer et al., 1993, 323)

A number of physicians involved in the treatment of infertility have asked whether they are exploiting couples (Blackwell, 1987). Equally justifiable is the question as to whether socially and economically disadvantaged women are being exploited; for example, in the context of surrogate mothering. Most eco-nomically disadvantaged women, often from racial minorities, could never afford the costs of IVF for the treatment of their infertility. However, relatively affluent infertile couples have turned to economically disadvantaged fertile women for surrogacy services. Is a black single mother of a three-year old girl, a mother who has already had two prior miscarriages and two stillbirths, being favoured or exploited when a couple (the wife, Filipino, the husband, Caucasian) offers her $10,000 to be a surrogate mother for them? An isolated case? A study of forty-four cases of surrogate pregnancy found that women from low socioeconomic groups were most likely to consider and undertake a surrogate pregnancy, at least during the early 1980s. Financial compensation for surrogacy services seems to attract the most disadvantaged groups of women (Reame, 1990, 1222).

A number of feminist thinkers, and others as well, would probably endorse the claim that the contribution of the reproductive technologies to the general autonomy of women seems to be largely negative (Sherwin, 1992, 134). This claim, in the light of the few and selected observations of this section, merits serious considerations.

SURROGATE MOTHERING: CONDITIONAL, PROVISIONAL, AND MONITORED ETHICAL TOLERATION?

Refusal to reject outright a reproductive practice is not equivalent to whole-hearted and unqualified acceptance. Surrogate motherhood offers an example of provisional, conditional, and monitored ethical toleration of a reproductive arrangement. The particular arrangement under consideration here uses only the technology of artificial insemination, and the surrogate mother is both genetic and gestational mother of the child. This particular form of surrogate mothering, though quite common in the mid-1980s, is now in decline in Canada and the United States, in part because some of the concerns expressed below proved to occur altogether too painfully in real life.

Concerns and Reservations

Any thinking person should have concerns about surrogate mothering. Though this reproductive arrangement has worked harmoniously for some, it has been the occasion of intense personal and emotional suffering for others. This practice demonstrates a profound *ambiguity*, requiring an ethical evaluation based upon experience of the comprehensive impact of this practice on all persons involved. Though the social experiment of surrogate motherhood is not yet completed, enough evidence has accumulated to indicate that the following concerns, identified by many observers over the past few years, are not theoretical, but very likely to become reality for some who try the experiment:

- Some women who have offered to be surrogate mothers have passed through a period of grief and mourning after giving up the child to the commissioning couple. A single woman about to enter pregnancy for the first time, and indeed, as a surrogate mother, may well come to experience new emotions she has never had before, emotions of strong attachment to her child. She is not protected by corporeal and temporal distance, as is the sperm donor in artificial insemination, from potential strong involvement with the child. The pain of separation, if she honours the surrogate agreement, may be intense.

- Moreover, a surrogate mother, depending on her socioeconomic circumstances, could be commercially seduced to do for money what normally brings fulfilment only when it is done for love, for oneself, for one's loved spouse, and for one's own family. Exploitation of poor women is a real danger in surrogate mothering, as we have already noted above in the section on power, control, and the good of women.

- The babies born in a surrogate-motherhood arrangement may be harmed in a number of ways. Perhaps the most tragic happening is when such a baby is born with handicaps, and is rejected by both the surrogate and the commissioning couple. Payment of large sums of money for the surrogate service may well motivate parents to look upon a handicapped infant as "damaged goods."

- The commissioning couple may well be harmed emotionally and financially if the surrogate mother refuses to give the child over to them after birth. Their social life may be disrupted by months of wrangling before the courts, and the outcome of a judicial process in this matter is never certain. The legal status of surrogate motherhood is still uncertain in many jurisdictions.

- For all practical purposes, a child born in a surrogate-motherhood arrangement will be intentionally barred from socially realizing bonds to his or her genetic-gestational mother and to her extended family. Some adopted children suffer deeply over the split between their genetic and social identities. Surrogate-mothered children may also experience similar suffering.

These are only a few of the concerns identified by many working groups in their reflection on surrogate motherhood.

Conditional and Monitored Ethical Toleration

The American Fertility Society report represents the position of provisional, conditional, and monitored ethical toleration of surrogate-motherhood arrangements. The Ethics Committee did not find sufficient reasons to recommend legal prohibition of surrogate-motherhood arrangements. It recommended, however, that this practice be considered experimental and be kept under intense scrutiny. That scrutiny should take the form of methodologically sound research on a range of factors that will deliver empirical evidence to gauge the effect of this practice on all persons involved.

The Ethics Committee identifies some of the conditions for ethically tolerating the practice, conditions such as:

- informed, comprehending, and voluntary consent of all persons involved is essential;
- surrogate motherhood should only be undertaken for medical reasons, not for the simple convenience of the commissioning woman;
- the surrogate mother and the sperm donor husband of the commissioning couple should be screened for infectious diseases and the surrogate mother should be screened for genetic defects;
- surrogate mothers should not receive payment for the surrogacy service, only financial compensation for expenses and inconvenience (Ethics Committee, 1990, 67S).

The American Fertility Society's emphasis on intense scrutiny and research implies that the accumulated evidence may, in the future, necessitate saying "no" where the *Ethical Considerations* once said a very reserved "yes."

An Unconditional No

The U.K. *Report of the Committee of Inquiry into Human Fertilization and Embryology*, more commonly known as the Warnock Committee because it was chaired by Dame Mary Warnock, said "no" to surrogate motherhood in its report. The "no" was unconditional.

The Warnock Committee recommended legislation to render criminal the creation or the operation in the United Kingdom of agencies whose purposes include the recruitment of women for surrogate pregnancy, or making arrangements for individuals or couples who wish to utilize the services of a carrying mother. The Committee also recommended provision by legal statute that all surrogacy agreements are illegal contracts and, therefore, unenforceable in the courts (Warnock, 1984, 47).

Regulation Rather Than Prohibition

The Ontario Law Reform Commission has proposed legislation to regulate, rather than to prohibit, surrogate-motherhood arrangements. It has outlined a regulatory scheme in thirty-two proposals. The starting point of this scheme is required approvals by the Provincial Court (Family Division), or by the Unified Family Court, of any proposed surrogate-motherhood arrangement (Ontario Law Reform Commission, 1985).

RESEARCH ON THE HUMAN EMBRYO

Research on and with the human embryo was impossible, as long as fertilization took place exclusively within the woman's body. Today, in vitro fertilization procedures may produce more embryos than needed to treat the donors' infertility, or these procedures may be used to fashion embryos explicitly for research.

A wide range of research projects, considered by a number of scientists to be highly important both for basic science and for the eventual prevention and cure of disease, would require the study of the human embryo in ways that would disrupt its normal course of development, render the embryo unfit for implantation, or entail the embryo's destruction. Though the question of the moral status of the human embryo arises in the setting of laboratory fertilization and embryo transfer for the treatment of infertility, the ethical issue about the degree of respect and protection due to the human embryo is most acute in the setting of research.

Categories of Possible Human Embryo Research

Several years ago, the Royal Society of England outlined the kinds of research that would necessitate experimental work on the human embryo. Most, if not all, of the research to be outlined below could not be successfully undertaken on animal embryos, since the human embryo is dramatically different in many ways from the embryos of other mammalian species, the primates included. Because of these differences, one could not simply do the research envisaged below on animal embryos, and then assert that the results obtained are also true of human embryos. Some kinds of research have to be done with the human embryo, or not done at all.

The *first category* covers research directly relevant to the improvement of in vitro fertilization and embryo transfer. Why do so many embryos created by laboratory fertilization fail to implant in the uterus? Is this failure due to the medium in which the embryos are maintained prior to transfer? Is the failure due to the timing of the transfer? Do these embryos undergo growth abnormalities, while maintained in the laboratory prior to culture? These and other questions dealing, for example, with frozen storage of embryos cannot be answered without research on the human embryo.

A *second category* of research would focus on advancing scientific understanding of the causes of infertility and of the problem of inherited genetic disease. Why is it that human sperm fails to penetrate and fertilize the human ovum? In vitro fertilization procedures could be used to elucidate this aspect of infertility. Another direction of research would involve embryo biopsy (removal of a few cells from the embryo), to develop the technology for preimplantation genetic diagnosis of the embryo.

The *third category* would comprise studies in basic research that could have long-range scientific significance. These studies could focus on advancing understanding about: the development of the embryo, how genes are expressed in the early embryo; the possibility of developing specific body tissues from the culture of embryonic stem cells, this with a view to eventual transplantation; the role of viruses and chemicals in the causation of congenital malformations; and the possibility of developing techniques for genetic manipulation of early embryos (Royal Society, 1983, 5-9).

The kinds of experimental manipulations involved in these research projects could range from simple observation to manipulation of the embryo, including: developing part of the embryo in culture; dividing the embryo; forming hybrids and chimeras by interspecies fertilization or intraspecies fusion of embryos; inserting genes or chromosomes into the embryo; transplanting the cell nucleus; freezing and thawing the embryo; and treating the embryo with various kinds of agents.

At the inauguration of the Center for Bioethics of the Clinical Research Institute of Montréal in 1976, René Dubos, one of the great scientists of this century, spoke of the responsibility a human being experiences when the moment comes to interfere with the natural order of things, and especially when the moment comes to intervene in the determinisms of life. This is what research on the human embryo is, really: an intervention into, possibly an interference with, human life in its beginnings. Whether such research should be undertaken is inescapably an ethical question. It must not be answered only by a small group of people, regardless of whether they are scientists or representatives of any other discipline.

Is Research on the Human Embryo Acceptable in Principle?

The argument will be developed, in the chapter on research ethics, that it is both scientifically and ethically necessary to validate the safety and efficacy of new therapies. In a similar vein, the Anglican Archbishop of York in England has argued that it is immoral not to conduct research on the new reproductive technologies, if we continue to use these technologies: imperfect techniques without a backing in research are bad practice medically and wrong morally (U.K. Hansard, 1989). However, much of this needed research will have to be carried out with and on the human embryo, or not at all.

Discussion about the ethical acceptability of conducting research on the early human embryo turns, in part though not exclusively, around the issue of whether the early human embryo is biologically and morally an individual human being. The Roman Catholic *Instruction* affirms the moral statement that a human being must be respected as a person from the first moment of his or her existence (Congregation, 1987, 17). The debate here is about when individual existence as a human being really begins.

The *Instruction* asserts that recent findings of biological science indicate that the zygote resulting from fertilization has the biological identity of a new human individual, so that a unique and individual human being exists once the fertilization process is completed. However, quite to the contrary, the findings of biological science cast serious doubt on the assertion that the fertilized ovum or zygote is biologically an individual organism. While the cells, after fertilization, each contain a unique and new genome, individuation of these cells into a single unique organism occurs later in the development of the early embryo.

A number of scientists and commissions distinguish between the *early embryo* and the *definite embryo*, and the similar distinction between the *preembryo* and the *embryo* is now regularly made, to account for scientific facts and to guide policy on research with human life in its earliest stages of development. During the first two weeks of development after fertilization, most of the dividing cells deriving from the fertilized ovum are destined to form tissues and membranes, such as the placenta, that will provide supporting and nourishing connections of the future embryo to the mother. Towards the end of this preembryonic phase of development, up to 99% of the cells coming from the fertilized ovum are destined to form these extraembryonic tissues, and only a small group of cells deriving from the fertilized ovum will go on to form the embryo that will develop into the fetus and the baby. It happens often enough that no embryo at all forms from the preembryonic cells, or that twin embryos emerge from these cells (Royal Society, 1983, 3; McLaren, 1989, 470). The "primitive streak" is a longitudinal band of cells, forming from the preembryonic cells about 13 to 16 days after fertilization. This is the latest stage at which twinning can take place, and the formation of the primitive streak marks the emergence of an individual embryo (McLaren, 1986, 11).

Individuals are differentiated one from another if it is impossible to combine two to produce a third, or to divide one to make two individuals of a kind. On this understanding, the early embryo cannot yet be an individual organism, because division of these early cells can and does produce identical twins. If one group of human cells can, and does at times, split within the first 14 days after fertilization to form two individuals, then it is difficult to argue that this group of cells was one human individual prior to the split.

A different phenomenon, the converse of twinning in humans, is perhaps even more significant as an indicator of *delayed individuation* in human embryological development. The reference here is to "six case studies in which multiple zygotic origin seems incontrovertible" for six cases of human *whole-body-chimerism* (Bernirscke, 1969, 41; Myre, 1965).

A spontaneous human *whole-body-chimera* arises when the groups of cells resulting from more than one fertilization combine within the mother's body to form one individual. The coexistence within one individual of both XX and XY chromosomes, of two different populations of red blood cells, of two different tissue types, and the presence of heterochromia (different colours) of the eyes are criteria for human whole-body-chimerism. If two early human embryos can fuse within the first days of development to form one individual human being, *it is difficult to argue that these early embryos are individual human beings* prior to the fusion.

This discussion of *biological individuality* is morally highly significant, since we generally assume that the wrongfulness of killing or injuring is due to the fact that it is human individuals, all morally equal, who are killed or harmed. But the individual status of the early human embryo is seriously doubtful. There is also a long history of expressions of this doubt within the Roman Catholic tradition (Tauer, 1984). This doubt has motivated Karl Rahner, one of the leading theologians of that tradition, to state: "The reasons in favour of experimenting might carry more weight, considered rationally, than the uncertain rights of a human being whose very existence is in doubt." (Rahner, 1972, 236)

Human Embryo Research: Conditional Acceptance

Most who hold that research on the human embryo is acceptable in principle do not propose that such research is acceptable under any and all circumstances. Among others, the following conditions have been mentioned.

The *first* condition regards the acceptability of the goal of research. Research directed towards a procedure that would be immoral or impermissible is itself immoral and impermissible (Law Society, 1983, 5).

A *second* condition is that research should be for clinical or therapeutic purposes. This is required by a number of groups.

A *third* condition is that the research be for important scientific purposes. Some take the position that research on the human embryo is ethically acceptable only if undertaken to obtain important scientific knowledge that cannot be won by research on embryos of any other species.

A *fourth* condition centres on consent. Only those embryonic cells may be used that have come from men and women who have been adequately informed, who comprehend the nature and objectives of the research, and who approve of the research.

Some groups insist on a *fifth* condition, namely, that research on the early human embryo is acceptable only if it is done with spare embryos, and not with embryos constructed specifically for research purposes.

A *last* condition to be mentioned here is a *condition of time*. Many groups have stipulated that no early human embryo should be subjected to research beyond the period after fertilization that corresponds to the end of the implantation period, or to the stage, already mentioned, at which the primitive streak is formed. This last condition, then, would limit research on the early human embryo to the period of 14 to 17 days after fertilization.

Some believe this 14-day limit to be arbitrary. Others believe there are good reasons for setting this limit. Ann McLaren has summarized the argument in its favour:

> This 14-day limit was chosen advisedly. It is early enough to antedate the development of the embryo itself, as opposed to that of the extraembryonic membranes, so is well before even the beginnings of a heart, nervous system or other organs; it is late enough to allow the type of research that led to the development of IVF as a therapeutic procedure, and that is now required to improve the procedure; and it corresponds to an important landmark in embryological development, namely the appearance of the primitive streak. (McLaren, 1989, 469)

THE REPRODUCTIVE TECHNOLOGIES IN CANADIAN LAW

Canadian law on the reproductive technologies is difficult to state in any comprehensive way, because it exists at a provincial and territorial level in written legislation of the twelve jurisdictions, and in declarations of law made by courts on the particular facts of individual cases. A general statement of background legal principles can be proposed, however, that indicates the approach the law tends to take to the technologies in question. Criminal law, which is of federal origin, is rarely implicated in reproductive matters. Legal issues tend to centre on the acquisition and use of gametes, what prospects patients have of achieving legal recognition of childbirth, and what protective duties professionals bear to patients, children resulting from treatments, and others (Combined Ethics Committee, 1990).

Therapeutic Donor Insemination

The law accommodates therapeutic donor insemination reasonably well, particularly when the woman is married. Tenacious legal presumptions show that a husband is father of his wife's child, and sperm donors may rely with great (but not complete) confidence on not being considered in law to be fathers of children born of TDI. They will have neither maintenance responsibilities nor access rights concerning their biological offspring. Declining to preserve records of donors' identities would be ill-advised, however, because in an exceptional case, it may be necessary to trace the biological parent of a child, or the children of a parent. Further, the law may, in time, recognize that children are entitled to genetic information of their parentage. The law requires that sperm donors be adequately screened for risk of transmission of harmful genetic and other conditions, such as HIV infection. Sperm donors are distinguishable, however, from men whose sperm are applied to specific women, such as wives or "surrogate mothers," and who intend to act as fathers to the resultant children.

Selection of Recipients of Therapeutic Donor Insemination and Discrimination

The rendering of TDI services to unmarried women is governed by provincial law and standards of professional conduct, and provincial health plans determine whether this is covered as a "medically necessary service." Single women usually cannot be rejected on the sole ground that they are unmarried. Provincial human rights legislation often prohibits discrimination on grounds of marital status and, in several provinces, sexual orientation. In each case, the matter turns, not on marital status, but on the potential of a couple or single woman to offer a child an adequate nurturing environment.

Ovum and Embryo Donation

Practices and principles applicable to sperm donors are applicable in principle to egg donors. Properly informed consent must be acquired before a woman acts as a donor. When another woman becomes pregnant or gives birth following donation, the donor may not be considered in law to be the mother. Historically, motherhood was evidenced by gestation and delivery of a child, and the presumption that a woman who carries a child is its mother is likely to endure. The presumption may be rebutted, however, in cases of ovum or embryo transfer when the carrying mother intends not to rear the child, but the genetic mother intends also to be the child's social or psychological parent after birth. A Canadian court has approved the birth registration of children gestated by a surrogate mother, showing the name of the genetic/social parent as mother, when the surrogate mother voluntarily surrendered the children on birth.

Cryopreserved Embryos

Control of gametes or preembryos in vitro or in cryopreservation is likely to be governed by the arrangements made between the human sources and the agencies storing the gametes or preembryos. If the sources of materials intend their deployment only for their own health or reproductive use, any use departing from that approved would be legally actionable for, for instance, breach of contract or conversion of property. A U.S. federal court has held that preembryos are governed by principles like those of property law, and parties' agreements regarding cryopreservation, and Canadian courts are likely to take this approach.

Surrogate Mothering

Professional involvement in surrogate-motherhood transactions has been legally unregulated, except through health professionals' obligations to observe standards of conduct enforced by provincial licensing authorities. Such agreements are not unlawful, but are probably unenforceable by judicial order of surrender of the child by its birth mother. Where the husband of a commissioning couple is the biological father, he has claims on the child, notably to access by visitation, if not to full custody. If the wife of the couple is also the biological mother, however, her status is liable to be legally unrecognized unless a court rules otherwise. When all parties comply with the agreement, the law is likely to recognize its consequences.

The bodily autonomy of a surrogate mother is not compromised by the terms of any agreement she has made. Her prior agreement to submit, for instance, to prenatal care and diagnosis of the child's genetic status is not legally enforceable, and she cannot be compelled to comply with any course of conduct she opposes. Breach of an agreement may be judicially remedied by orders of financial adjustment, but not by a court ordering compliance. This is the sense in which the agreement is legally unenforceable. Nevertheless, surrogate-motherhood agreements are not currently illegal, even when concluded on a commercial basis. Professionals' involvement is governed more directly by ethics than law, although ethical precepts may be invoked when provincial licensing authorities exercise legal powers of discipline for professional misconduct.

Research on Human Embryos

Research on embryos is likely to be acceptable under professional licensing authorities' legal powers to regulate professional conduct, if it conforms to guidelines such as are laid down by the Medical Research Council of Canada. These guidelines permit research up to 14 days gestation, and up to a short later period in studies into preembryonic failure of implantation. The MRC guidelines accommodate appropriate research up to 17 days gestational age. Further, when the goal is the survival and continued gestation of the very preembryo or embryo affected, no time limit is set, since the experiment is designed to achieve full gestation and birth of a specific child.

CLOSING REFLECTION

The influx of new powers into society nearly always challenges established orders and ways of doing things. This chapter has recounted some of the challenges to the traditional reproductive order that resulted from the influx, during the latter half of this century, of enormous new powers to control human reproduction. The search for a new reproductive order is ongoing, and will reach well into the next century. This is particularly true if science continues to innovate, as it likely will, and particularly true also if the world population continues its expansion, as it likely will, towards an estimated eight billion people on the planet by the year 2030. If roughly 95% of the estimated three billion increase of people over the next thirty to thirty-five years are destined, as it seems will be the case, to live in the underdeveloped and disadvantaged regions of the world, the search for a new reproductive order may well have to confront issues of greater urgency and difficulty than the ones we have been considering in this chapter.

REFERENCES

Advisory Committee to the Minister of National Health and Welfare (Canada) *Storage and Utilization of Human Sperm.* Ottawa: Health and Welfare Canada, 1982.

Asch R.H. et al. "Gamete Intrafallopian Transfer: International Cooperative Study of the First 800 Cases." In: H.J. Jones and C. Schrader, eds. "In Vitro Fertilization and Other Assisted Reproduction." *Annals of the New York Academy of Sciences.* Vol. 541. New York: The New York Academy of Sciences, 1988:722-727.

Bernirscke K. "Spontaneous Chimerism in Mammals. A Critical Review." *Current Topics in Pathology* 1969;1:1-61.

Blackwell R.E. et al. "Are We Exploiting the Infertile Couple?" *Fertility and Sterility* 1987;48:735-739.

Case Conference "Lesbian Couples: Should Help Extend to AID?" *Journal of Medical Ethics* 1978;4:91-95.

CECOS Federation, Le Lannon D. and **Lansac J.** "Artificial Procreation with Frozen Donor Semen: Experience of the French Federation CECOS." *Human Reproduction* 1989;4/7:757-761.

Clément J.L., Decoret B. and **Houel A.** "Les enfants conçus par insémination artificielle avec donneur." *Le Concours médical* 1987;109:2387-2391.

Collins J. et al. "Treatment-Independent Pregnancy Among Infertile Couples." *The New England Journal of Medicine* 1983;309:1201-1206.

Combined Ethics Committee of the Canadian Fertility and Andrology Society and the Society of Obstetricians and Gynaecologists of Canada *Ethical Considerations of the New Reproductive Technologies.* Toronto: Ribosome Communications, 1990.

Congregation for the Doctrine of the Faith *Instruction on Respect for Human Life in its Origin, and on the Dignity of Procreation. Replies to Certain Questions of the Day.* Sherbrooke, Québec: Les Éditions Paulines, 1987.

Creighton, P. and **Task Force on Human Life, The Anglican Church of Canada** *Artificial Insemination by Donor. A Study of Ethics, Medicine, and Law in our Technological Society.* Toronto: The Anglican Book Centre, 1977.

David G. and **Lansac J.** "The Organization of the Centers for the Study and Preservation of Semen in France." In: G. David and W.S. Price, eds. *Human Artificial Insemination and Semen Preservation.* New York, London: Plenum Press, 1980:15-26.

Editorial "Conception in a Watch Glass." *The New England Journal of Medicine* 1937;217/17:678.

Editorial *Lancet* 1974;1:203-204.

Ethics Committee of the American Fertility Society "Ethical Considerations of the New Reproductive Technologies." *Fertility and Sterility* 1990;53:Supplement 2, 1S-109S.

Fuller Torrey E. "Artificial Insemination: A Problem in Medical Ethics." *McGill Medical Journal* 1963;32:4-14.

Gemmette E.V. "Selective Pregnancy Reduction: Medical Attitudes, Legal Implications, and a Viable Alternative." *Journal of Health Politics, Policy, and Law* 1991;16:383-395.

Glass B. "Introduction to R.G. Edwards. Fertilization of Human Eggs In Vitro: Morals, Ethics and The Law." 50th Anniversary Special Issue. *The Quarterly Review of Biology* 1974;49:367-391.

Guirgis R.R. and **Craft I.L.** "Gamete Intrafallopian Transfer in Women Who Had Ectopic Pregnancy Previously." *Obstetrics & Gynecology* 1992;79:586-588.

Handyside A.H. et al. "Pregnancies from Biopsied Human Preimplantation Embryos Sexed by Y-Specific DNA Amplification." *Nature* 1990;344:768-770.

Hanscombe G. "The Right to Lesbian Parenthood." *Journal of Medical Ethics* 1983; 9:133-135.

Hummel W.P. and **Luther L.M.** "Current Management of a Donor Insemination Program." *Fertility and Sterility* 1989;51:919-930.

Kerin J.F. et al. "Incidence of Multiple Pregnancy after In Vitro Fertilization and Embryo Transfer." *Lancet* 1983;2:537-540.

Law Society's Standing Committee on Family Law *Human Fertilization and Embryology. A Memorandum.* London: The Law Society's Hall, 1983.

Lobo G. *Current Problems in Medical Ethics.* Allahabad: St. Paul, 1975.

Lutjen P. et al. "The Establishment and Maintenance of Pregnancy Using In Vitro Fertilization and Embryo Donation in a Patient with Primary Ovarian Failure." *Nature* 1984;307:174-175. (The authors speak of a "donated embryo," however, the donated ovum was inseminated with the infertile woman's husband's sperm. In this chapter's terminology, this was a case of a donated ovum, not a donated embryo.)

Macklin R. "Artificial Means of Reproduction and our Understanding of the Family." *Hastings Center Report* 1991;21:5-11.

McEwan K.L., Costello C.G. and **Taylor P.J.** "Adjustment to Infertility." *Journal of Abnormal Psychology* 1987;96:108-116.

McLaren A. "IVF: Regulation or Prohibition." *Nature* 1989;342:469-470.

McLaren A. "Prelude to Embryogenesis." In: The CIBA Foundation. *Human Embryo Research. Yes or No?* London, New York: Tavistock Publications, 1986:5-23.

Medical Research International, Society for Assisted Reproductive Technology (SART) and **American Fertility Society** "In Vitro Fertilization-Embryo Transfer (IVF-ET) in the United States: 1990 Results from the IVF-ET Registry." *Fertility and Sterility* 1992;57:15-24.

Menken J., Trussell J. and **Larsen U.** "Age and Infertility." *Science* 1986;233:1389-1394.

Moghissi K.S. "Reflections on the New Guidelines for the Use of Semen Donor Insemination." *Fertility and Sterility* 1990;53:399-400.

Myre B. et al. "Two Populations of Erythrocytes Associated with XX-XY Mosaicism." *Transfusion* 1965;5:501-505.

Office of Technology Assessment, Congress of the United States *Artificial Insemination Practice in the United States.* Washington, D.C.: Government Printing Office, 1988.

Ontario Law Reform Commission *Report on Human Artificial Reproduction and Related Matters*, Vol. II. Toronto: Ministry of the Attorney General, 1985, 218-272, 281-285.

Overall C. *Ethics and Human Reproduction: A Feminist Analysis.* Boston: Allen and Unwin, 1987.

Overall C., ed. *The Future of Human Reproduction.* Toronto: The Women's Press, 1989.

Page H. "Calculating the Effectiveness of In Vitro Fertilization. A Review." *British Journal of Obstetrics and Gynecology* 1989;96:334-339.

Pfeffer N. "The Uninformed Conception." *New Scientist* July 20, 1991:40-41.

Piatelli-Palmarini M. "Biological Roots of the Human Individual." In: *Law and Ethics of A.I.D. and Embryo Transfer*. Ciba Foundation Symposium 17. Amsterdam, London, New York: Elsevier, Excerpta Medical, North-Holland, 1973:19-25.

Rahner K. "The Problem of Genetic Manipulation." In: K. Rahner. *Theological Investigations*. New York: Seabury, 1972.

Reame N.E. and **Parker P.J.** "Surrogate Pregnancy: Clinical Features of Forty-Four Cases." *American Journal of Obstetrics and Gynecology* 1990;162:1220-1225.

Robertson J.A. "Technology and Motherhood: Legal and Ethical Issues in Human Egg Donation." *Case Western Reserve Law Review* 1988-1989;39:1-38.

Royal Society *Human Fertilization and Embryology*. London: The Royal Society, 1983.

Rubin B. "Psychological Aspects of Human Artificial Insemination." *Archives of General Psychiatry* 1965;13:121-132.

Sauer M.V. and **Paulson R.J.** "Human Oocyte and Preembryo Donation: An Evolving Method for the Treatment of Infertility." *American Journal of Obstetrics and Gynecology* 1990;163:1421-1424.

Sauer M.V. et al. "Pregnancy after Age 50: Application of Oocyte Donation to Women After Natural Menopause." *Lancet* 1993;341:321-323.

Sauer M.V. et al. "Reversing the Natural Decline in Human Fertility." *Journal of the American Medical Association* 1992;268:1275-1279.

Sauer M.V. et al. "Survey of Attitudes Regarding the Use of Siblings for Gamete Donation." *Fertility and Sterility* 1988;49:721-722.

Sauer M.V. et al. "A Preliminary Report on Oocyte Donation Extending Reproductive Potential to Women Over 40." *The New England Journal of Medicine* 1990;323:1157-1160.

Seibel M.M. and **Taymor M.L.** "Emotional Aspects of Infertility." *Fertility and Sterility* 1982;37:137-145.

Sherwin S. *No Longer Patient: Feminist Ethics and Health Care*. Philadelphia: Temple University Press, 1992.

St. Clair Stephenson P. and **Wagner M.G.** "Turkey-Baster Babies: A View from Europe." *The Milbank Quarterly* 1991;69:45-50.

Swainson G. "For Quints' Parents, There's no Magic Formula: Raising Brood of Five Is as Much Art as Science." *The Gazette* (Montréal) February 7, 1993:A6.

Tan L.T. et al. "Cumulative Conception and Live Birth Rates after In Vitro Fertilization." *Lancet* 1992;339:1390-1394.

Tauer C.A. "The Tradition of Probabilism and the Moral Status of the Early Embryo." *Theological Studies* 1984;45:3-33.

Testart J. "À la recherche du cobaye idéal." *Le Monde diplomatique* juillet 1990:19.

Trounson A. and **Mohr L.** "Human Pregnancy Following Cryopreservation, Thawing and Transfer of an Eight-Cell Embryo." *Nature* 1983;305:707-709.

U.K. Hansard, House of Lords *Official Report.* 7th December 1989. We have cited the Archbishop in A. McLaren "IVF: Regulation or Prohibition?" *Nature* 1989;242:470.

Utian W.H. et al. "Preliminary Experience with In Vitro Fertilization-Surrogate Gestational Pregnancy." *Fertility and Sterility* 1989;52:633-638.

Wagner M. and **St. Clair P.A.** "Are In Vitro Fertilization and Embryo Transfer of Benefit to All?" *Lancet* October 28, 1989:1027-1030.

Walters L. "Ethical Aspects of the New Reproductive Technologies." In: H.W. Jones and C. Schrader, eds. "In Vitro Fertilization and Other Assisted Reproduction." *Annals of the New York Academy of Sciences.* Vol. 541. New York: The New York Academy of Sciences, 1988:646-663.

Warnock M. (Chairman) Department of Health and Social Security *Report of the Committee of Inquiry into Human Fertilization and Embryology.* London: Her Majesty's Stationery Office, 1984.

Wikler D. and **Wikler N.J.** "Turkey-Baster Babies: The Demedicalization of Artificial Insemination." *The Milbank Quarterly* 1991;69:5-40.

Wolf D.P. et al. "In Vitro Fertilization-Embryo Transfer in Nonhuman Primates: The Technique and its Applications." *Molecular Reproduction and Development* 1990;27:261-280.

Wright J. et al. "Psychosocial Distress and Infertility: A Review of Controlled Research." *International Journal of Fertility* 1989;34:126-142.

7

WHEN PEOPLE FEAR GIVING BIRTH TO A MALFORMED CHILD: GENETIC COUNSELLING, PRENATAL DIAGNOSIS, AND FETAL THERAPY

The first systematic attempts to diagnose a pathologic condition in the unborn, by analyzing samples of the amniotic fluid surrounding the fetus in its mother's womb, date back nearly forty years. In its earliest phase, prenatal diagnosis was linked to treatment of the fetus affected by severe anemia, resulting from Rh incompatibility with its mother. In the mid-1950s, Dr. Bevis discovered that an analysis of amniotic fluid offered a basis for predicting the severity of this anemia, and several years later, Dr. Liley reported the first successful intrauterine transfusion of blood to the fetus in danger of dying from Rh-incompatibility anemia. Amniocentesis — the extraction of samples of amniotic fluid from the amniotic sac enveloping the fetus — became a routine method in the care of Rh-immunized pregnant women, and many fetuses, who would have died before birth, were saved.

If emphasis in the early days of prenatal diagnosis was on timely detection and treatment of the fetus for anemia, by the late 1960s attention, interest, and emphasis had shifted to early detection of fetal anomalies and abortion (Powledge, 1974, 11). The shift was due, in part, to scientific advances and, in part, to changes of attitudes towards abortion. The discovery, in the late 1950s, of diseases due to defects in the chromosomes, progress in identification of metabolic disorders based on defects in genes, and the development of more refined methods to detect these defects increased the scope of prenatal diagnosis (Fraser, 1979). Selective abortion — an abortion sought because of fetal defects, as contrasted with abortion requested when the pregnancy as such is unwanted — became socially possible, after attitudes towards abortion and abortion law in several countries became less restrictive through the 1970s. Early tentative linkings of prenatal diagnosis to abortion gradually gave way to the realization that abortion requested after prenatal diagnosis would be a societal reality for many years to come (Motulsky, 1974, 659).

Nothing, however, stands still for very long where science and technology are involved, and societal attitudes and trends of thought are also continuously on the move. Discussions of prenatal diagnosis in the 1990s inevitably occur on a higher turn of the spiral of control over reproduction, on a higher turn also of the spiral of ethical complexity. The basic ethical choice, in Joseph Fletcher's phrase of twenty years ago, remains that of chance versus control (Fletcher, 1974, 36). In the preceding chapter, the issue of control was over whether a woman became pregnant or not; in this chapter, control versus chance centres on the quality of the fetus, and on whether it will be allowed to be born. In the past, prospective parents had little choice. Chance ruled over the entire period of pregnancy, and a couple, often with great anxiety, had to wait until birth to know if their baby was normal or not; if not, parents then had to live with the consequences.

Developments over the last several years now allow prospective parents to have their fetus monitored for defects at earlier and earlier moments in the reproductive process: around the tenth week of pregnancy, if chorionic villus sampling (to be discussed below) is used; and even before implantation in the uterus, if IVF and preimplantation diagnosis (also to be discussed below) are used. Prenatal and preimplantation diagnosis are several more of those steps, as A. Motulsky observed over twenty years ago, with which human beings, unconsciously or consciously, grasp the reins of their own genetic destiny (Motulsky, 1971, 31). As work progresses on the human genome project (Chapter 18), more and more diagnostic tests will become available, and the issue of human control over genetic destiny will become even more prominent than it is now.

In this chapter, we centre attention on genetic counselling, on prenatal and preimplantation diagnosis, and on the emerging possibilities for treating the fetus while it is in the mother's body. We open the discussion with two stories, one about an individual family, the other about a specific community. These stories identify two directions of control over reproduction, and they will be taken up again in the chapter's last section, on eugenics. A scientific and medical overview of the technologies involved in prenatal and preimplantation diagnosis, and in fetal therapy, follow the opening stories. We then identify and analyze the ethical issues that are the main concern of this chapter.

GENETIC COUNSELLING AND PRENATAL DIAGNOSIS: FOR THE FAMILY? FOR THE POPULATION?

At an interdisciplinary meeting held in Berlin in December 1990, on the multiple relationships between bioscience and society, Marcus Pembrey, an English specialist in paediatric genetics, emphasized that the proper focus of genetic counselling and prenatal diagnosis is in family medicine, not in public health. The goal is to help prospective parents, in the face of known genetic risks, to achieve their desired family of healthy children. The goal should not be to reduce the numbers of babies born with genetic or congenital defects in the population. Genetic counselling and prenatal diagnosis could become discredited as state-inspired eugenics, were they to become instruments for the achievement of the goal of public health, social economics, or population engineering. Reduction of the birth incidence of genetic or congenital diseases or disorders may be a consequence, but should not, in Pembry's view and in the view of many other medical geneticists, be the aim of genetic counselling and prenatal diagnosis (Pembrey, 1991, 53-54).

Two stories illustrate the possible ends for which genetic counselling and prenatal diagnosis may be employed as means. A brief preliminary discussion of genetic diseases and disorders will set the stage for these stories and the rest of the chapter.

Genetic and Congenital Diseases and Disorders

The terms *genetic* and *congenital* are often confused, in their use as adjectives to qualify diseases and disorders. *Genetic* means present at conception, and *congenital* means evident at birth or, with the use of the imaging and diagnostic techniques, evidenced in utero. Genetic disease results from derangements of the hereditary material (chromosomes and the genes they carry), in its transmission from one generation to the next (Edwards, 1988, 211-212). Congenital diseases or disorders may result from chromosome or gene defects, from environmental influences (such as maternal use of tobacco, alcohol, or drugs), or from a combination of both.

Hereditary disorders may be due to large-scale chromosomal defects. The normal human cell has 46 chromosomes, grouped into 23 pairs, of which one pair, the sex chromosomes, determine whether an embryo will be born as a girl or a boy. Broken or structurally disordered chromosomes, as well as a deficiency or an excess in the number of chromosomes, may cause early death or severe disability. *Down's syndrome*, a disorder people used to call *mongolism* — a racial term that is no longer used — arises from the presence of three, rather than the normal two, chromosomes in the twenty-first group of chromosomes. The risk of giving birth to a child with Down's syndrome is what most frequently motivates women to consult genetic counsellors and to request pre-natal diagnosis.

In other cases, several defective genes, rather than a defect in chromosome number or structure, are the cause of hereditary disease or disorder. These are called *polygenic* diseases. Diseases due to single-gene defects are called *monogenic*.

Gene products, such as enzymes, hormones, and other proteins, are essential for life and health. Single-gene defects frequently result in the human body's deficient production of these substances. When single-gene defects cause an enzyme deficiency, human metabolism may be seriously disrupted. The consequences are usually devastating, and often fatal, for the affected individual.

In some cases, a genetic disease requires the presence of two defective genes (one from the mother, the other from the father) at the same place on a chromosome. Such diseases are said to be recessive and transmitted in Mendelian fashion, after the monk, Gregor Mendel, who worked out the patterns of hereditary transmission of inherited characteristics in the last century. A person carrying both defectives genes is said to be homozygous, and has the disease arising from the gene defects. A person who has only one of the defective genes involved in a recessive disease is said to be heterozygous, or a carrier of the defective gene. Such persons do not have the disease itself.

A genetic disease is said to be dominant when it results from derangement or defect in only one of the two genes at the same place on the chromosome. *Huntington's disease*, which usually appears in middle age and progresses from loss of motor control through mental derangement to death over a number of years, is an example of a dominant genetic disease.

Some genetic diseases or disorders are linked to one or another of the two sex chromosomes. *Duchenne muscular dystrophy*, for example, is linked to the X chromosome. Boys are affected with the disease if their single X chromosome carries the gene defect for this form of muscular dystrophy. Duchenne muscular dystrophy is marked by the appearance of symptoms of muscular weakness early in life. The diseases progresses to relatively early death in young adulthood.

Tay-Sachs disease is an example of an hereditary disorder arising from a single-gene defect. In this case, the single-gene defect leads to the deficient or zero production of a particular enzyme, called hexosaminidase A. Without that one enzyme, fatty substances in the brain are not broken down or metabolized. The resultant buildup of these substances in the brain of an affected newborn child creates very severe neurologic problems, causes great suffering to child and family, and leads to early death, usually between the ages of two and four years of age.

Beta thalassemia is another example of a disease resulting from defect in a single gene. This disease, in its most severe form, leads to severe anemia, because of the body's inability to produce one of the important constituents of blood. This disease, left untreated, occurs at an early age. Treatment consists of regular blood transfusions, but these cause a dangerous buildup of iron in the body. So the second arm of treatment involves administration of a drug, desferrioxamine, to reduce levels of iron. Despite this treatment, death usually occurs in young adulthood.

These last two recessive genetic diseases are background for the two following stories that illustrate the workings and consequences of genetic counselling and prenatal diagnosis.

Towards a Healthy Family

Mr. and Mrs. M.-L. gave birth to a baby boy, their first child, after they had postponed pregnancy for many years after marriage, so that they could finish their university studies and launch their careers. This child, their first baby, had Tay-Sachs disease. He deteriorated rapidly and died at 18 months of age. Mrs. M.-L. was at the hospital every day during the baby's last six months of life. She was terribly upset, had to stop work, and knew she could never go through such emotional suffering again.

Mrs. and Mr. M.-L. wanted children very much. So they went to a genetic counsellor to learn all they could about Tay-Sachs disease, and they learned they faced a pretty high risk of producing another child with this disease. But the counsellor told them that prenatal diagnosis was available and could detect this genetic defect, or the lack of the enzyme, early enough in pregnancy to permit Mrs. M.-L. to request an abortion if the fetus was found to carry the defect. Had prenatal diagnosis not been available, Mr. and Mrs. M.-L. would not have dared try another pregnancy. They may have tried to adopt a child, but without too much chance of success, given their age, current adoption practice, and the fact that the husband was physically handicapped as the result of an auto accident. Prenatal diagnosis was available, so the M.-L.s went ahead with pregnancy. The result? The fetus had Tay-Sachs disease and Mrs. M.-L. requested an abortion. Mrs. M.-L. then became pregnant again. Once again prenatal diagnosis revealed that the fetus carried the defect for Tay-Sachs disease. Mrs. M.-L. requested a second abortion. Finally, at the end of her fourth pregnancy, Mrs. M.-L. gave birth to a normal healthy baby girl.

This story illustrates how genetic counselling and prenatal diagnosis, based upon astounding advances in molecular biology and human genetics over the past several years, increase a couple's reproductive alternatives when they face the risk of transmitting hereditary defects to their future child. As Marcus Pembrey emphasized, genetic counselling and prenatal diagnosis enabled this couple to have their desired family.

Reducing the Birth Rate of Babies with Genetic Disease: A Consequence or a Goal of Genetic Counselling and Prenatal Diagnosis?

Dr. Marcus Pembrey stated above, as do many clinical geneticists involved in delivering counselling and genetic services to families, that reducing the number of births of babies with genetic diseases in the population may well be a consequence, but it is not, or should not be, the goal of genetic counselling and prenatal diagnosis. The workings of programmes to control beta thalassemia in the Cypriot population in London, and in Cyprus, raise the title question of this subsection of the chapter. The beta thalassemia story is complex, but easy enough to follow if we follow it step by step.

First, *the disease*. There are many forms of thalassemia, but the worst form of beta thalassemia, mentioned briefly in the preceding subsection, is a lethal condition. Worldwide, it is one of the most frequently occurring of lethal inherited diseases among human beings. The normal fetus produces haemoglobin during its development in the womb, but that process switches off about the time of birth and is naturally replaced by a second process of haemoglobin production, called adult haemoglobin synthesis. This replacement fails to occur in babies affected with the lethal form of thalassemia. They suffer severe anemia which, if untreated, leads to early death (Modell, 1982, 146-147).

Second, *the treatment*. Treatment, as explained in the previous subsection, exists, but the combination of blood transfusions and drug treatment for transfusion-linked iron build-up is expensive. As Dr. B. Modell has observed, the disease can be a trap for families who cannot afford treatment for their affected child or children. They are trapped between misery and distress: misery of and with their untreated child, and distress because a treatment is available for which they do not have the resources. When treatment is effective, people with the disease do not die early and the population of beta thalassemia people needing treatment increases. As Dr. Modell points out, effective and costly treatment has political implications when the costs are carried by society, for instance, societies having a national health service (Modell, 1982, 148).

Third, *the mode of inheritance*. Beta thalassemia is a monogenic recessive disease. If both the prospective father and mother carry the defective gene leading to this disease, they have a one-in-four chance of giving birth to a baby affected with beta thalassemia. However, relatively simple tests are available, to determine if both the prospective parents are carriers of the beta thalassemia gene. This is called carrier testing.

Fourth, results of *the thalassemia control programme*. Before carrier testing and prenatal diagnosis were available, Cypriot couples tended to have pregnancies quite frequently, and fewer than half of the children born were healthy and unaffected with thalassemia. After couples came to know of their risk of giving birth to a beta thalassemia child, and before prenatal diagnosis was available, they greatly delayed any attempt at pregnancy, and 70% of pregnancies that did occur ended in abortions motivated by parental anxiety over giving birth to a thalassemic child. After both carrier testing and prenatal diagnosis were available, pregnancy rates, which had dropped when couples knew of the risk and prenatal diagnosis was not available, rose again when 98% of Cypriot couples opted for the use of prenatal diagnosis (Modell, 1982, 151-152).

The availability of carrier testing, genetic counselling, prenatal diagnosis, and nearly universal screening for beta thalassemia has resulted in a greater than 40% reduction of thalassemia-related abortions, as compared to the number of abortions requested by anxious couples before prenatal diagnosis was available (Modell, 1982, 152). The thalassemia control programme has also led to the virtual disappearance of births of beta thalassemia babies in Cyprus since 1986 (Modell, 1992, 552).

Screening came to be universal, or nearly so, in the following way. The Greek Orthodox Archbishop of Cyprus, concerned that prenatal diagnosis alone left women little other choice than abortion if results were positive, passed a ruling requiring, as a condition for church marriage, that couples present a certificate attesting that they had undergone carrier testing for thalassemia. The reasoning behind the ruling was that carrier testing before marriage would give women and couples more options, such as marrying another partner if both tested positive as carriers, or turning to adoption rather than to pregnancy, prenatal diagnosis, and selective abortion. As the great majority of Cypriots wanted church marriage, carrier testing became nearly universal. However, 98% of Cypriot couples, as already noted, chose to attempt pregnancy, and to use prenatal diagnosis and selective abortion if the diagnosis indicated an affected fetus (Modell, 1992, 553).

Fifth, *the interpretation of these results*. The dramatic reduction, over a decade, of the number of babies born with beta thalassemia in Cyprus seems to have been the cumulative consequence of individual couples pursuing the family goal of having healthy children. There are no indications whatsoever that individual Cypriot couples were, in their reproductive decisions, seeking to do their part to bring about a beta thalassemia-free population. Yet the goals of those who establish and offer genetic counselling, and the goal of those who financially support these services, may be different from the goals of individual couples. Dr. Modell has spoken of the European programmes that have been set up "with the aim of decreasing the incidence of thalassemia major," the form of thalassemia we have been discussing (Modell, 1982, 145). Moreover, in reference to the perception of some people that the aim of prenatal diagnosis is to eliminate the handicapped from society, Dr. Modell observed that genetic counselling and prenatal diagnosis can be as much a service for patients as for the rest of the population.

We shall return to the issue raised in the title question of this subsection when we consider eugenics, towards the end of this chapter.

GENETIC COUNSELLING: CAN IT REALLY BE NONDIRECTIVE?

Genetic counselling involves communication between professionals who are knowledgeable about genetics, and persons who face risks of transmitting hereditary disease to the children they want to have. This counselling has, basically, three dimensions: information about hereditary disease and its risks of recurring in a family; exploration of reproductive options in the presence of such risks; and offering the support individuals or couples may need to arrive at a reproductive decision, for example, to undergo prenatal diagnosis and possibly selective abortion, and to live with this decision once it has been made (Sorenson, 1979, 85). Genetic counsellors have been seen from a number of perspectives: as information-givers (Hsia, 1979); as facilitators in the decision process (Antley, 1979); as psychotherapists (Kessler, 1979); and as moral advisors (Twiss, 1979).

A number of these perspectives on genetic counselling correspond only partially to the way medical geneticists and genetic counsellors in Canada view their role and work. Respondents to a study of ethics and medical genetics in Canada saw themselves primarily as information-providers and support-givers. They emphasized two goals of genetic counsellors as being essential; helping prospective parents understand their reproductive options, and then helping them to live in peace with their reproductive choices (Roy, 1989, 134).

Medical geneticists and genetic counsellors in Canada do not tend to pontificate on matters of reproductive right and wrong. They tend to be nonjudgmental. They do not see it as their responsibility to help parents to evaluate ethically their reproductive choices, nor would they ethically question the reproductive decisions of the parents they counsel. The maxims that seem to govern genetic counsellors in Canada are; inform accurately and honestly, support sensitively but do not advise, dictate or criticize parents' reproductive decisions.

One medical geneticist characterized the relationship of the genetic counsellor to parents as: "I am, in a sense, their servant." Respecting and promoting the autonomy of individual parents seem to be the dominant value professed by the majority of medical geneticists and genetic counsellors in Canada (Roy, 1989, 134).

To sum things up, most medical geneticists approach ethical issues in a non-analytical, nondirective, and nonjudgmental way. They do not seem to consider the *analysis* of ethical issues associated with their practice to be one of their prime responsibilities. They respond in a practical and pragmatic way, guided by the maxim just mentioned, to the ethical issues they face on a nearly daily basis in their work.

Genetic counsellors encounter a wide range of ethical issues in their every-day contacts with couples who face the risk of transmitting hereditary diseases, when they plan to have children. Though a discussion of these issues would require more space than is available for this chapter, we draw attention to three recurring kinds of ethical problems.

The ideal of nondirectiveness in genetic counselling can be challenged in a very specific way, when parents request prenatal diagnosis to learn only the sex of the fetus, so that they can request an abortion if the fetus is not of the sex they desire. Counsellors and geneticists are divided about how they should respond to such requests, when the requests have nothing at all to do with the risk of passing on a sex-linked disease, like X-linked Duchenne mus-cular dystrophy, to the child (Roy, 1989, 128). There is intense ethical con-troversy about sex-selection uses of prenatal diagnosis, for reasons having nothing to do with the transmission of hereditary diseases (Wertz, 1989; Dickens, 1986).

A *second ethical issue* centres on telling the truth. Telling the whole truth can be difficult for genetic counsellors, when that truth may psychologically disturb the person seeking counselling, or when the truth may even disrupt that per-son's self-image and life. Imagine having to tell a woman, who is married and has been unable to conceive a child, that tests show she is chromosomally male, not female. This person looks like a woman, feels like a woman, has always thought of herself as a woman, and the counsellor must now tell her that, chro-mosomally, she is a male and will never be able to conceive a child. Must the counsellor tell the whole truth to the woman? Sixty-eight percent of respon-dents in the study of ethics and medical genetics in Canada answered affirma-tively; other respondents preferred to tailor the truth, according to what they perceived the woman could tolerate (Roy, 1989, 125).

A *third ethical issue* deals with confidentiality. Are genetic counsellors ever justified in disclosing confidential information to third parties? Generally, the answer is no. Counsellors should not divulge confidential information. But the principle is not absolute. The Canadian College of Medical Geneticists (CCMG), for example, directs counsellors to keep information obtained from patients in confidence, unless patients have given written permission to release this infor-mation to others, or unless it can be shown that nondisclosure of this informa-tion is likely to cause significant harm to the health of other persons (Canadian College, 1986).

An example will illustrate the difficulty of the confidentiality dilemma. Consider Huntington's disease. A person with the genetic defect for this disease usually leads a normal life, often unaware that he has the condition, until dis-turbing symptoms begin to appear somewhere between the ages of 30 and 45.

The subsequent deterioration is physically and mentally devastating, until death occurs several years after first symptoms. Siblings of a person who has been diagnosed as having Huntington's disease face a 50% chance of carrying that gene themselves. If the person diagnosed refuses to tell his brothers and sisters about his diagnosis, should the genetic counsellor do so?

Some Canadian geneticists would safeguard confidentiality; others would utilize the CCMG exception clause cited above (Roy, 1989, 126).

The *fourth and central issue* appears in the title question of this section. Can genetic counselling really be nondirective, and should it try to be so?

The cross-cultural study of ethics and human genetics showed that nondirectiveness is the most widely ingrained approach to genetic counselling (Fletcher, "Ethics and Human Genetics," 1989, 459). That approach is epitomized in the statement, cited above, of one Canadian medical geneticist who said of the relationship of counsellor to prospective parents: "I am, in a sense, their servant."

One geneticist, setting about critically to examine the widespread assumption that genetic counselling can and should be nondirective, has called nondirective counselling in connection with prenatal diagnosis a sham (Clarke, 1991, 998). The offer of prenatal diagnosis, in his view, implies a recommendation to couples to accept the offer, and the offer also entails an unspoken agreement with, if not a recommendation for, abortion, if prenatal diagnosis reveals abnormality in the fetus. This sequence is built into the genetic counsellor-prospective parent encounter, and is present whatever the counsellor's personal thoughts or feelings may be. The very existence of prenatal diagnostic technology, and its expansion in the current social context, carry a tacit but powerful influence towards selective abortion, an influence stronger than any nondirective posture genetic counsellors may adopt (Clarke, 1991, 1000).

Genetic counsellors, however, generally are utterly sincere and genuine in their professional commitment to nondirectiveness, particularly when they single-mindedly anchor their practices to the goals of family medicine. The intention of genetic counsellors to honour the autonomy and freedom of reproductive choice of prospective parents is not emptied of value and meaning, just because social pressures may diminish the reproductive freedom of couples more significantly than is often appreciated by counsellors and couples themselves. However, nondirectiveness does become little more than a posture when genetic counsellors are committed to the population goal and public-health objectives of ever more effectively reducing the birth rates of babies afflicted with prenatally diagnosable genetic diseases and disorders. Dr. Clarke's charge is that it is impossible sincerely to maintain a nondirective approach to genetic counselling, while simultaneously pursuing the goal of preventing the birth of those afflicted with genetic abnormalities (Clarke, 1991, 999).

PRENATAL DIAGNOSIS: SCOPE, TECHNOLOGIES, AND GOALS

Death and suffering early in human life are largely due to the devastating impact of chromosomal disorders, Mendelian disorders and congenital malformations (Scriver, 1982, 493). The preceding sections cited examples of these disorders that can be diagnosed in the fetus. However, the few examples given, such as Down's syndrome (trisomy 21), beta thalassemia, Tay-Sachs disease, and Duchenne muscular dystrophy, give only a very feeble idea of the range of inherited diseases, and of the power of prenatal diagnostic technology. Continuing progress in the development and refinement of these technologies has advanced the timing and extended the scope of prenatal diagnosis. Does prenatal diagnosis suffer from a wealth of means and a poverty of ends or goals?

The Scope and Power of Prenatal Diagnosis

Women's risk of having a fetus affected by one or another of the devastating disorders caused by abnormality of chromosome number (more or less than two chromosomes in any of the 23 pairs of chromosomes), increases quite dramatically after women pass age 40 (Evans, 1989, 19). Down's syndrome has already been mentioned, and trisomy 13 or 18, conditions marked by severe mental retardation and early death, are additional examples of chromosome disorders occurring more frequently the older a pregnant woman is.

Practically all abnormalities of chromosome number and their related disorders can be diagnosed in the fetus early or midway in pregnancy, by application of standard chromosome study techniques to the fetal cells obtained by chorionic villus sampling (CVS) or amniocentesis, both of which we shall discuss below. Many of the fetal disorders due to chromosome instability, or due to deletions of parts of a chromosome, can also be diagnosed before birth.

Fetal disorders due to chromosome abnormality are only part of the story. Many of the more than 4,000 single gene defects listed in McKusick's famous catalogues of Mendelian inheritance in humans show up as either dominant, recessive, or X-linked inherited disease (McKusick, 1990; McKusick, 1991). More than 200 such disorders were already diagnosable in the fetus over ten years ago (Stephenson, 1981). Refinements in ultrasound imaging of the fetus, and in the technologies for gene or DNA analysis, over the last decade have added many more fetal disorders to the list of what can be diagnosed before birth.

The fetal body, though still inside the mother's body, is no longer hidden and inaccessible. Disorders affecting nearly every organ system and part of the fetal body can now be diagnosed prenatally, whether these be diseases of the vital organs, like the heart, kidney, liver, or brain; or diseases of skin and blood;

or deformities of the skeletal structure. The fetus now conceals fewer and fewer of its tragic secrets.

Evidence is required for a prenatal diagnosis. The evidence may be a picture of the fetus, as in ultrasound imaging, or a sample of fetal tissue, fetal blood, or fetal cells. Ultrasound images require interpretation to become evidence of a fetal disorder, and fetal cells will reveal disorder only when examined by highly sophisticated chromosomal, biochemical, or DNA analytic techniques. We now offer an overview of these diagnostic technologies.

The Technology of Prenatal Diagnosis

Amniocentesis and *chorionic villus sampling* (CVS) both deliver fetal cells that can be studied by the methods of biochemical, chromosomal, or DNA analysis. *Amniocentesis*, used in prenatal diagnosis for many years now, involves needle aspiration of amniotic fluid under ultrasound guidance. Fetal cells are obtained from these amniotic fluid samples. This procedure is often performed around the sixteenth week of pregnancy (and even earlier in some cases), and test results, depending on the work load of laboratories, may not be available until the twentieth week of pregnancy or even later. *Chorionic villus sampling* has been used clinically since 1984. The sampling procedure removes bits of chorionic villi, filament-like tissue surrounding the amniotic sac. The cells in this tissue contain the chromosomes and genes of the fetus, and they can be studied by the same methods used to analyze fetal cells contained in amniotic fluid samples.

The most striking feature of chorionic villus sampling, a feature highly valued by many, is that it is performed much earlier in pregnancy than is amniocentesis. CVS is performed between eight and nine weeks of pregnancy, and new rapid methods to study the fetal cells can often deliver a diagnosis of genetic or chromosomal status within days. If a fetal abnormality is diagnosed, the early timing of the diagnosis that is possible with CVS enables a woman to request an abortion in the first trimester of pregnancy, often before family or friends would ever detect that she is pregnant.

However, the advantages of chorionic villus sampling have to be balanced against its higher risks, as compared with amniocentesis. Chorionic villus sampling may provoke more spontaneous abortions of normal fetuses than amniocentesis, and may even cause malformations, such as limb malformations, in otherwise healthy fetuses. The relative safety of CVS is still subject to uncertainty and controversy (Firth, 1991; Halliday, 1992; MRC Working Party, 1991; Jackson, 1992).

Ultrasound or *ultrasonography* produces highly refined images of fetal soft tissue, such as fetal organs. The images are somewhat like X-ray images of the body's bones, and also like X-rays, require expert interpretation to deliver reliable diagnostic information. Ultrasound is routinely used to monitor pregnancies in many countries. As an instrument of prenatal diagnosis, ultrasound imaging can deliver reliable diagnosis of a wide range of fetal abnormalities. Because this technology is used so widely during pregnancy, and at a time when the fetal brain is developing rapidly, concerns have been expressed about the long-term safety of ultrasound. A recent study found that the reading and writing skills of 8- and 9-year-old children whose mothers had received ultrasound examination during pregnancy were no worse that those of children whose mothers had not undergone such examination (Salvesen, 1992, 85). The issue of whether ultrasound is being overutilized in the monitoring of pregnancy is now under study by Canada's Royal Commission on the Reproductive Technologies, due to submit its report in the summer of 1993.

Since the early 1980s, commercial kits have been available for *maternal serum alpha-fetoprotein (MSAFP)* screening of pregnant women. High levels of alpha-fetoprotein in a pregnant woman's blood may indicate that the fetus she is carrying has a neural tube defect, such as anencephaly (no brain), or spina bifida with myelomeningocele (lesion in the spine leading to paralysis and varying degrees of mental handicap). MSAFP screening may produce false positive results, causing a number of women high levels of anxiety and distress until a more specific diagnosis, for example, by ultrasound, shows the fetus to be unaffected. So discussion of the accuracy of MSAFP screening is linked to discussions of the ethics of this technique (Madlon-Kay, 1992; Walters, 1989).

Of all the methods used to analyze fetal cells obtained by amniocentesis and chorionic villus sampling, the most rapid progress has been made in developing and refining the methods for *gene or DNA analysis*. Basically, there are two methods. When the specific genetic defect responsible for a genetic disease or disorder and the exact location of the defective gene are known, the *direct method of genetic or DNA diagnosis* utilizes sensitive probes (cloned genes) to find and identify this defect in one or another of the chromosomes in the fetal cell. This direct method can now be used to find the defective gene for Duchenne muscular dystrophy on the X chromosome. When the exact location of a gene responsible for a genetic disease is not known, the *indirect method of genetic or DNA diagnosis* uses markers, such as the length of the chromosome fragment cut by a specific enzyme, that can be detected and that are known, with varying degrees of probability, to be associated with the gene responsible for a given disease. This is called *linkage analysis*. It requires comparison of markers in the fetal cell with markers in the cells of family members who have, and who have not, had the disease in question. The probability of an accurate diagnosis can vary considerably when the indirect method of DNA analysis is used to analyze fetal cells (Bell, 1990).

In theory, these new methods of DNA analysis open horizons for the eventual prenatal diagnosis of nearly all diseases and disorders arising from single gene defects. The genetic knowledge needed to explore these horizons is accumulating at an astounding speed, as evidenced in work now in progress on the human genome project (Chapter 18).

If the fetal body now conceals fewer and fewer of its tragic secrets, the fetal cell is revealing more and more of the basic genetic plan, according to which the fetal body develops through pregnancy.

The Goals of Prenatal Diagnosis

From its very beginnings, prenatal diagnosis had a link to fetal therapy, and that link may well be strengthening as we approach the end of this century. There are, of course, no effective treatments available for most of the genetic diseases and disorders that have been, and are being, prenatally diagnosed. Prospective parents regularly request selective abortion, after positive (a fetal abnormality is found) prenatal diagnoses. However, prenatal diagnosis delivers negative results in the overwhelming majority of prenatal diagnoses. This information dissuades prospective parents from the abortions they would have demanded, rather than face an even small chance of having an abnormal child. Prenatal diagnosis is also regularly used to guide clinical decisions on the best approaches to care, for fetuses with various kinds of disorders. It is not possible honestly and fairly to characterize prenatal diagnosis as a "search and destroy mission," as some have claimed. Prenatal diagnosis serves many, at times, conflicting goals. They may be summarized as: to have a normal child; to care; to prevent, treat, and cure disease; and to control the quality of the population.

To Have a Normal Child

Parental desire for a normal child, reproductive liberty, freedom from suffering and reproductive disappointment, and familial independence from the burdens of lifelong care of a severely handicapped child are the values now determining one of the governing purposes of prenatal diagnosis, as currently practised. Protection of families from suffering they perceive as unbearable is judged as sufficiently high in the hierarchy of values to morally balance the sacrifice of fetal life, particularly if the fetus is severely defective, fated to suffer much, and destined to die early in life. This position is captured in Dr. Benzie's statement: disaster can be redeemed by love; but, if disaster can be avoided, abortion may be justified (Benzie, 1979, 686).

To Care

A currently less-governing view holds that prenatal diagnosis serves the purpose of giving parents the information they can use to better prepare themselves to care for their disabled child after, or even prior to, birth. This purpose rests upon the value judgment that suffering is not the greatest evil in human life, and that the physical and mental quality of a child is a lesser value than the child itself. Moreover, the destruction of the unborn deprives these developing human beings of every possibility of human experience and fulfilment, in order to permit parents the fulfilment of one among many human desires and goals. Some believe the value sacrificed in this situation, namely, the life of the fetus, far outweighs the value protected by selective abortion.

To Prevent, Treat, and Cure Disease

If medicine, as Dr. J. Lejeune affirms, is essentially and by nature working against natural selection (Lejeune, 1973, 19), then prevention, treatment, and cure, not abortion, should be the aim of prenatal diagnosis (Benzie, 1979, 687). The values serving this prime purpose are compassion for the ill, whatever their condition, aggressive zest in affirming, extending, and enhancing life, and loyalty to the welfare of individual patients, whatever their presumable social utility (Dyck, 1971, 726). If prenatal diagnosis fails to serve these values, it may, as Arthur Dyck claims, threaten to erode them. The difficulty here is that, until recently, very few treatments were available for most of the fetal problems that could be diagnosed before birth. We shall discuss emerging fetal therapy later in this chapter, and Chapter 18 will describe the current state of gene therapy. So we are moving into a new era in which this goal of prenatal diagnosis, its therapeutic goal, may well be increasingly achievable.

To Control the Quality of the Population

Well-organized genetic counselling and prenatal diagnostic programmes, and the workings of parental choice, can lead to dramatic reductions in the birth rates of babies with various kinds of genetic diseases and disorders. With continuing progress in developing the methods of prenatal diagnosis, the Royal College of Physicians in England estimates that the birth prevalence of dominant and X-linked severe disorders might be reduced by up to 50%, and that the birth prevalence of recessively inherited disorders could be drastically reduced by population screening of carriers (Royal College, 1989, 217). Is maintenance of the quality, and not only the quantity, of the population within reasonable limits a goal of prenatal diagnosis? Some believe it is (Morison, 1973, 211).

PREIMPLANTATION DIAGNOSIS

Prenatal diagnosis focuses on the fetus in the woman's womb. Preimplantation diagnosis focuses on the embryo, resulting from in vitro fertilization, before it ever enters the womb.

A combination of in vitro fertilization techniques with the techniques for detecting single gene defects now sets the stage for achieving diagnosis at the preembryonic stage, in the development of the human fertilized ovum. When the gene defects that can now be detected at this stage would lead to very serious, and eventually lethal, diseases in the future child, parents can decide against transfer of such embryo from the IVF laboratory to the uterus. Preimplantation diagnosis is possible, because IVF gives access to human embryos.

Because a discussion of the various approaches to preimplantation diagnosis would exceed the scope of this chapter (Hardy, 1992; Grifo, 1992; Critser, 1992), we limit our observations to the fact that one of three possible approaches involves removal of one or two cells from the six-cell to ten-cell human embryo (preembryo) created by IVF procedures. One or two cells can be removed without damaging the remaining cells of the early embryo, and without negatively affecting continuing embryonic development after the diagnosis. A recently developed method, called polymerase chain reaction (PCR), can rapidly increase or amplify the amount of DNA extracted from even one embryonic cell, so that enough DNA will be available for diagnosis (Mullis, 1990).

As of 1993, preimplantation diagnosis has been used for a number of severe abnormalities and diseases known to be caused by gene defects, including abnormalities that are linked to the X chromosome, such as hemophilia and Duchenne muscular dystrophy, and diseases, such as cystic fibrosis, that are caused by mutations in a single gene.

Cystic fibrosis, a quite common disease with a frequency of about 1 in 2,000 births in Canada, is a monogenic recessively inherited disease that people acquire when they receive two copies, one from their mother, the other from their father, of the gene defect causing the disease. There are both mild and severe forms of the disease. When there is a complete absence of channels through which chloride ions (salt molecules) pass in and out of cells, thick mucus builds up in the lungs and digestive tracts, and severely affected cystic fibrosis patients usually die at a fairly early age. A recent study shows how complex this disease is, and that complexity can lead to ambiguity in the interpretation of prenatal diagnostic tests. The tests may not give a clear prognosis of how severely affected a future child will be (Sheppard, 1993).

In early 1990, three English couples, who were carriers of the gene defect for cystic fibrosis, entered the IVF programme at Hammersmith Hospital in London. Preimplantation diagnosis of the IVF embryos permitted transfer of two embryos, one normal, the other carrying only one of the cystic fibrosis genes, to the wife of one of these couples. She then gave birth to a normal baby girl (Handyside, 1992).

Preimplantation diagnosis allows couples, who face risks of giving birth to children with some kinds of genetic disorders, to bypass in utero diagnosis, and the difficult decision about abortion if fetal diagnosis detects abnormalities. However, in vitro fertilization and embryo transfer are only moderately successful in establishing pregnancy, and IVF combined with preimplantation diagnosis is quite costly (Simpson, 1992, 953). Though many would find it difficult to formulate a persuasive ethical argument against preimplantation diagnosis, this new diagnostic approach will undoubtedly contribute to the survival, and perhaps an intensification, of ethical controversy over the status of the fetus and over eugenics (Robertson, 1992; Warnock, 1992).

FETAL THERAPY: WHEN THE PATIENT IS INSIDE ANOTHER HUMAN BEING

Fetal Therapy: The Possibilities

In the early 1960s, Dr. Liley successfully administered intrauterine blood transfusions to fetuses who, otherwise, would have died from severe anemia resulting from rhesus incompatibility with the mother (Liley, 1963). This form of prenatal treatment, with improved methods and more successful results, continues today (Weiner, 1991; Ney, 1991). However, during the 1970s and 1980s, parents generally had few real choices, after prenatal diagnosis of a severe condition in the fetus. Most of the time, the choice was either abortion or birth of a severely handicapped or dying child.

Four approaches now increase the range of parental options. The *time of delivery can be advanced*, to permit early treatment of some conditions that would cause severe damage or death to the fetus, were these conditions to be left untreated through the full course of pregnancy. The *mode of delivery can be changed* from vaginal to cesarean delivery, when vaginal delivery would threaten the child, or both the mother and the child. The *third* approach, guided by adequate prenatal diagnosis, involves assembly of the medical or surgical expertise needed for immediate treatment of the baby after birth. The *fourth* approach, now possible and successful for some conditions, and still quite experimental for other conditions, is prenatal treatment: treatment of the fetus before birth.

Drug treatment of the fetus may, as some claim, prove to be a mainstay of fetal therapy (Schulman, 1990, 197-198). Doctors have now successfully prevented a most distressing birth defect in human fetuses carrying a genetic defect that affects the adrenal gland. The condition is called congenital adrenal hyperplasia. Female fetuses affected by this condition undergo masculinization of the genital organs due to abnormal adrenal gland production of male hormones, called androgens. After receiving the drug dexamethasone, from the tenth week of pregnancy, a woman pregnant with a female fetus affected by the genetic defect associated with this condition gave birth to a baby girl with normal external genital organs. The drug, which passed the placenta, had successfully suppressed the fetus's abnormal production of male hormones and preserved her genital organs from masculinization (Evans and Shulman, 1989, 404-405).

Advances in ultrasound imaging are particularly indispensable for the prenatal diagnosis and treatment of fetal conditions requiring *surgical correction.* Hydrocephaly is one such condition. Fluid builds up within the fetal skull, and the increasing pressure causes brain damage and severe mental retardation. The surgery involves implanting a shunt, so that this fluid can drain from the fetal skull into the amniotic sac within which the fetus nests. As of July 1, 1989, 45 attempts of this experimental procedure were reported to the International Registry set up to track and monitor prenatal surgery.

Results of this surgery were not very successful for fetuses affected by multiple congenital problems. Thirty-eight infants survived these 45 attempts at prenatal shunt surgery. Of these, only the 14 who did not have multiple congenital problems were normal at a year or so after birth. The remaining 24 all had varying degrees of mental handicap. In 18 cases, the handicap was severe (Evans et al., 1989, 1432).

A number of these now-severely handicapped babies would most likely have died, had prenatal shunt implantation not been tried. Some would say these babies would have been better off dead than alive, with such terrible brain damage (Fletcher, "Ethics in Experimental Fetal Therapy," 1989, 440). This brief story of prenatal treatment of fetal hydrocephalus underlines one important lesson: it is essential to determine, as precisely as possible, who among the unborn will truly benefit and who will suffer from experimental prenatal treatment.

Surgery on the fetus has been done to correct a number of conditions that would, without an operation, prove to be highly damaging or even fatal to the fetus before birth, or to the child shortly after birth. These operations are performed on the fetus while it is still within the mother. Fetal surgery, of necessity, means the mother must be operated on also: once to open her abdomen and uterus, so the surgeon can partially remove the fetus from the uterus; and often a second operation, a cesarean section, is necessary to deliver the child at the end of the pregnancy.

Some of the first cases of prenatal surgery involved two fetal conditions: congenital diaphragmatic hernia (8 cases) and severe bilateral hydronephrosis (7 cases). Many fetuses with congenital diaphragmatic hernia die despite the best possible treatment after birth, while others survive after such treatment. Consequently, there is some controversy about which fetuses really require surgery before birth. Clearly, some fetuses can benefit from prenatal surgery for this condition. When a hole (the hernia) in the fetal diaphragm fails to close, the stomach, intestines, and other organs squeeze up into the fetal chest. The fetal lungs can become so compressed that they fail to grow and the baby dies from an inability to breathe. When fetuses are affected by congenital bilateral hydronephrosis, the tubes transporting urine are blocked and this can result in lethal damage to the fetal kidneys and lungs.

A 1991 report reviewing these first cases of fetal surgery focused on the issue of safety of in utero surgery for the mother. None of these pregnant women died or suffered serious injury as a result of the surgery performed on the fetuses within their bodies. However, there are some complications, such as premature labour resulting from these operations, that are still unsolved problems (Longaker, 1991). A number of these women who underwent surgery on their fetuses were later able to become pregnant again and give birth to healthy children. So fetal surgery does not seem to endanger a woman's future reproductive potential.

Are prenatal operations safe and effective treatments for the fetuses involved? Pregnancies have continued, fetuses have been born alive, and some have progressed well after fetal surgery. Fetal surgery, however, is still at an experimental stage, and demonstration of its relative safety and efficacy, as compared with ordinary or conventional treatment, awaits the conduct of controlled clinical research (Harrison, 1990).

Fetal Therapy: Ethical Reflections

The fetus, though an individual organism, has often been perceived as simply part of the pregnant woman's body. Some believe this perception is bound to change in the light of advances in fetal therapy and surgery, procedures that clearly differentiate the fetus from the mother for purposes of treatment (Rosner, 1989, 83).

Physicians and surgeons who treat human fetuses in utero quite certainly regard these fetuses as patients (Harrison, 1982). However, many normal human fetuses of the same or even higher gestational age than those treated prenatally are aborted. This clash of perceptions has provoked a number of questions.

Now that the fetus is a visible, vivid object of diagnosis and therapy, is it a "patient"? And if it is a patient, is it also thereby a person with rights to treatment? Are such rights overriding, if the mother rejects this new therapy? Does the fetus have a new moral status, by virtue of the new therapeutic options available to it? If so, will physicians who currently perform abortions find themselves in a moral bind?(Ruddick, 1982)

John Fletcher has responded to at least two of these questions. He believes that the innovative prenatal fetal therapies will enhance the "much debated moral status of the fetus," and with that enhancement will come a "much stronger ethical argument" for a duty to perform therapy (Fletcher, "Ethics in Experimental Fetal Therapy," 1989, 442). Will fetal need for prenatal therapy override a woman's right to bodily integrity?

Pregnancy, as such, is not a disease and pregnant women, as such, are not patients. However, fetal surgery, requiring surgical opening of the pregnant woman's abdomen and uterus, definitely turns the pregnant woman into a patient, and places her at risk for the sake of her fetus.

As long as prenatal therapy is experimental, and not sufficiently validated as safe and effective to be recognized as a standard of medical practice, the generally dominant view is that pregnant women would not be legally or ethically obligated to consent to such treatment. However, would the legal or ethical status of the pregnant woman's right to refuse be different if it were medically established that a particular treatment, for example a fetal operation, would protect the fetus from severe damage or death? Answers to this question depend upon at least three additional considerations.

First, has the mother decided against abortion, and for continuance of the pregnancy? A woman's legal freedom not to have a child is distinct from her freedom over her body if she decides to have a child. This latter freedom may be limited, both by legal and ethical considerations, when the fetus, destined for birth, can be protected from harm, serious damage, or death. *If* a fetal therapy has been *established* as *safe* for mother and fetus, and *effective* for the condition affecting a fetus, the pregnant woman who has chosen not to abort "may be legally obligated" in some countries to accept fetal therapy (Robertson, 1989, 434).

Second, how intrusive and potentially harmful would fetal therapy be for the pregnant woman? The more intrusive and risky to the pregnant woman an act of fetal therapy would be, the less likely it is that any court would order such treatment over her refusal of consent. The guideline also makes ethical sense. But would the guideline hold, regardless of the nonviability or viability of the fetus?

With this *third* consideration, we enter into the thicket of abortion law. And that law varies from country to country. It is difficult to imagine that courts, in jurisdictions having few legal restraints on the abortion of previable fetuses, would try to force a woman to undergo fetal therapy against her consent. She could simply decide for an abortion, and might be reduced to doing so by such pressure. However, several courts in the United States have already forced women to undergo cesarean delivery, an act of surgery on the pregnant woman, to permit immediate treatment of an endangered viable fetus (Robertson, 1982, 356-357). This preference of the near-term fetus's health and life over the mother's interest in bodily integrity could, in some countries, lead to far-reaching intrusions into the mother's body in the context of established fetal therapies. This is particularly true if the principle is accepted that a woman may not choose a course of action "that will lead to the death of the viable or near-term fetus any more than she can once the child is born."(Robertson, 1982, 354). This tendency to prefer the fetus over the mother, however much suffering the mother may have to endure as a result of this preference, may weaken considerably after the tragic Angela Corder case (Annas, 1988, 23).

Some people opposed to this way of thinking emphasize the necessity of the voluntary and informed consent of the pregnant woman, prior to the performance of fetal research or therapy. The right to make a mistake should continue to be the pregnant woman's, not the physician's or the judge's (Elias, 1983).

EUGENICS: A GOAL OR A CONSEQUENCE OF PRENATAL DIAGNOSIS?

Some would reject the binary thinking implicit in this section title's question. Canadian medical geneticists, responding to the study mentioned earlier in this chapter, gave low ranking to eugenics as a future ethical concern (Roy, 1989, 136). Indeed, there is little evidence to support the possible suspicion that genetic counsellors and medical geneticists are motivated by any eugenic goal in their daily work, particularly if eugenics refers to efforts to improve the quality of the human species. The individual-family perspective, not the population or species perspective, sets the framework generally for genetic services in Canada.

Discussions of eugenics are complex and fraught with pitfalls, because the term has many meanings and is heavy with historical associations to programmes of racially inspired and extraordinary evil (Kevles, 1985; Adams, 1990; Proctor, 1988; Roll-Hansen, 1988). Discussion in this section will focus on two dimensions of eugenics, and we see these as linked in the contemporary context of genetic counselling and prenatal diagnosis. One dimension is eugenics as the cumulative effect of the free workings of parental choice, in response to the availability of prenatal diagnosis technology. The other dimension is eugenics, pursued as an aim by those who see the reduction of birth rates of those with genetic diseases in the population, and a related reduction of societal costs involved in the cure of genetically and congenitally disabled people, as the goal of prenatal diagnosis.

Some would define eugenics as any effort to interfere with individuals' procreative choices, in order to attain a societal goal (Holtzman, 1989, 223). Eugenics, however, can result from the free workings of parental choice. There is no need for a state-inspired and state-organized and, by implication, coercive eugenics programme, if voluntary parental uptake and utilization of prenatal diagnosis, with selective abortion of fetuses found to be defective, will, for all practical purposes, achieve the same result.

It is difficult to avoid recognizing that the cumulative effect of individual parental decisions for selective abortion, on the basis of fetal indications, amounts to a eugenic trend in modern societies (Roy, 1989, 136). In this sense, eugenics, as E.A. Murphy has written, seems to be used more and more to refer to short-term gains, namely avoidance of genetic disease in the current generation (Murphy, 1978).

The term "avoidance of genetic disease in the current generation" merits a moment of reflection. Ethics requires the very careful use of language, particularly, a scrupulous refusal to use words and terms that mask the reality of which we are trying to speak, or that cover with a mantle of respectability actions we know are morally dubious, or at least morally controversial in society. "Prevention of disease" is a highly respectable term used for an often-neglected, but high-priority, medical and social goal. People have often spoken of prenatal diagnosis as leading to the prevention of genetic disease, when what they are really talking about is selective abortion after prenatal diagnosis, to avoid the births of babies affected with genetic disorders and congenital anomalies. Real prevention of genetic disorders is only possible by reducing the rate of mutations that cause genetic defects, and this kind of prevention is limited to mutations that have not yet occurred (Edwards, 1988, 213).

The "now-generation" eugenics we are talking about results from the free working of parental choice, and of parental desire for a normal, healthy child. But the notions of "quality control," of "lives not worth living," and of "thresholds of intolerable differences among human beings" are tacitly operative in the free workings of parental choice responding to prenatal diagnosis. Prenatal diagnosis, as Abby Lippman observes, *is* a means of separating fetuses we wish to develop from those we wish to discontinue. Are children, in this context, not seen as consumer objects, subject to quality control? (Lippman, 1991)

Ruth Hubbard, while not questioning a woman's right to have an abortion, detects an important difference between decisions about what *kind* of baby to bear and decisions about *whether* to bear a baby at all. The former decisions, in her view, are bedeviled by unspoken judgments about which lives "are worth living," and about "who should and who should not inhabit the world." (Hubbard, 1985; Hubbard, 1986)

The first lesson of genetics, Albert Jacquard has emphasized, is that individuals are all different, and cannot be classified, evaluated, or placed on a hierarchy (Jacquard, 1984). That is not the first lesson of prenatal diagnosis, as it has functioned in Western societies over the last quarter-century. The practice of prenatal diagnosis has taught that there are differences between human beings, differences in quality and value that some people find intolerable and that, in their view, justify selective abortion. Leaving all decisions to the discretion of parents, Angus Clarke stresses, indicates the low value our society places upon those with genetic disorders and handicaps (Clarke, 1991). The justification of this charge rests with the question of how free parental choice for selective abortion after prenatal diagnosis can really be, if we have societally decided that the costs of caring for those who differ from the normal are too much to bear. Cost-efficiency considerations seem to make it advisable, as Benno Müller-

Hill has perceived, for both parents and state, to destroy the cost-intensive embryo and fetus (Müller-Hill, 1987).

How will those with genetic diseases and congenital disorders, if they escape spontaneous or selective abortion, come to be seen in our society? Leon Kass fears they may be seen as persons who need not have been, and who would not have been, if only someone would have gotten to them on time (Kass, 1973, 189). It may well be true that only constant reinforcement of tolerance for differences will prevent such tragic eugenic devaluation of human beings (Holtzman, 1989, 228). But who will reinforce this tolerance for differences, if no one has the perception and the social courage to define the threshold beyond which selective abortions are intolerable? (Clarke, 1991, 998, 1000)

REFERENCES

Adams M.B., ed. *The Wellborn Science: Eugenics in Germany, France, Brazil, and Russia.* New York: Oxford University Press, 1990.

Annas G.J. "She's Going to Die: The Case of Angela C." *Hastings Center Report 1988*;18:23-25.

Antley R.M. "The Genetic Counselor as Facilitator of the Counselor's Decision Process." In: **A.M. Capron** et al., eds. *Genetic Counseling: Facts, Values, and Norms.* The National Foundation - March of Dimes Birth Defects: Original Article Series 1979:XV. New York: Alan R. Liss, 1979:137-168.

Bell J. "Prenatal Diagnosis: Current Status and Future Trends." In: Ciba Foundation Symposium *Human Genetic Information: Science, Law and Ethics.* Chichester, New York, Toronto: John Wiley & Sons, 1990:18-36.

Benzie R.J. "Antenatal Genetic Diagnosis: Current Status and Future Prospects." *Canadian Medical Association Journal* 1979;120:685-692.

Canadian College of Medical Geneticists *Professional and Ethical Guidelines.* Ottawa: CCMG, 1986.

Clarke A. "Is Nondirective Genetic Counselling Possible?" *Lancet* 1991;338:998-1001.

Critser E.S. "Preimplantation Genetics." *Archives of Pathology and Laboratory Medicine* 1992;116:383-387.

Dickens B.M. "Prenatal Diagnosis and Female Abortion: A Case Study in Medical Law and Ethics." *Journal of Medical Ethics* 1986;12:143-144, 150.

Dyck A.J. "Ethical Issues in Community and Research Medicine." *The New England Journal of Medicine* 1971;284:725-726.

Edwards J.H. "The Importance of Genetic Disease and the Need for Prevention." *Philosophical Transactions of the Royal Society of London* 1988;B319:211-227.

Elias S. and **Annas G.J.** "Perspectives in Fetal Surgery." *American Journal of Obstetrics and Gynecology* 1983;145:807-812.

Evans M.I. and **Shulman J.D.** "Medical Fetal Therapy." In: M.I. Evans et al., eds. *Fetal Diagnosis and Therapy. Science, Ethics, and the Law.* Philadelphia: J.B. Lippincott, 1989:403-412.

Evans M.I. et al. "Fetal Surgery in the 1990's." *American Journal of Diseases of Children* 1989;143:1431-1436.

Evans M.I. "Prenatal Diagnosis of Chromosomal and Mendelian Disorders." In: M.I. Evans et al., eds. Fetal Diagnosis and Therapy. Science, Ethics, and the Law. Philadelphia: J.B. Lippincott, 1989:17-36.

Firth H.V. et al. "Severe Limb Abnormalities after Chorion Villus Sampling at 55-56 Days' Gestation." *Lancet* 1991;337:762-763.

Fletcher J. *The Ethics of Genetic Control.* New York: Anchor Press/Doubleday, 1974.

Fletcher J.C. "Ethics and Human Genetics: A Cross-Cultural Perspective." In: D.C. Wertz and J.C. Fletcher, eds. Ethics and Human Genetics. A Cross-Cultural Perspective. New York: Springer-Verlag, 1989:457-490.

Fletcher J.C. "Ethics in Experimental Fetal Therapy: Is There an Early Consensus?" In: M.I. Evans et al., eds. *Fetal Diagnosis and Therapy. Science, Ethics and the Law.* Philadelphia: J.B. Lippincott, 1989:438-446.

Fraser F.C. "Introduction: The Development of Genetic Counseling." In: A.M. Capron et al., eds. *Genetic Counseling: Facts, Values, and Norms.* The National Foundation - March of Dimes Birth Defects: Original Article Series 1979:XV. New York: Alan R. Liss, 1979:5-15.

Grifo J.A. et al. "Preimplantation Genetic Diagnosis. In Situ Hybridization as a Tool for Analysis." *Archives of Pathology and Laboratory Medicine* 1992;116:393-397.

Halliday J.L. et al. "Importance of Complete Follow-up of Spontaneous Fetal Loss after Amniocentesis and Chorion Villus Sampling." *Lancet* 1992;340:886-896.

Handyside A.H. et al. "Birth of a Normal Girl after In Vitro Fertilization and Preimplant-ation Diagnostic Testing for Cystic Fibrosis." *The New England Journal of Medicine* 1992;327:905-909.

Hardy K. and **Handyside A.H.** "Biopsy of Cleavage Stage Human Embryos and Diagnosis of Single Gene Defects by DNA Amplification." *Archives of Pathology and Laboratory Medicine* 1992;116:388-392.

Harrison M.R. "Successful Repair in Utero of a Fetal Diaphragmatic Hernia after Removal of Herniated Viscera from the Left Thorax." *The New England Journal of Medicine* 1990;322:1582-1584.

Harrison M.R. "Unborn: Historical Perspective of the Fetus as Patient." *Pharos* 1982;45:19-24.

Holtzman N.A. *Proceed with Caution: Predicting Genetic Risks in the Recombinant DNA Era.* Baltimore, London: The Johns Hopkins University Press, 1989.

Hsia Y.E. "The Genetic Counselor as Information Giver." In: A.M. Capron et al., eds. *Genetic Counseling: Facts, Values, and Norms.* The National Foundation - March of Dimes Birth Defects: Original Article Series 1979:XV. New York: Alan R. Liss, 1979:169-186.

Hubbard R. "Eugenics and Prenatal Testing." *International Journal of Health Services* 1986;16:227-242.

Hubbard R. "Prenatal Diagnosis and Eugenic Ideology." *Women's Studies International Forum* 1985;8:567-576.

Jackson L.G. et al. "A Randomized Comparison of Transcervical and Transabdominal Chorionic Villus Sampling." *The New England Journal of Medicine* 1992;327:594-598.

Jacquard A. *In Praise of Difference. Genetics and Human Affairs.* New York: Columbia University Press, 1984. Translation by M.M. Moriarty of the French original: *Éloge de la différence.* Paris: Éditions du Seuil, 1978.

Kass L.R. "Implications of Prenatal Diagnosis for the Human Right to Life." In: B. Hilton et al., eds. *Ethical Issues in Human Genetics. Genetic Counseling and the Use of Genetic Knowledge.* New York: Plenum Press, 1973:185-199.

Kessler S. "The Genetic Counselor as Psychotherapist." In: A.M. Capron et al., eds. *Genetic Counseling: Facts, Values, and Norms.* The National Foundation - March of Dimes Birth Defects: Original Article Series 1979:XV. New York: Alan R. Liss, 1979:187-200.

Kevles D.J. *In the Name of Eugenics: Genetics and the Uses of Human Heredity.* New York: Alfred A. Knopf, 1985.

Lejeune J. "General Discussion." In: B. Hilton et al., eds. *Ethical Issues in Human Genetics.* New York: Plenum Press, 1973:17-22.

Liley A.W. "Intrauterine Transfusion of Fetus in Hemolytic Disease." *British Medical Journal* 1963;2:1107-1109.

Lippman A. "Prenatal Genetic Testing and Screening: Constructing Needs and Reinforcing Inequities." *American Journal of Law and Medicine* 1991;XVII:15-50.

Longaker M.I. et al. "Maternal Outcome after Open Fetal Surgery. A Review of the First 17 Human Cases." *Journal of the American Medical Association* 1991;265:737-741.

Madlon-Kay D.J. et al. "Maternal Serum Alpha-Fetoprotein Testing: Physician Experience and Attitudes and their Influence on Patient Acceptance." *The Journal of Family Practice* 1992;35:395-400.

McKusick V.A. "Current Trends in Mapping Human Genes." *Faseb Journal* 1991; 5:12-20.

McKusick V.A. *Mendelian Inheritance in Man: Catalogs of Autosomal Dominant, Autosomal Recessive, and X-Linked Phenotypes.* 9th Edition. Baltimore: The John Hopkins University Press, 1990.

Modell B. "Ethical Aspects of Genetic Screening." *Annals of Medicine* 1992;24:549-555.

Modell B. "Social Aspects of Prenatal Monitoring for Genetic Disease." In: H. Galjaard, ed. *The Future of Prenatal Diagnoses.* Edinburgh, London, Melbourne, New York: Churchill Livingstone, 1982:145-159.

Morison R.S. "Implications of Prenatal Diagnosis for the Quality of, and Right to, Human Life: Society as a Standard." In: B. Hilton et al., eds. *Ethical Issues in Human Genetics.* New York: Plenum Press, 1973:210-211.

Motulsky A.G. "Brave New World?" *Science* 1974;185:653-663.

Motulsky A.G. "Public Health and Long-Term Genetic Implications of Intrauterine Diagnosis and Selective Abortion." *Birth Defects: Original Article Series* April 1971;7:22-32.

MRC Working Party on the Evaluation of Chorion Villus Sampling "Medical Research Council European Trial of Chorion Villus Sampling." *Lancet* 1991:337:1491-1499.

Mullis K.B. "The Unusual Origin of the Polymerase Chain Reaction." *Scientific American* 1990;262:56-65.

Müller-Hill B. "Genetics after Auschwitz." *Holocaust and Genocide Studies* 1987;2:3-20.

Murphy E.A. "Eugenics: An Ethical Analysis." *Mayo Clinic Proceedings* 1978;53:655-664.

Ney J.A. et al. "Perinatal Outcome Following Intravascular Transfusion in Severely Isoimmunized Fetuses." *International Journal of Gynecology and Obstetrics* 1991;35:41-46.

Pembrey M. "Prenatal Diagnosis: Healthier, Wealthier, and Wiser?" In: D.J. Roy, B.E. Wynne and R.W. Old, eds. *Bioscience — Society.* Chichester, New York, Toronto: John Wiley & Sons, 1991:53-66.

Powledge T.M. and **Sollitto S.** "Prenatal Diagnosis - The Past and The Future." *Hastings Center Report* 1974;4:11-13.

Proctor N. *Racial Hygiene: Medicine under the Nazis.* Cambridge, Mass.: Harvard University Press, 1988.

Robertson J.A. "Ethical and Legal Issues in Preimplantation Genetic Screening." *Fertility and Sterility* 1992;57:1-11.

Robertson J.A. "Legal Issues in Fetal Therapy." In: M.I. Evans et al., eds. *Fetal Diagnosis and Therapy. Science, Ethics, and the Law.* Philadelphia: J.B. Lippincott, 1989: 431-437.

Robertson J.A. "The Right to Procreate and In Utero Fetal Therapy." *Journal of Legal Medicine* 1982;3:333-366.

Roll-Hansen N. "The Progress of Eugenics: Growth of Knowledge and Change in Ideology." *History of Science* 1988;26:295-331.

Rosner F. et al. "Fetal Therapy and Surgery. Fetal Rights Versus Maternal Obligations." *New York State Journal of Medicine* 1989;89:80-84.

Roy D.J. and **Hall J.G.** "Ethics and Medical Genetics in Canada." In: D.C. Wertz and J.C. Fletcher, eds. *Ethics and Human Genetics. A Cross-Cultural Perspective.* New York: Springer-Verlag, 1989:119-140.

Royal College of Physicians "Prenatal Diagnosis and Genetic Screening. Summary and Recommendations of a Report of the Royal College of Physicians." *Journal of the Royal College of Physicians of London* 1989;23:215-220.

Ruddick W. and **Wilcox W.** "Operating on the Fetus." *Hastings Center Report* 1982;12:10-14.

Salvesen K.A. "Routine Ultrasonography In Utero and School Performance at Age 8-9 Years." *Lancet* 1992;339:85-89.

Schulman J.D. "Treatment of the Embryo and the Fetus in the First Trimester: Current Status and Future Prospects." *American Journal of Medical Genetics* 1990;35:197-200.

Scriver C.R. "Window Panes of Eternity. Health, Disease, and Inherited Risk." *The Yale Journal of Biology and Medicine* 1982;55:487-513.

Sheppard D. et al. "Mutations in CFTR Associated with Mild-Disease-Form Cl-channels with Altered Pore Properties." *Nature* 1993;362:160-164.

Simpson J.L. and **Carson S.A.** "Preimplantation Genetic Diagnosis." *The New England Journal of Medicine* 1992;327:951-953.

Sorenson J.R. and **Culbert A.J.** "Professional Orientations to Contemporary Genetic Counseling." In: A.M. Capron et al., eds. *Genetic Counseling: Facts, Values, and Norms.* The National Foundation - March of Dimes Birth Defects: Original Article Series 1979:XV. New York: Alan R. Liss, 1979:85-102.

Stephenson S.R. and **Weaver D.D.** "Prenatal Diagnosis - A Compilation of Diagnosed Conditions." *American Journal of Obstetrics and Gynecology* 1981;141:319-343.

Twiss S.B. "The Genetic Counselor as Moral Advisor." In: A.M. Capron et al., eds. *Genetic Counseling: Facts, Values, and Norms.* The National Foundation - March of Dimes Birth Defects: Original Article Series 1979:XV. New York: Alan R. Liss, 1979:201-212.

Walters L. "Ethical Issues in Maternal Serum Alpha-Fetoprotein Testing and Screening: A Reappraisal." In: M.I. Evans et al., eds. *Fetal Diagnosis and Therapy. Science, Ethics and the Law.* Philadelphia: J.B. Lippincott, 1989:54-60.

Warnock M. "Ethical Challenges in Embryo Manipulation." *British Medical Journal* 1992;304:1045-1049.

Weiner C.P. et al. "Management of Fetal Hemolytic Disease by Cordocentesis. II. Outcome of Treatment." *American Journal of Obstetrics and Gynecology* 1991;165:1302-1307.

Wertz D.C. and **Fletcher J.** "Fatal Knowledge? Prenatal Diagnosis and Sex Selection." *Hastings Center Report* 1989;19:21-27.

8

WHEN PEOPLE DO NOT WANT A CHILD: ABORTION

Abortion can be defined as the deliberate termination of a pregnancy, resulting in the intentional death of the fetus, prior to normal or spontaneous delivery. It has been the most controversial ethical and legal issue in Canada and the United States during the past twenty-five years, and there is little sign that this is about to change. In this chapter, we will identify the major ethical and legal aspects of abortion, and describe the range of positions on this issue in contemporary Canadian society. The purpose of this chapter is not to argue for any one of these positions against the others, but to provide you with the information you need to develop and defend your own position.

HISTORY

Ancient and Medieval Times

Abortion has been practised since the beginning of human history. A recipe for an abortifacient potion is contained in a Chinese text from approximately 2600 B.C.E.. In ancient Greece and Rome, both abortion and infanticide were widely accepted. The two most influential Greek philosophers, Plato (427-347 B.C.E.) and Aristotle (384-322 B.C.E.), recommended abortion as a way of limiting the population. On the other hand, the famous Greek physician Hippocrates, whose teachings

form the basis of the Hippocratic Oath, which is still upheld by many doctors, for-
bade participation in abortion by medical practitioners (Carrick, 1985).

From the beginning of the common era until the twentieth century, the
debate over the morality of abortion in the Western world was conducted predominantly by religious scholars and organizations. Philosophers, physicians,
and other health care workers contributed relatively little to this discussion from
their academic and professional experience. Any historical account of abortion
must, therefore, concentrate on religious teachings.

In the Hebrew Bible (the Christian Old Testament), there is no direct mention
of abortion. Jewish scholars in the first centuries of the Christian era argued among
themselves whether certain scriptural passages could be applied to abortion, but
they never came to a consensus on this matter. The Jewish faith has always permitted a range of interpretations about the morality of abortion (Feldman, 1978).

The early Christians took quite a different view. They were repelled by the
prevailing Greek and Roman attitudes to sexuality and reproduction, and they
developed a strict code of ethics to regulate their own behaviour on these matters. One of the earliest Christian documents, the *Didache* or *Teachings of the
Twelve Apostles*, prohibited the following deeds: killing, adultery, sexual relations
with young boys, fornication, stealing, magic, and abortion. Other condemna-
tions of abortion can be found in the writings of early Church authorities, such
as Clement of Alexandria, Tertullian, and Augustine (Noonan, 1970, 7-18).
These and later Christian leaders associated abortion with contraception and
other non-procreative sexual practices, and condemned them all for the same
reason: the sole legitimate purpose of sex was reproduction. The sixth-century
Bishop of Arles, Caesarius, makes this very clear in a text that was to exercise
great influence on subsequent Church teaching:

> ... no woman may take a potion so that she is unable to conceive ... As often as
> she could have conceived or given birth, of that many homicides she will be
> held guilty, and, unless she undergoes suitable penance, she will be damned by
> eternal death in hell. If a woman does not wish to have children, let her enter
> into a religious agreement with her husband; for chastity is the sole sterility of a
> Christian woman (Harrison, 1983, 293).

Despite this severe condemnation of non-procreative sex, abortion was not a
major preoccupation of the Christian Church for the first fourteen centuries of
its existence. One reason for this may be that there is no reference to it in the
New Testament.

Transition to Modern Times

When Christian moralists did begin to consider abortion seriously, beginning in
the fifteenth century, they did not condemn it unequivocally. Among the factors
to be taken into account when judging the morality of a particular abortion deci-

sion or act, two were, and still are, of special importance: (a) the stage of development of the fetus, and (b) the medical condition of the mother. Until the nineteenth century, it was believed that the fetus did not receive its human soul until some time after conception (generally considered to be forty days for males and eighty days for females). Abortion before this point was wrong, but no more so than contraception, which was now judged much more leniently than in previous times. After "ensoulment," however, it was far more serious. Nevertheless, even in the later stages of pregnancy, it could still be justified in order to save the life of the mother.

The Nineteenth Century: Abortion Under Attack

During the nineteenth century, the Protestant churches did not consider abortion to be a significant moral issue. With the development of biological science, however, the Roman Catholic Church's understanding of ensoulment changed, and so did its teaching on abortion. From the time of Pope Pius IX (1846-78) onwards, this church has taught that ensoulment takes place at conception. Consequently, it has condemned abortion, at any stage, as equivalent to murder. The only exceptions that might be justified are in those cases where both the fetus and the mother will die unless the fetus is killed (for example, if the pregnancy is ectopic* or if the uterus is cancerous). Such procedures have been justified by invoking the principle of "double effect," according to which a bad result (or "effect") of an action can be tolerated, if it is an unavoidable and unintended consequence of an attempt to achieve a good result. In the case of these abortions, the goal of the procedures is to save the life of the pregnant woman, not to kill the fetus. Since there is no other way to achieve this goal, and failure to act will result in the death of both mother and fetus, the operations are not immoral even though the fetus is killed in the process (McCormick, 1981, 413-429).

The Roman Catholic Church was not the only source of the growing opposition to abortion in the nineteenth century. In England, the U.S.A., and Canada, increasingly restrictive legislation was passed, which prohibited abortion at all stages of pregnancy, except when the life of the mother was endangered. Such legislation was encouraged by the medical profession, which, during this period, was attempting to extend its domain to include all aspects of human reproduction. The American Medical Association, in particular, was strongly opposed to abortion, and was instrumental in convincing most states to introduce laws against this practice (Melton, 1989, xxi). Both law and medicine concurred with the Roman Catholic Church's association of abortion with contraception. Since

---

*An ectopic pregnancy occurs when a fertilized ovum, instead of passing through the fallopian tube and descending into the uterus, is trapped in the tube and begins to grow there. If the embryo continues to develop, the tube will eventually burst, resulting in the death of the embryo, and possibly of the mother as well.

these practices were considered to be immoral and unhealthy, it was not surprising that they, too, were made illegal.

The Twentieth Century: Pluralism and Conflict

This religious, legal, and medical consensus on abortion began to weaken in the
first half of the twentieth century, and it has been almost completely destroyed
since the 1960s. The emergence of women as a major political force in the 1920s
and 1930s brought about rapid changes in social policies on family planning. The
medical profession began to support birth control, and most Protestant churches
adopted a similar position. In the 1960s, the introduction of the birth control
pill confirmed the separability of sexual intercourse and reproduction. Along with
other social factors, this medical advance contributed to a rapid relaxation of the
standards of sexual behaviour throughout the Western world.

Contrary to popular expectations, the birth control pill and other methods
of contraception did not eliminate, or even diminish, the problem of unwanted
pregnancies. Consequently, there arose in the 1960s a powerful movement in
favour of abortion. Among the arguments put forth to support its legalization
were the following:

- women should have the *right* to control their fertility; restrictions on abortion are no more justified than laws that discriminate against individuals on
  the basis of race or colour;

- thousands of women suffer injury, or even death, while undergoing illegal
  abortions;

- abortion is primarily a *moral* issue; in a pluralistic society individuals should
  be free to make their own moral decisions, as long as they do not infringe
  the rights of other individuals.

Although the Roman Catholic Church, some conservative Protestant
churches, and Orthodox Jews and Muslims lobbied against the legalization of
abortion for any reason other than to save the life of the mother, this position
was rejected by most Protestant churches, women's organizations, and medical
and legal associations. In 1967, the Parliament of the United Kingdom passed a
law permitting abortion upon request, if the continuation of the pregnancy
would involve risk to the life or the health (mental or physical) of the woman.
Canada followed suit in 1969, with its own abortion law (see below) and, in
1973, the Supreme Court of the U.S.A. ruled, in *Roe v. Wade*, that the government had no authority to restrict abortion during the first three months of pregnancy, and in the next three months could only regulate it to protect the
woman's health. Most other Western countries adopted comparable laws during
the 1970s and 1980s. The principal exceptions are Belgium, which changed its
law only in 1990, and Ireland, where the ban against abortion was incorporated

into the nation's constitution in 1983 (Law Reform Commission, 1989, 67-77).

The legalization of abortion had the predictable consequence of increasing the reported number of abortions in the first few years after the changes in the law. In Canada, there were 11,152 abortions reported in 1970, the year the new law came into force. This number increased to 30,923 in 1971, and climbed steadily to 75,071 in 1982. During the next few years, the total declined slightly (to 72,693 in 1988). However, after the 1988 Supreme Court decision that is described in the next section, abortions increased once again (to just over 94,000 in 1990).

In Canada, as in almost every Western country, the availability of legal abortion has been welcomed by the medical and nursing professions, by most Protestant churches, and by large segments of the general public. Although none of these groups favours abortion for its own sake, they all see it as, in many instances, the lesser of two evils, the other one being the continuation of an unwanted pregnancy. Individuals differ sharply on what they consider to be acceptable reasons for abortion in specific cases. Most are in favour when the pregnancy poses a serious danger to the life or the health of the mother, when conception takes place as a result of rape or incest, when the mother is in her early teens, or when the fetus has been diagnosed as having a severe and untreatable illness. There is less agreement on abortion for socioeconomic reasons, when there is a possibility of a handicapped child, or in cases of contraceptive failure. In the Western world, there is great resistance to abortion because the child is not of the desired gender, although this is a major factor in some cultural groups. The Roman Catholic Church and conservative Protestant groups reject abortion for all these reasons, although an exception may be made in cases where the mother is likely to die if the pregnancy is not terminated.

Despite the widespread legalization and practice of abortion, its opponents have not given up. They hope that, by promoting public recognition of the fetus as a human being with the same right to life as those who have been born, they will be able to convince legislators to reverse the permissive laws that have been adopted during the past twenty-five years. As a result of their efforts, abortion continues to be a hotly debated moral and legal issue in most Western countries. It is impossible to predict what the outcome of this debate will be in another twenty-five, or even ten, years from now.

ABORTION AS A LEGAL ISSUE

The 1969 Canadian Abortion Law

As mentioned above, the Canadian abortion law was revised in 1969. The previous law had been in force since 1892. It made abortion punishable by life imprisonment, unless it was performed to save the mother's life or permanent health. In the late 1960s, the Government of Canada decided to revise those sections of the *Criminal Code* that dealt with homosexuality, divorce, contraception, and abortion. After several years of parliamentary debate and public hearings, the proposed changes were adopted in August 1969. The new abortion law (section 251 of the *Criminal Code*) retained the penalty of life imprisonment for anyone who tried to perform an abortion, and a two-year sentence for women seeking to be aborted. In legal terms, the reforms were more apparent than real (Dickens, 1981), but conditions were created to establish the legality of abortion before it was performed. These conditions were the following:

- the abortion had to be performed by a qualified medical practitioner in an accredited or approved hospital;
- it had to be approved by the therapeutic abortion committee of the hospital;
- the sole grounds for approval were that the continuation of the pregnancy would or would be likely to endanger the life or health of the woman seeking abortion.

Soon after the law was passed, problems arose in its application. To begin with, many hospitals that were eligible to do so refused to establish therapeutic abortion committees, and so abortions were not performed there. Secondly, some committees interpreted the phrase, "would or would be likely to endanger the life or health of the woman," quite strictly and, as a result, approved very few requests for abortion. Other committees took a much more permissive approach, and almost always granted the requests. Finally, the committee system usually produced delays that resulted in more complex and dangerous abortion procedures being used. All these problems were described in the 1977 *Report of the Committee on the Operation of the Abortion Law* (Badgeley, 1977), which was established by the federal government to recommend changes in the application of the law. However, no changes were implemented in the decade following the publication of this report.

Challenges to the Law

Henry Morgentaler

Dissatisfied with the government's failure to revise what they considered to be a bad law, both proponents and opponents of legalized abortion in Canada decided to challenge the law in the courts. The first major confrontation took place in Montréal in 1970, when Dr. Henry Morgentaler established a clinic solely for performing abortions. This was in clear opposition to the provision of the law that restricted the procedure to hospitals with therapeutic abortion committees.

Dr. Morgentaler was arrested and tried three times on charges of performing an illegal abortion, and each time he was found not guilty by a jury. In an appeal following the first jury acquittal, the Québec Court of Appeal reversed the acquittal and convicted; the Supreme Court of Canada ruled in 1975 that power to do that existed, and Dr. Morgentaler was imprisoned. When courts' power to convict following jury acquittal was removed, Dr. Morgentaler was released and ordered retried, resulting in a third jury acquittal. After the third acquittal in 1976, the Québec government allowed his clinic to operate in open violation of the law.

In 1983, Dr. Morgentaler set up an abortion clinic in Toronto, and was promptly arrested and charged, along with two other doctors, with conspiracy to perform illegal abortions. Once again, a jury found the defendants not guilty. This decision was appealed and, on October 1, 1985, the Ontario Court of Appeal overturned the decision of the jury and ordered a new trial. Dr. Morgentaler then appealed this ruling to the Supreme Court of Canada. On January 28, 1988, in a five-to-two decision, this Court overturned the Court of Appeal decision, and restored the original jury acquittal of the three defendants. At the same time, the Supreme Court declared that the abortion law, as amended in 1969, was unconstitutional and, therefore, no longer in effect.

The Court based this ruling on the 1982 *Canadian Charter of Rights and Freedoms*, especially section 7: "Everyone has the right to life, liberty and security of the person and the right not to be deprived thereof except in accordance with the principles of fundamental justice." Chief Justice Dickson found that the requirement of the law that abortions can only be performed in certain hospitals, and only with the approval of a therapeutic abortion committee

> clearly interferes with a woman's bodily integrity in both a physical and emotional sense. Forcing a woman, by threat of criminal sanction, to carry a fetus to term unless she meets certain criteria unrelated to her own priorities and aspirations, is a profound interference with a woman's body and thus a violation of security of the person ... the operation of the decision-making mechanism set out in s. 251 [of the *Criminal Code*] creates additional glaring breaches of security of the person. The evidence indicates that s. 251 causes a certain amount of delay for women who are successful in meeting its criteria. In the context of abortion, any unnecessary delay can have profound consequences on the woman's physical and emotional well-being. (*R. v. Morgentaler*, 1988, 402)

For various reasons, the Court concluded that the abortion law offended against the principles of fundamental justice and, therefore, its restrictions on the security of the pregnant woman's person were not justified.

Although the Court declared the abortion law inoperative in its entirety, it did suggest that Parliament might formulate a new law that could restrict the availability of abortion in the interests of the fetus. However, it declined to deal with the question as to whether a fetus is included in the word "everyone" in section 7 of the *Charter*, so as to have a right to "life, liberty and security of the person."

Joe Borowski

The Supreme Court of Canada has also dealt with challenges to the abortion law from opponents of abortion. In 1981, the Court allowed Joe Borowski, a well-known campaigner against abortion from Winnipeg, to challenge the abortion law on behalf of the unborn child. The case was argued before the Saskatchewan Court of Queen's Bench in 1983, shortly after the *Charter* came into effect. In its judgment, the Court rejected Joe Borowski's contention that the fetus is a person and, therefore, falls within the definition of "everyone" in the *Charter*. The judgment states:

> Although rapid advances in medical science may make it socially desirable that some legal status be extended to fetuses, irrespective of ultimate viability, it is the prerogative of Parliament, and not the courts, to enact whatever legislation may be considered appropriate to extend to the unborn any or all legal rights possessed by living persons. Because there is no existing basis in law which justifies a conclusion that fetuses are legal persons, and therefore within the scope of the term "everyone" utilized in the Charter, the claim of the plaintiff must be dismissed (*Borowski v. Attorney General Canada*, 1983, 131).

This judgment, upheld by the provincial Court of Appeal, was also appealed to the Supreme Court of Canada, which heard the case in 1988, nine months after its decision in the Morgentaler case. The Supreme Court held that there was no longer an issue to decide under the *Criminal Code*'s provision on abortion, because the Court had held it inoperative in the earlier case.

Jean-Guy Tremblay

In August 1989, the Supreme Court dealt with a third abortion-related case, this one having to do with a father's right to prevent an abortion. On July 7, 1989, Jean-Guy Tremblay, the ex-boyfriend of Chantal Daigle, obtained a temporary injunction from a Québec Superior Court judge, preventing her from having an abortion. Ms. Daigle, who was eighteen weeks pregnant at the time, reappeared before the Québec Superior Court on July 17, at which time another judge maintained the injunction. He stated that, according to the Québec *Charter of Rights* and sections of the *Civil Code* of Québec, a fetus is a human being with legal rights, and is entitled to protection under the law. Ms. Daigle then appealed this judgment to the Québec Court of Appeal. On July 26, in a three-to-two decision, this Court reaffirmed the injunction, with each of the judges giving separate reasons for decision. A request was then made to the Supreme Court of

Canada to allow an appeal. The request was granted and, on August 8, the full Court heard the case and rendered their unanimous verdict, which was to quash the injunction. The reason given for this decision was that, in neither the *Charter* nor the *Code*, is the fetus included within the term "human being." In this respect, the legal status of the fetus is the same in Québec as elsewhere in Canada, where a child must be born alive to enjoy rights.

A New Law?

As a result of these decisions, Canada has been without a criminal abortion law since January 1988, and has no penal sanction to protect the fetus. The federal government proposed three alternative laws to Parliament in July 1988, but none of them received a majority vote, and the issue was set aside until after the fall-1988 federal election.

In order to guide Parliament in formulating a new abortion law, the Law Reform Commission of Canada published a document entitled *Crimes Against the Fetus* in January 1989. The Commission recommended that abortion be, once again, made a criminal offence for both the pregnant woman and the one performing the procedure. Exceptions would be allowed under certain conditions, and the document provided three different proposals to legalize abortion. The majority position was that the crime of destroying a fetus should not apply to acts done before the twenty-second week of pregnancy to protect the mother's physical or psychological health, or after the twenty-second week to save her life or to protect her against serious physical injury, or because the fetus suffers from an incurable and terminal medical condition. The second position was identical to the first, except that abortion would be allowed for any reason up to twelve weeks. The third position would have permitted abortion only to save the pregnant woman's life, or to protect her against serious and substantial danger to her health.

When the federal government did finally introduce its proposed abortion legislation, in the fall of 1989, it did not adopt the Law Reform Commission's recommendation, to make abortion easier to obtain in the earlier stages of pregnancy and harder in the later ones. Instead, abortion would be permitted at any stage, as long as it was performed by a doctor "who is of the opinion that, if the abortion were not induced, the health or life of the female person would be likely to be threatened." Health was defined as including physical, mental, and psychological aspects. All other abortions would be illegal, and punishable by a prison term of up to two years. On May 29, 1990, the House of Commons approved this bill by a vote of 140 to 131. It was then sent to the Senate, which gave it lengthy consideration. On January 31, 1991, the bill was put to a vote, and the result was a tie, 43 to 43. Under Senate rules, a tie is considered not to be approval of a bill. The government's reaction was to declare that it would not introduce any new abortion legislation during the remaining two to three years of its current mandate.

ABORTION AS AN ETHICAL ISSUE

Few, if any, people today are indifferent to abortion. There is widespread agreement that it is an ethical issue, a matter of right or wrong, both at the individual level and at the level of law and public policy. It involves a great many ethical questions, only some of which can be dealt with here. We will begin by examining the relationship of law and ethics, insofar as this affects the evaluation of abortion. Next, we will deal with the status of the fetus. We will then discuss and evaluate the reasons why women seek abortion. A fourth important question is who should make decisions about this matter. Finally, we will investigate alternatives to abortion.

Law and Ethics

In Chapter 3, we discussed the relationship of law and ethics in general. There we saw that not every immoral action should be illegal. The Law Reform Commission of Canada, in its document, *Crimes Against the Fetus*, proposed a set of criteria for acts that should be prohibited by the *Criminal Code*:

- such an act should seriously harm other people, or so seriously contravene our fundamental values in some other way as to be harmful to society;

- the enforcement measures necessary for using criminal law against the act should not themselves seriously contravene our fundamental values;

- criminal law should make a significant contribution to dealing with the problem (Law Reform Commission, 1989, 32)

According to these criteria, the Commission believed that abortion should be criminalized, but not absolutely. In some situations, for example, where the life, health, or safety of the pregnant woman is endangered, use of the criminal law against abortion may seriously contravene fundamental values of life, liberty, and security of the person.

Many Canadians accept these criteria, but come to quite a different conclusion on abortion than the Law Reform Commission. They are not convinced that legalized abortion seriously contravenes our fundamental values. They point to the absence of a criminal abortion law in Canada since January 1988, and see no evidence that society is any worse off as a result. Moreover, they note that the Supreme Court struck down the 1969 abortion law because it was not equitable, and they feel that any such law is bound to be inequitable, in that it will be easier for wealthy women to have abortions (if necessary, by going to another country) than for poor women. Finally, they argue that the criminalization of abortion will give rise to even greater evils, namely unsafe illegal abortions or unwanted children.

It is possible to be opposed to abortion on *moral* grounds, and yet not be in favour of its criminalization. On the other hand, advocates of unborn children are convinced that society must state, in the strongest possible terms, that abortion is no more justifiable than the killing of children or adults, and that criminal sanctions are needed to enforce this conviction. These two extreme positions are rejected by many individuals and groups, as by the Law Reform Commission. They believe that abortion should not, or can not, be outlawed altogether, but the law should indicate that society regards abortion with disfavour and should allow it only under certain specified conditions. This lack of agreement on the role of law in a pluralistic society such as Canada is a major obstacle to the formulation of public policy on abortion. It is by no means the only such obstacle, however. As we shall see, the Canadian public is divided on almost every aspect of this issue.

Status of the Fetus

It is an oversimplification to say that the ethical problem of abortion is the conflict between the rights of the fetus and those of the pregnant woman. Nevertheless, the debate has often taken this form, with advocates of fetal rights being opposed to abortion and advocates of women's rights being in favour. The goal of ethics is to enhance the rights of all parties, and then to balance them if they are in competition. We will begin here with the fetus.

The principal right that is in question is the right of the fetus to life, or more precisely, its right not to be killed. Whether the fetus actually has such a right depends, to a large extent, on what sort of being it is. There are three principal positions on this matter:

- the fetus is a human being from conception, with the same right to life as any other living human being;
- the fetus gradually develops as a human being; as it does, its right to life comes into existence and increases until it is equal to that of living human beings (either at birth or when it becomes capable of independent survival outside the mother);
- the fetus only becomes a human being at birth; before that, it has no rights (this is the traditional Common law definition).

The third ethical position is almost universally regarded as unsatisfactory today. The major debate is between proponents of the first and second positions. As we saw earlier, this debate has been going on since the beginning of the common era. Although the issue is no longer the time of ensoulment, there is still fundamental disagreement about what it means to become fully human, and when that occurs.

Proponents of the first position believe that conception marks the beginning of an individual human being that has all the necessary genetic material to develop into a living human person. They can see no point in the growth of the fetus where it "becomes" the possessor of the right to life; therefore that right must be there from conception.

Those who hold the second position believe that the union of a human sperm and ovum is not enough to constitute a fully human person, with the same right to life as one who has been born. In the first two weeks after conception, a large percentage of conceptuses (possibly over 50%) perish of natural causes; others divide into twins, and sometimes two of them fuse together to make a single individual. Even after the fetus is fully formed (at eight weeks), it cannot survive on its own until at least twenty weeks after conception. For these reasons, many people believe that the right to life of the fetus, while not nonexistent, is still not equal to that of those who have been born.

All efforts to settle this debate have, so far, been unsuccessful. Both sides use scientific, philosophical, and theological arguments to support their positions. But, with rare exceptions, the arguments on one side have failed to convince those who are on the other side. Both groups have managed to make new converts from the previously undecided, and so the disagreement continues, with no resolution in sight.

Why Women Want Abortion

For those who consider the right to life of the fetus to be absolute, there are no acceptable reasons for abortion. For all others, however, the woman's feelings about her pregnancy are an important, if not a decisive, factor in judging the morality of abortion. What, then, are the reasons why it is sought by so many women?

The overriding reason, of course, is that the pregnancy is unwanted. Here, it is important to distinguish between the pregnancy and the child. If it were simply a matter of not wanting to have a child, it would still be possible to continue the pregnancy, give birth, and then give the child up for adoption. The decision to abort involves not just the rejection of parenthood, but also of gestation. Among the reasons for making this choice are the following:

- the act of sexual intercourse was contraceptively guarded, but all contraceptive methods suffer failures;

- the act of sexual intercourse that resulted in conception was itself unwanted; instances of this would be pregnancy as a result of rape or incest;

- the woman is likely to suffer severe punishment if it is discovered that she has become pregnant;
- the woman is incapable of providing a child with a decent upbringing; this may be because of her youth, her family situation, her economic circumstances, or other factors;
- the woman's health is likely to be damaged by the continuation of the pregnancy;
- the woman's education, career, or personal relationships will be disrupted by the pregnancy;
- others for whom the woman is responsible, such as her dependent children or elderly relatives, would be harmed by her pregnancy or rearing of a young child;
- the fetus suffers from a serious genetic disease or other abnormality.

It is difficult, if not impossible, to evaluate these reasons in the abstract, since each case is different and often involves a combination of factors. The 1969 Canadian abortion law attempted to impose objective medical standards for deciding which reasons should be regarded as valid, but this proved to be a failure, since the definition of "health" is capable of many different interpretations. As noted above, if the right to life of the fetus were given absolute priority over the right of the mother to decide whether or not to continue her pregnancy, it would be easy to resolve all disagreements. However, when fetal rights are regarded as just one factor among others, to be balanced against the rights of the woman, then there is no obvious solution to the problem (Churchill, 1982). The tendency, then, is to allow the woman's desires to take precedence.

Even when a woman does not want to continue her pregnancy, however, there are several reasons for not having an abortion. Like any medical procedure, abortion involves certain physical dangers, such as infection, although statistically it is safer than childbirth. Perhaps more serious is the psychological aftermath. There have been many reports of grief, depression, and regret from women who have had abortions, although it is not known how widespread such reactions are (Parthun, 1985). Thus, even for those who are unconcerned with the well-being of the fetus, abortion is not the perfect solution to an unwanted pregnancy.

Who Should Decide?

Since there is so much disagreement about the *reasons* for abortion, much of the current legal and ethical debate centres on the *procedures* for deciding whether or not an abortion should take place. The various candidates for decision-making authority are the pregnant woman, other family members (spouse or parents), doctors, and independent third parties.

The 1969 Canadian law required the approval of a therapeutic abortion committee, for an abortion to be performed. It was felt that an independent committee of doctors would consider all factors objectively, and would render fair and consistent decisions in all cases. This procedure could have succeeded only if the committees were given a clear set of criteria to apply in each case. As we saw above, the 1969 law did not provide such criteria; the committee was required to base its decision on its opinion of whether the continuation of the pregnancy would, or would be likely to, endanger the life or health of the pregnant woman, but no definition of health was included. As a result, the Supreme Court struck down this provision of the law, on the grounds of vagueness and unfairness.

The law that was introduced into Parliament in the fall of 1989 also assigned decision-making authority to doctors. They would have been permitted to perform abortions if, in their opinion, the continuation of the pregnancy would be likely to threaten the health or life of the woman. This proposal was criticized for being so broad that abortion for any reason would be permitted. Others felt that it was too restrictive, since a doctor might decide, for whatever reason, that a woman should not have an abortion, no matter how strongly she felt about it. If this law had been passed, it is likely that it would have been applied just as inconsistently as was the 1969 version.

The role of spouses or sexual partners in abortion decisions has been hotly contested, as we saw in Jean-Guy Tremblay's case against Chantal Daigle. There have been many other instances of men trying to prevent women from having abortions. In almost every case, the courts have left the final decision to the woman. There is no way of knowing how many similar cases occur that are not taken to court, but are resolved in other ways. Nor is it always the woman who wants the abortion; often women are pressured by their male partners to have abortions that they do not want. All this is a sign that abortion is just one part of a much larger social issue today: the relationship between men and women.

Another difficult conflict in abortion decision-making arises when a young adolescent becomes pregnant. Sometimes she wants to have the baby, but her parents coerce her into having an abortion. In other situations, the girl seeks abortion, with or without her parents' consent. No matter what the outcome, these cases are always tragic, and demonstrate that the only appropriate solution to the problem is the prevention of unwanted pregnancy before it occurs.

Even if other decision-makers could operate fairly and consistently in all cases, the most obvious candidate for authority in this matter would seem to be the pregnant woman. She knows, far better than anyone else, why she does or does not want to continue the pregnancy, and she is the one most affected by the decision. Why, then, is there a debate over who should decide this matter?

The principal reason, though not generally admitted, is that women are not regarded as reliable moral agents, in anything to do with sexuality and reproduction. In the words of Beverly Wildung Harrison:

> Much discussion of abortion betrays the heavy hand of misogyny or the hatred of women. We all have a responsibility to recognize this bias — sometimes subtle — when ancient negative attitudes toward women intrude into the abortion debate. (Harrison, 1982, 210)

Opponents of abortion would reply that women are naturally biased, when they do not want to continue a pregnancy. There is another party whose interests need to be represented — the fetus. Therefore, women should not have sole decision-making authority. If necessary, they should be forced to subordinate their own desires to the welfare of the fetus.

At a time when most Western institutions are coming to realize, and attempting to remedy, the devastating effects of sexism at all levels of society, it is difficult to oppose women's decision-making authority in abortion without being accused of perpetuating misogyny. Opponents of abortion are challenged to demonstrate, better than they have up to the present, that it is possible to be advocates both of the unborn and of women, particularly those who are unwillingly pregnant.

Alternatives to Abortion

A decision or act can only be moral or immoral if it is the result of a choice between two or more alternatives. If there is just one way for us to act in a situation, then we cannot be blamed or praised for what we do. In many situations of unwanted pregnancy, the women involved feel that there is no real alternative to having an abortion, or else the available alternatives are much worse. The opponents of abortion have, therefore, to suggest or provide realistic alternatives, if they wish to convince others that abortion is not the answer. The problem of unwanted pregnancies needs to be dealt with at two levels: prevention, and when that fails, other solutions.

There is probably nobody who does not consider it preferable to avoid an unwanted pregnancy than to end it by abortion. The controversy centres on how this goal is to be accomplished. According to the official teaching of the Roman Catholic Church, every act of sexual intercourse should be open to the possibility of conception. Therefore, if a child is not wanted, intercourse should not take place. This is always the case outside of marriage, and even within marriage, where "natural" methods of birth control are permitted, the couple must be ready to accept the consequence of intercourse, i.e., a child, if they wish to perform the act.

This understanding of the interrelatedness of sexual intercourse and parenthood is not widely accepted outside of the Roman Catholic Church. Instead, a wide variety of techniques are recommended for preventing unwanted pregnancies. First of all, early and comprehensive sex education is encouraged, so that young people will learn how conception takes place, and how it can be prevented. Secondly, contraceptive measures are considered essential for any act of sexual intercourse where pregnancy is not intended. Finally, efforts must be made to eradicate sexism, so that women will not be coerced to have intercourse when they find it not to be in their interest.

If, in spite of efforts to the contrary, an unwanted pregnancy does occur, or because of a change in circumstances, a wanted pregnancy becomes unwanted, what alternatives are there to abortion? Unfortunately, at present there are very few. The social stigma attached to women having abortions is generally less severe than it is for unmarried pregnant teenagers and mothers. Abortion is far easier to obtain in many communities than social services to support a mother and child. And since many families require two salaries to get by, if a woman has to interrupt her career to bear and raise another child, it can cause severe hardship to the family. All these problems must be addressed, if abortion is not to be regarded as the only practicable solution to an unwanted pregnancy.

ABORTION AS A THEOLOGICAL AND PHILOSOPHICAL ISSUE

As we saw in Chapter 1, abortion was one of the principal issues that gave rise to the birth of bioethics, in the late 1960s and early 1970s. The legal accommodation of abortion in Canada and other Western countries was preceded and accompanied by a large number of books and articles on this subject by philosophers and religious scholars, which often represented their first entry into the field of bioethics. Despite the continued popularity of this topic in the literature, scholars have attained no greater a consensus on the ethical aspects of abortion than is found in the general public. Their one major accomplishment has been to set forth the major alternative positions on this topic, from which others can choose.

A defence of the extreme pro-choice approach to abortion has been offered by several prominent philosophers, including Judith Jarvis Thompson, Michael Tooley, Peter Singer and H. Tristram Engelhardt, Jr. The principal justification that they provide for abortion is the negligible moral status of the fetus. Engelhardt's view is typical in this regard: "Fetuses, infants, the profoundly mentally retarded, and the hopelessly comatose provide examples of human nonpersons." (Engelhardt, 1986, 107) According to these philosophers, human rights, including the right to life, do not belong to all members of the species *homo sapiens*, but only to persons. A person is defined in various ways, but a common element is the capacity to reason. Since fetuses cannot reason, they are not persons and have no intrinsic right to continued existence. Thus, women are fully justified in having abortions for any purpose.

A completely different evaluation of abortion is defended by philosophers such as Baruch Brody, and by many religious scholars. They argue that the fetus is a developing human being, and has its own value and accompanying rights, including the right to life. Brody examines the arguments in favour of abortion that are set forth by their proponents, and rejects each one of them. He concludes that, once a fetus becomes a human being, i.e., develops a functioning brain (which, he claims, occurs some time between two and twelve weeks after conception), abortion can be justified in only one situation — when the alternative would be the death of both mother and fetus (Brody, 1975). Theologians who support the official Roman Catholic position on abortion generally agree with Brody's arguments, with one exception: for them, the right to life of the fetus begins at conception, not later in its development.

Between these two extreme approaches to the morality of abortion can be found a variety of intermediate positions. Most of them are based on a "developmental" understanding of the fetus, according to which it gradually acquires both the status of human personhood and the rights that accompany this status, including the right to life. Philosophers who espouse this approach include Wayne Sumner and Eike-Henner W. Kluge (Sumner, 1981, 124-160; Kluge, 1992, 275-300); they are joined by the majority of Protestant, and a minority of Roman Catholic, moral theologians. Most of these scholars hold the view that the woman's interests outweigh those of the fetus in the early stages of pregnancy but, after viability, the fetus attains equal or near-equal status with the mother. At that point, abortion should be performed only if there is serious danger to the life or health of the woman, or if it seems to be in the best interests of the fetus (e.g., because of serious genetic disease).

Which of these approaches to abortion is philosophically or theologically superior to the others? As we stated above, there is no greater consensus on this matter than there was twenty-five years ago. Despite an avalanche of literature on the topic, along with widespread political and legal activity, proponents of each position on abortion have generally failed to convince others. Abortion has become a prime example of the moral pluralism that holds forth in countries such as Canada. As such, it has been increasingly relegated to the sphere of private, or personal, morality, despite its obvious social implications. Since reasonable people cannot agree on when, if ever, abortion is morally permissible, or to what extent it should be legally available, Canadian policy-makers have decided to leave it up to individual citizens to decide whether to have abortions. Whether this state of affairs is to be applauded or deplored is a matter of dispute. In any case, it is a *fait accompli*, and indeed one that may well be replicated with regard to other controversial bioethical issues, such as euthanasia.

NEW DEVELOPMENTS

Three recent advances in medical science threaten to complicate even further the ethical dilemmas of abortion. A new drug, known as RU-486, has been developed, which prevents a fertilized ovum from attaching itself to the wall of the uterus. The drug can be taken between fifteen days and ten weeks after ovulation, whether or not the woman knows she is pregnant. Despite great opposition from anti-abortion groups, it is now widely used in France and the United Kingdom, and will likely be made available in other countries in the future.

RU-486 has been welcomed by advocates of abortion, because it is considered to be much more desirable than other abortion techniques, such as surgery. Some feel that it eliminates, or at least reduces, the moral problem of abortion, since it works in the very early stage of pregnancy, before the fetus is fully formed. On the other hand, those who believe that the fetus is fully human from conception are worried that the use of this drug will simply increase the number of abortions, since those women who might have continued their pregnancies for the sake of the children may no longer feel such an obligation.

The second new technique is known as selective reduction in multiple pregnancy. By means of prenatal diagnosis, it is possible to determine that one fetus among twins or triplets is affected by a serious, perhaps fatal, condition whereas the other one(s) are perfectly healthy. A related situation is where a woman is carrying four or more fetuses, none of which will survive unless something is done to reduce their number. It is now possible to kill one or more fetuses in the womb, in order to preserve the lives of the others. Pregnant women in these situations, and their doctors, are faced with the decision of whether to do nothing, and leave the lives of all the fetuses in danger, or to choose to terminate the lives of some, in order to save the lives of others.

The third new technique is still in its research phase. It involves transplanting fetal brain cells into patients suffering from Parkinson disease, and perhaps other neurological conditions that may be relieved by the brain's potential to grow new cells, a quality that fetal neural cells can introduce. Cells from spontaneous abortuses cannot be used, because they may have genetic flaws. Cells must be of a particular gestational age, rendering them suitable for recovery from scheduled abortions. Fetal brain-cell transplantation may persuade women who are ambivalent about whether to have an abortion, as many women are, that a benefit to others gives added weight to reasons to abort. A risk to women is that they may be asked to consider delaying or risking an abortion decision, in order to maximize the utility of resulting fetal tissues, and to have any abortion they decide to have by a technique that permits identification of fetal cells, rather than by another technique that may be more suited for them. The prospect of recovery and use of fetal cells raises bioethical questions of autonomy, exploitation, and disclosure of the risks and potential benefits of medical choices.

CONCLUSION

Despite over twenty-five years of intense ethical and legal debate, abortion is still one of the most contentious and divisive bioethical issues in countries such as Canada. It involves substantial, and apparently unresolvable, conflicts at the level of ethos and of morality, among groups for whom a particular approach to abortion has become a badge of identity. As we noted in Chapter 2, there is no easy solution to such conflicts. All that can be hoped for, at least in respect to public ethics, is a policy that sets the conditions under which a morally disputed behaviour will be, at least, socially tolerated by most people, even if it may not be socially championed.

In the Canada of the early 1990s, we are fortunate that such tolerance seems to prevail. The lack of any criminal law regulating abortion has not caused great social tension. Those who wish to avail themselves of abortion services are generally free to do so, and those who oppose the practice are not forced to take part. The truce between these two viewpoints may be temporary but, given the unlikelihood of Parliament taking up this issue in the foreseeable future, the present solution may come to be regarded by all parties as normal.

The abortion issue, for clinical ethics, is considerably more contentious. The legal freedom to obtain an abortion does not do away with the need to make an ethical decision about whether abortion is the best way to deal with an unwanted pregnancy. Unlike many other bioethical decisions, such as whether or not to withdraw life-sustaining treatment, abortion is often decided by the pregnant woman alone. Physicians and nurses are needed to carry out the procedure, but they generally play little, if any, role in the decision to abort. Insofar as abortion is a matter of clinical ethics, then, it is not primarily an issue for clinicians, but for patients. The abortion issue thus serves as a reminder that bioethics education must be aimed not just at health professionals, but at all members of society.

REFERENCES

Badgeley R.F. *Report of the Committee on the Operation of the Abortion Law.* Ottawa: Ministry of Supply and Services Canada, 1977.

Borowski v. Attorney General Canada (1983), 4 Dominion Law Reports (4th) 112.

Brody B. *Abortion and the Sanctity of Human Life.* Cambridge, MA: M.I.T. Press, 1975.

Carrick P. *Medical Ethics in Antiquity: Philosophical Perspectives on Abortion and Euthanasia* (Philosophy and Medicine 18). Dordrecht/Boston/ Lancaster: D. Reidel, 1985, 99-125.

Churchill L.R. and **Siman J.J.** "Abortion and the Rhetoric of Individual Rights." *Hastings Center Report* 1982;12/1:9-12.

Dickens B.M. "Legal Aspects of Abortion." In: P. Sachdev, ed. *Abortion: Readings and Research*. Toronto: Butterworths, 1981, 16-29.

Engelhardt H.T. Jr. *The Foundations of Bioethics*. New York: Oxford University Press, 1986.

Feldman D.M. "Abortion: Jewish Perspectives." In: W.T. Reich, ed. *Encyclopedia of Bioethics*. Vol. 1. New York: The Free Press, 1978, 5-9.

Harrison B.W. *Our Right to Choose: Toward a New Ethic of Abortion*. Boston: Beacon Press, 1983.

Harrison B.W. "Theology of Pro-Choice: A Feminist Perspective." In: E. Batchelor Jr., ed. *Abortion: The Moral Issues*. New York: The Pilgrim Press, 1982, 210-226.

Kluge E.-H.W. *Biomedical Ethics in a Canadian Context*. Toronto: Prentice Hall, 1992.

Law Reform Commission of Canada *Crimes Against the Fetus*. Ottawa, 1989.

McCormick R.A. *How Brave a New World? Dilemmas in Bioethics*. New York: Doubleday, 1981.

Melton J.G., ed. *The Churches Speak on: Abortion*. Detroit: Gale Research Inc., 1989.

Noonan J.T. Jr. "An Almost Absolute Value in History." In: J.T. Noonan Jr., ed. *The Morality of Abortion: Legal and Historical Perspectives*. Cambridge, MA: Harvard University Press, 1970, 1-59.

Parthun M. "The Psychological Effects of Induced Abortion." In: Human Life Research Institute Reports. *No. 2. Abortion's Aftermath*. Toronto: Human Life Research Institute, 1985, 7-31.

R. v. Morgentaler (1988), 44 Dominion Law Reports (4th) 385.

Sumner L.W. *Abortion and Moral Theory*. Princeton, NJ: Princeton University Press, 1981.

9

WHEN PEOPLE ARE UNABLE TO PARENT: STERILIZATION OF THE INTELLECTUALLY DISABLED

THE PROBLEM UNDER DISCUSSION IN THIS CHAPTER

This chapter, perhaps more than any other in this book, with the possible exception of Chapter 8 on abortion, centres attention on the sometimes tense relationships between law and ethics. For this reason, we should be clear from the very beginning about what we are, and what we are not, going to study in the following pages.

We are *not* going to discuss *voluntary sterilization for contraceptive purposes*. Of their own accord, men request vasectomies and women request tubal ligations quite frequently today, when they do not want to have any more children and other contraceptive methods are unsuitable for them. Some cultural and religious groups strongly oppose the morality of contraceptive sterilization, and certain medical questions are being raised about vasectomy. But these matters are *not* the focus of discussion in this chapter.

Neither are we discussing *sterilization that results as a by-product from surgical operations required to protect health or life*. This is often called *therapeutic sterilization*. For example, sterility or inability to conceive a child of one's own results from surgery to remove cancerous ovaries or cancerous testicles. This sterilization does not pose a significant moral or ethical problem. You should, however, refer back to Chapter 6 on the reproductive technologies, for a discussion of the ethical issues raised by ovum and embryo donation and by surrogate motherhood. A woman who becomes unable to conceive or bear a child, because of therapeutic sterilization, may want to use one of the reproductive technologies in her attempt to have a child.

It is most important to understand that this chapter is also *not discussing eugenic sterilization*, though we will have to draw attention to the history of prejudice, discrimination, and error that has plagued sterilization for eugenic purposes in this century. *Eugenic sterilization*, to give a brief definition, is enforced sterilization of individuals who would not want to be sterilized. These enforced sterilizations have been called "eugenic," because they were done, often on the basis of a very poor and faulty understanding of genetics and heredity, to protect society from the burden of caring for defective and retarded children of apparently (intellectually) impaired parents. Eugenic sterilization is proposed for the interests of society, not for the best interests of intellectually impaired persons.

What, then, *are* we really discussing in this chapter? First of all, we are talking about *persons*. If we forget that, we lose our bearings completely. Secondly, we are talking about persons who have *serious intellectual and mental impairment*. If we forget that, we will not understand what the ethical problem is. The three real-life cases to be presented below will give a clearer picture of the ethical and legal issue of this chapter. In general terms, we are talking about intellectual impairments of the following severity. These persons will never understand or be able to fulfil the responsibilities of caring for a child. They themselves have the mental capacities of a child. However, these people have sexual desires, just like everyone else. Some of these persons, though unable to care for a child, can understand marriage and can, with social help and support, lead a married life. Others cannot even do that, but do desire and seek sexual love and affection.

We are discussing persons who should not have children, because they will never be able to care for children, and any they might have will have to be taken from them and placed in foster care or for adoption. Moreover, the persons under discussion do not have the required intellectual understanding and discipline to practise contraception. Nor are these persons able to give a valid consent to, or a valid refusal of, sterilization, since they do not understand the link between sexual relations, pregnancy, and the birth of a child.

It is for these and similar persons that the difficult ethical and legal question of *non-consensual, non-therapeutic* sterilization arises. The sterilization in question is *non-therapeutic*, since it will not arise as a by-product of any surgical operation to correct a health- or life-threatening condition. It is under consideration strictly as a way of preventing pregnancy. This sterilization is being considered *for contraceptive purposes*, and is called *non-consensual* or *involuntary* because it is under consideration for persons whose intellectual impairment is severe enough that they cannot give informed, comprehending, and voluntary consent.

The following *central questions have to be asked*. Is sterilization ever in the best interests of the persons just described in the general terms above? Is such sterilization ever ethically and legally justified? If so, under what conditions? Who should authorize such sterilization, presuming that it can be justified in individual cases?

These are the *main questions of this chapter*. As you will see in a moment, thoughtful people are far from being in agreement about how these questions should be answered. Law and ethics in Canada are not in agreement on this issue, and the law established by Canada's Supreme Court differs from the legal judgment of the highest court of the United Kingdom.

It is essential, in discussing this issue of sterilization of mentally impaired persons, to pay close attention both to *legal* and *ethical* reasoning. This chapter's discussion will help you to gain a deeper and more precise understanding of the *relationship between ethics and law*, a relationship we have already examined together in a more general way in Chapter 3. This chapter, as well as Chapter 8 on abortion, should help you to think more clearly about two difficult situations: the circumstances under which *it may be ethically wrong to do what the law permits*; and the circumstances under which *it may be ethically justified to do what the law prohibits* or refuses to authorize.

WHY WE BEGIN BY CONSIDERING CASES THAT HAVE COME BEFORE THE COURTS OF LAW

One of the best ways to think clearly about the many complex issues raised by proposals to sterilize mentally retarded persons, who are incapable of consent, is to consider carefully how the courts have handled requests for authorization to perform such sterilizations. We select three cases to guide our reflection: the case of *Eve* in Canada, and the cases of *B* and *D* in England.

We begin this way because we want to emphasize several very important lessons, by the very way we open discussion of this legally and ethically thorny issue.

Lesson One
The question of sterilization of the mentally retarded always has to be particularized. The real question is whether *this particular person* needs sterilization for personal development, and how involuntary sterilization can be harmonized with *this particular person's* basic rights. This question can never be adequately answered simply by comparing general philosophical and moral arguments, as important as these are. So we do not begin this chapter by presenting and criticizing such arguments.

Lesson Two

The question of whether *this particular person's* best interests and personal development require involuntary sterilization can never be answered adequately or fairly simply on the basis of this person's having been labeled, however justifiably, as "mentally retarded." People may be retarded in some areas of life's activities, and yet, quite capable of performing adequately in other areas of life's ordinary activities, including parenthood. *The particular person's whole biography has to be considered.* So we begin by observing how courts of law have carefully considered individual biography, to reach a judgment about how the sterilization question should be answered when a particular person's needs are in conflict with her basic rights.

Lesson Three

In pluralistic societies, such as our own, law is not morality and morality is not the law. We all know that. The important lesson, though, is that careful ethical reflection on controversial social issues can have an impact on what the law will become. Moreover, models of such ethical reflection are often exhibited within the reasoning judges follow, to arrive at decisions in particularly difficult and contentious cases. Judicial reasoning is also often a prime source of ethical clarification. Ethicists, philosophers, and theologians are not the only ones who "do ethics."

Lesson Four

Though law is distinct from morality, the reasoning followed by the judges in the three cases we are about to consider demonstrates one of the close similarities between legal and ethical thinking. That similarity is found in the need to consider the particular circumstances and specific problems of each case, a need that can never be fulfilled by resting content with citing and analyzing general principles (Perelman, 1980, 116).

THE CASE OF *EVE*: CANADA

The case of *Eve* (so named to protect privacy) has appeared before three courts in Canada: first, before the Family Division of the Supreme Court of Prince Edward Island, judgment delivered in 1979; second, before the appeal tribunal of the Supreme Court of Prince Edward Island, judgment delivered in 1981; and finally, before the Supreme Court of Canada, judgment delivered in 1986. These lengthy deliberations began when Eve's mother, referred to as Mrs. E., applied to the court for authorization to have her daughter sterilized by tubal ligation. The judges on these courts differed principally about two issues: (1) whether the court had the power to grant authorization for contraceptive sterilization; and (2) whether contraceptive sterilization served Eve's best interests or violated her rights.

The Courts Accept the Fact of Eve's Mental Incompetency

Eve was twenty-four years of age when her mother applied to the court to have her daughter declared mentally incompetent, and to obtain authorization to consent to Eve's undergoing an operation for tubal ligation. Born in 1955, Eve was gradually diagnosed as affected by a condition called extreme expressive aphasia. A doctor who cared for Eve for many years explained that Eve's incapacity to express herself made it impossible for anyone ever to know what she really did or did not understand. At age 16, Eve could repeat the letters of the alphabet up to "G," she could not read simple words, and her I.Q. was scored at 37.

The judges of the three courts substantially agreed that Eve could not validly consent to sterilization; that her mental condition would never likely improve; that she did not understand the link between sexual relations, pregnancy, and birth; that she would not be able to fulfil the responsibilities of motherhood; that she was incapable of practising alternative means of contraception; and that it was unlikely that Eve would suffer emotionally or psychologically from an operation for tubal ligation. The courts also accepted the description of Eve as being an affectionate person who was physically adult, as well as capable of being attracted to, and attractive to, the opposite sex.

Do the Courts Have the Right to Grant Authorization for Non-Consensual Contraceptive Sterilization?

In the trial judgment of the case of *Eve*, Justice Charles McQuaid, of the Family Division of the Prince Edward Island Supreme Court, concluded that the court *"does not have either the authority or the jurisdiction to authorize a surgical procedure on a mentally retarded person, the intent and purpose of which is solely contraceptive — sterilization for the sake of sterilization."* (*E.* [P.E.I.], 1979, 329)

This judge declared his sympathy for, and understanding of, Mrs. E.'s real concern for her daughter's well-being. He did not believe she was requesting her daughter's tubal ligation for her own sake, rather than for her daughter's best interests. However, Justice McQuaid emphasized the *irreversibility of the sterilization*, and alluded to the *possibility of some medical advance* that might enable Eve, one day, to exercise the right and responsibility of motherhood. He agreed with an English judge that the principle the court should follow is "not to risk the incurring of damage to children which it cannot repair, but rather to prevent the damage being done." (*E.* [P.E.I.], 1979, 326)

Basically, Justice McQuaid refused to grant Mrs. E. authorization for her daughter's tubal ligation, because he believed the court had no authority or jurisdiction to grant such authorization. And he believed this because of the following view:

> The Eves of this world, regardless of how retarded, are nevertheless persons with rights which the courts must preserve and protect. One of these rights is the inviolability of their persons from involuntary trespass. This right supersedes … the right to be protected from pregnancy. While the preservation of this right might well, and even predictably, result in no little inconvenience and expense and indeed even hardship to others, the court must, regardless of its own natural sympathy to those others, ensure that the law have the care of those who are not able to care for themselves and ensure the preservation of the higher right. (*E.* [P.E.I.], 1979, 328)

Mrs. E. appealed to the Prince Edward Island Supreme Court for a reversal of Justice McQuaid's decision. Two of the three judges of this court, Justices Large and Campbell, *differed* from Justice McQuaid, and affirmed that the court *did have* the authority and jurisdiction to authorize Eve's sterilization. Their interpretation of what Eve's best interests required was the basis for their reversal of Justice McQuaid's decision.

Would Sterilization Serve Eve's Best Interests?

Both Justice Large and Justice Campbell found that tubal ligation would, indeed, serve Eve's best interests. They *disagreed* with Justice McQuaid's view that the "inviolability of the person from involuntary trespass" overrides or supersedes the right to be protected from pregnancy.

Justice Large did not consider that sterilization, which would deprive Eve of the possibility of pregnancy, could be described as depriving her of the possible fulfilment of one of the great powers and privileges of her life.(*Eve* [P.E.I.], 1981, 392) All the judges agreed that Eve would never be able to understand motherhood or care for a child. Justice Campbell emphasized that the need to protect Eve from pregnancy would, in the absence of a tubal ligation, lead to intolerable restrictions upon her freedom of action:

> Her social contacts, her privileges in a group home, even the modest privileges of attending a movie, taking a stroll or making use of public transit are in prospect of limitations, controls and restrictions for the very reason that she is more vulnerable to sexual abuse and pregnancy. I am of the opinion that without the protection of a permanent sterilization the protected environment will become a guarded environment and the loss to Eve in terms of her social options and her relative freedom would cause substantial injury.…(*Eve* [P.E.I.], 1981, 320)

Having found jurisdiction to approve sterilization, the two majority judges subsequently gave their approval to hysterectomy, which is a considerably more invasive surgical procedure than tubal ligation.

The Supreme Court of Canada on the Case of *Eve*

The majority decision of the Prince Edward Island Supreme Court to approve contraceptive hysterectomy was appealed to the Supreme Court of Canada. In October 1986, Justice LaForest delivered the unanimous decision of the Court, a decision *denying* that provincial courts had the jurisdiction to authorize non-consensual, non-therapeutic sterilization, and *denying* that sterilization would be in Eve's best interest. The Supreme Court reasoned in the following way.

Regarding the Courts' Jurisdiction to Authorize Non-Consensual Sterilization for Contraceptive Purposes

Justice LaForest offered an extensive study of the Courts' parental or, as it is called, *parens patriae* jurisdiction. While the *origin* of this jurisdiction is lost in the mists of antiquity, the *scope* of the jurisdiction is recognized as unlimited, as covering everything necessary to protect those who cannot care for themselves. The *exercise* of this jurisdiction, however, is governed by its underlying principle, namely: that the *parens patriae* jurisdiction must be used only for the benefit of the person in need of protection, and not for the benefit of others.

The Supreme Court of Canada concluded:

> Sterilization should never be authorized for non-therapeutic purposes under the *parens patriae* jurisdiction. In the absence of the affected person's consent, it can never be safely determined that it is for the benefit of that person. The grave intrusion on a person's rights and the ensuing physical damage outweigh the highly questionable advantages that can result from it. The Court, *therefore*, lacks jurisdiction in such a case. (*Eve v. Mrs. E.*, 1986, 5)

We have given emphasis to the word *therefore* to draw your attention to the reasons Justice LaForest gave for denying the Courts' jurisdiction to authorize non-consensual, non-therapeutic sterilization. We will offer a commentary on these reasons later in this chapter.

Regarding Sterilization as Not Being in Eve's Best Interests

Justice LaForest brought forth many reasons to support the Supreme Court of Canada's refusal to grant authorization for the sterilization of Eve. These reasons bolster the Court's emphasis that the *parens patriae* jurisdiction must be exercised with great caution, "a caution that must be redoubled as the seriousness of the matter increases." (*Eve v. Mrs. E.*, 1986, 53) And no one really doubts that sterilization of someone unable to give consent is a very serious matter.

Reason 1

The judge referred to the sterilization laws of the provinces of British Columbia and Alberta, laws that were repealed in 1973 and 1972, respectively (Law

Reform Commission of Canada, 1979, 27-29; 42-45). Justice LaForest cited the influence of eugenic theories on these laws, theories that are now discredited, but that encouraged the perception of intellectually handicapped people as being somewhat less than human. The implication is that these eugenic ideas may still cloud and distort our judgment about what is in a mentally retarded person's best interests, and influence thinking about the effects their reproduction might have on society.

Reason 2
Sterilization deprives a person of the great privilege of giving birth, and is, in practice, irreversible.

Reason 3
Sterilization of a person unable to give consent may seriously damage that person's psychological well-being.

Reason 4
Omitting to perform a hysterectomy will not necessarily lead to an endangering of Eve's physical or psychological health. The judge gave no weight to the fear that pregnancy and birth could be traumatic for Eve.

In short, Justice LaForest found it difficult to imagine a case in which non-therapeutic *sterilization* could possibly be of benefit to the person on behalf of whom a court purports to act, let alone to imagine a case in which non-therapeutic sterilization is necessary for a person's best interests (*Eve v. Mrs. E.*, 1986, 59).

The Supreme Court of Canada concluded unanimously that the proposed hysterectomy would not be in Eve's best interests. Justice LaForest expressed that conclusion as follows:

> The grave intrusion on a person's rights and the certain physical damage that ensues from non-therapeutic sterilization without consent, when compared to the highly questionable advantages that can result from it have persuaded me that it can never safely be determined that such a procedure is for the benefit of that person. Accordingly, the procedure should never be authorized for non-therapeutic purposes under the *parens patriae* jurisdiction. (*Eve v. Mrs. E.*, 1986, 59)

IN ENGLAND: THE CASE OF *B*

As in the case of *Eve*, the English case of *B*, a mentally handicapped and epileptic seventeen-year-old girl, went through three courts. A local government authority responsible for the care of B applied, with B's mother's agreement, to the Family Division of the High Court, sitting in Newcastle-Upon-Tyne, for authorization to have B undergo a tubal ligation. Justice Bush granted the authorization, but the Official Solicitor, acting as B's guardian, appealed to the Court of Appeal. The Court of Appeal agreed with Justice Bush and dismissed the appeal. The Official Solicitor then appealed to the House of Lords, England's highest court.

Who Was B?

B was born on May 20, 1969, and had been in the care of a local government authority since 1973. When her case came to the courts (the judgments of each of these courts were all delivered between the months of January and April, 1987) B was a seventeen-year-old, but demonstrated a mental age of six. She had no understanding of the connection between sexual relations, pregnancy, and birth. She was seen as never being able to cope with the experience of birth, and as never being able to care for a child. She was incapable of consenting to marriage, or to a course of contraceptive treatment, or to sterilization, or to an abortion were she to become pregnant.

Possible pregnancy posed particular problems for this girl. First of all, she would never understand what her pregnant condition was. Secondly, if B did become pregnant, it was unlikely that those caring for her would notice the pregnancy in time to seek an abortion. This was because B was quite obese and was menstrually irregular. Third, because B would not understand what was happening to her, she would likely panic at the time of birth. Heavy sedation could damage the child, so delivery would probably have to be by caesarean section. However, B's behaviour in the past led those caring for her justifiably to believe that she would play with her sutures and scars, open the wound, suffer infection, and prevent healing.

There were many reasons to prevent B from becoming pregnant, but only two practicable contraceptive means were available, namely sterilization or daily intake of a pill over a period of twenty-five to thirty years. The pill did not merit real consideration. There were serious concerns about the health effects of taking a progesterone (contraceptive) pill for over twenty-five years. Secondly, medication generally upset B's behaviour and made her very aggressive. She displayed frequent episodes of aggressive behaviour following the medication she had to take for her epilepsy. These episodes, combined with B's lack of understanding and personal self-discipline, made it highly unlikely that she would be able to take a contraceptive pill daily and, indeed, over a long period of time.

The Decision of the House of Lords

The five members of the House of Lords hearing this case unanimously dismissed the appeal of the Official Solicitor, and supported the reasoning of the earlier judges in the case. These judges had decided that sterilization was the only possible decision that would protect the future welfare of the young woman B.

Lord Hailsham introduced a most important consideration. He emphasized that to place B in a strictly guarded environment, to protect her from sexual relations and pregnancy, *would drastically limit the little liberty this young woman would be able to enjoy.* This restriction would be "gravely detrimental to the amenity and quality of her life." (*B [a minor]*, 1987, 212)

Public comment on this case raised the spectre of eugenics, and a conflict between the welfare of B and the interest of B's mother. Lord Bridge stressed that "this case has nothing whatever to do with eugenic theory or with any attempt to lighten the burden which must fall on those who have the care of the ward. It is concerned, and concerned only, with the question of what will promote the welfare and serve the best interests of the ward." (*B [a minor]*, 1987, 213) Lord Oliver also stressed that this decision was for B's best interests and welfare, and had nothing to do with the eugenic goal of controlling the quantity or quality of the population.

Why the Case of *Eve* and the Case of *B* Differ from the Case of *D*

Judges in both the Canadian and English cases referred to the decision of Justice Heilbron in the case of *D*, a decision that was delivered in 1975 (Walters, 1976).

D was born in November 1963, affected by a condition diagnosed as Sotos Syndrome. The syndrome included accelerated growth during infancy, epilepsy, general clumsiness, an unusual facial appearance, emotional instability, and some impairment of mental function and intelligence. D's mother, fearing that D would become pregnant and give birth to an abnormal child, decided, with the agreement of the family's paediatrician, that it would be best to have D sterilized.

However, the facts of D's condition differed from the conditions of Eve and B in several very important respects. *First*, D was only approaching puberty when her mother requested the sterilization. *Second*, D had displayed remarkable improvement, when sent to a school specializing in learning difficulties. *Third*, all the evidence indicated that D would continue to improve, and that she had sufficient intellectual capacity to be able one day to consent to marry. She would also, presumably, one day be able to consent to, or refuse consent for, sterilization.

On this evidence, Justice Heilbron *refused to grant authorization for sterilization.* The main reason for the refusal was the high probability that D, in later years, *would be able to make her own choice*. That, on all evidence, would never be possible for either Eve or B (*D [a minor]*, 1976, 327).

THE HOUSE OF LORDS DIFFERS WITH THE SUPREME COURT OF CANADA

Though the House of Lords and the Supreme Court of Canada were dealing with comparable cases, Eve and B were two individual persons, with their own unique personal and biographical characteristics. For example, though each of these young women was intellectually handicapped, it was much more difficult for anyone to know just how profoundly handicapped Eve really was. Eve could not express herself, and this expressive aphasia was a barrier to knowing how much she understood of her circumstances. Nevertheless, the questions of welfare and protection of best interests, insofar as sterilization was concerned, were similar in the cases of Eve and B. Yet, the two courts arrived at diametrically opposed decisions. Why? We will understand this controversy more precisely and deeply if we pay close attention to the points on which the House of Lords differed from the Supreme Court of Canada.

The Absolute Prohibition of Contraceptive Sterilization

Lord Hailsham, in particular, found it impossible to accept Justice LaForest's position that contraceptive sterilization could *never*, on the basis of the court's *parens patriae* jurisdiction, be authorized for a person unable to give consent. Lord Hailsham found this position to be "totally unconvincing and in startling contradiction to the welfare principle which should be the first and paramount consideration in wardship cases." (*B [a minor]*, 1987, 213) Lord Bridge also criticized Justice LaForest's generalization: "This sweeping generalization seems to me, with respect, to be entirely unhelpful. To say that the Court can never authorize sterilization of a ward as being in her best interests would be patently wrong." (*B [a minor]*, 1987, 214)

The Distinction Between "Therapeutic" and "Non-Therapeutic" Sterilization

Justice LaForest placed great weight on the distinction between contraceptive sterilization, and sterilization resulting as a by-product of an operation to preserve health or life. Regarding the cases of Eve and B, Lord Hailsham found this distinction to be "totally meaningless, and, if meaningful, quite irrelevant to the correct application of the welfare principle." (*B [a minor]*, 1987, 213) Lord Bridge found that Justice LaForest's distinction was an invitation to enter an arid semantic debate, and to avoid facing the real issue. The real issue, in Lord Bridge's view, "is whether the operation is in the ward's best interest." (*B [a minor]*, 1987, 214) Yet, one should attend to the fact that quite different sterilization procedures were under consideration in each of these cases: tubal ligation in the case of B; and hysterectomy, a more serious operation, in the case of Eve.

Status of the Basic Right to Reproduce

Justice LaForest placed great emphasis on the right to reproduce as being basic, and a great privilege. Lord Hailsham did not agree that reproduction would be a great privilege for the two young women under discussion. He asserted: "To talk of the 'basic right' to reproduce of an individual who is not capable of knowing the causal connection between intercourse and childbirth, the nature of pregnancy, what is involved in delivery, unable to form maternal instincts or to care for a child appears to me wholly to part company with reality." (*B [a minor]*, 1987, 213) Once again, it is important to identify one of the differences between Eve and B. It was not clear or easy to determine, as it was in the case of B, that Eve could not grasp the connection between intercourse and childbirth, or that Eve was incapable of forming maternal instincts.

What is the legal or moral worth of emphasizing how basic the right to reproduce is, when the person in question will never be able to exercise this right? This is the point of Lord Bridge, when he states: "The sad fact in the instant case is that the mental and physical handicaps under which the ward suffers effectively render her incapable of ever exercising that right or enjoying that privilege. It is clear beyond argument that for her pregnancy would be an unmitigated disaster." (*B [a minor]*, 1987, 214)

ETHICAL CONDITIONS FOR CONTRACEPTIVE, NON-CONSENSUAL STERILIZATION

The judgments delivered in the court cases we have studied identify the main considerations to be balanced, in developing a reasonable and justifiable ethical position on this very difficult and controversial question. It is by appeal to one or several principles that an *absolutist ethics* would rule out (or permit) contraceptive sterilization of an intellectually disabled person, who cannot consent to such an operation. A *conditional ethics*, in contrast, may justify such a sterilization, but limits the justification to those personal situations in which a number of specified conditions are fulfilled. The *primary norm of a conditional ethics* of non-consensual contraceptive sterilization is the biography of the mentally retarded person. Will sterilization maximize or diminish this person's chances to achieve the fullest measure of personal development? That is the key question. If contraceptive sterilization may be ethically justified for a mentally retarded person who cannot give consent, then, indeed, it can only be on the basis of the following considerations, conditions and restrictions.

A Consideration of Rights Is Ethically Necessary but Insufficient

Human beings with mental handicaps have the same rights as other human beings have. Their rights deserve the same protection as is given to those of all other persons in society. Moreover, persons with *varying degrees* of intellectual disability have *different needs* (Thompson, 1978). There are some rights, such as the right to parenthood, that persons with mental handicap can exercise only if certain needs of theirs are given adequate attention. A society that respects the rights of mentally disabled people will offer them those kinds of service and supports they require, to meet their needs and exercise their rights.

However, *rights include responsibilities*. The exercise of rights demands corresponding capabilities. Persons with mental handicap may, in some cases, be utterly unable, even with optimal support and services, to fulfil the responsibilities linked to the exercise of some rights, for example the right to marry, or the even weightier right to have children.

Moreover, *persons*, not only *rights*, *deserve protection*. Persons living with mental handicap merit protection from burdens of responsibility they cannot carry, just as they merit the help they require to exercise those rights that correspond to their capabilities and to the responsibilities they *can* fulfil.

It must be recognized, however, that children whose natural parents cannot care for them may be adopted by others, and that proposing non-therapeutic, irreversible surgical solutions to forestall anticipated social difficulties may be objectionable, and violate the protection the *Canadian Charter of Rights and Freedoms* offers, of liberty and security of the person, and against discrimination on grounds of mental disability.

So, in arriving at a balanced ethical position on contraceptive sterilization of those with mental handicap, one has to think about rights, and also about needs, responsibilities, and capabilities.

Consideration of Capabilities Is Ethically Critical

Persons living with *varying degrees* of mental retardation *differ* in their capabilities to exercise their rights to love in a sexual relationship, to marriage, to reproduction, and to parenthood.

- Those persons with mental handicap who are capable of sexual relationship, marriage, reproduction, and parenthood merit the support and services they may require to exercise these rights. Moreover, anyone capable of marrying and caring for children, even if support and services are required, will be capable of consenting to, or refusing, contraceptive sterilization. Respect of such a person's consent or refusal is ethically mandatory.

- Some persons with mental handicap may desire, and be able to maintain, a sexual relationship and to marry, but may be unable, even with social help, to fulfil the responsibilities of reproduction and parenthood. These persons are *treated unfairly if they are prohibited, to prevent pregnancy, from expressing and receiving love and companionship in a sexual relationship or marriage.* Adequate contraception or suitable sterilization becomes a condition for their liberty to live a sexual or marital relationship.

- Persons unable to cope with the responsibilities of reproduction and parenthood may need special education and help, to choose and use the contraceptive method they require to live a responsible sexual or marital relationship. They have a right to this education and support. Sterilization may not be necessary for them (Gillon, 1987).

- If a person with mental handicap is able to consent to, or refuse, sterilization, that decision ethically belongs to that person, not to anyone else.

- Some persons with severe mental handicap are incapable of marriage, reproduction, and parenthood. They are also incapable of consenting to, or refusing, sterilization, when other contraceptive methods are also out of the question for them. But these persons do desire, as do most other people, sexual warmth, affection, and love. *The personal fulfilment of these persons will not be well served by an absolute prohibition of sterilization, when informed and voluntary consent is unobtainable.*

The Welfare of the Mentally Retarded Person

The authorization of contraceptive sterilization of a mentally handicapped person who is unable to give consent is *ethically unjustified when done for the good of someone else,* regardless of whether this "other" be the person's parents or society at large. The individual mentally handicapped person's welfare is the only, and the really decisive, ethical ground for such a decision.

Justice LaForest of the Supreme Court of Canada held that the court did not have jurisdiction or authority to authorize the contraceptive sterilization of Eve, *because* he could not imagine how such a sterilization could serve a mentally retarded person's welfare.

Justice LaForest failed to pay sufficient attention to the likely restrictions of liberty Eve would suffer, as a result of the understandable attempts people in charge of Eve would make to assure she would never become pregnant. Lord Hailsham, in the case of *B*, emphasized how placement of B in a closely guarded environment to protect her from sexual relations and pregnancy would drastically limit the young woman's liberty, and would gravely diminish the quality of her life. Justice LaForest paid little or no attention to this ethically critical and decisive consideration. On the other hand, Eve faced major abdominal surgery for hysterectomy, while B faced only the less invasive procedure of tubal ligation; the latter may be reasonably imposed in exchange for liberty, but not necessarily the former. Dr. Willard Gaylin has summarized the considerations that weigh heavily in conditional ethical justification of contraceptive sterilization of those who cannot consent:

> The price we make the retarded pay for their incapacity in one area is the sacrifice of capacity in certain other areas which could be compensatory if allowed to develop.

> Because we cast mentally retarded adults as children we are appalled, for example, at the thought of their having a sexual or even a social life. Deprived of the joy and privilege of parenthood, for which they have no capacity, they are punished further by being denied the privilege and pleasure of affection, tenderness, romance, and sexual contact for which they may indeed have a capacity (Gaylin, 1976).

Who Should Decide?

Contraceptive sterilization of mentally handicapped persons who cannot give consent can be ethically justified only if such decisions are based upon a careful examination of each person's situation, and sterilization is the least invasive measure feasible, and judged to be the measure of last resort required to serve the person's best interests. But who should make these decisions and judgments (Neville, 1978; Bayles, 1978)?

Decisions for non-consensual contraceptive sterilization of persons with mental handicap should not be left to the discretion of parents and guardians, relatives, physicians, or institutional administrators. This simple decisional procedure would open doors to conflicts of interest and abuses. Special societal and legal authorization is a necessary condition for the ethical justifiability of contraceptive sterilization of those who cannot consent. The Supreme Court of Canada said that legislation might permit Eve's sterilization. However, the Court's inherent parental jurisdiction, which dates from a time when sterilization was a common law maim, could not be the source of authorization for non-consensual contraceptive sterilization.

Determination of a mentally handicapped person's competency to consent, and determination of whether such a person's best interests require sterilization, should be entrusted to a judicial hearing. Lord Templeman, in his opinion in the case of *D* in England, summarized the reasoning in support of decision by judicial hearing as follows:

> A court exercising the wardship jurisdiction emanating from the Crown is the only authority which is empowered to authorize such a drastic step as sterilization after a full and informed investigation. The girl will be represented by the Official Solicitor or some other appropriate guardian; the parents will be made parties if they wish to appear and where appropriate the local authority will also appear. Expert evidence will be adduced setting out the reasons for the application, the history, conditions, circumstances and foreseeable future of the girl, the risks and consequences of pregnancy, the risks and consequences of sterilization, the practicability of alternative precautions against pregnancy, and any other relevant information. The judge may order additional evidence to be obtained. In my opinion, a decision should only be made by a High Court judge. In the Family Division a judge is selected for his or her experience, ability and compassion. No one has suggested a more satisfactory tribunal or a more satisfactory method of reaching a decision which vitally concerns an individual but also involved principles of law, ethics and medical practice. (*B [a minor]*, 1987, 214-215)

CONCLUSION

This chapter has argued that contraceptive sterilization of intellectually disabled persons, who cannot give consent, may be ethically justified. Yet, one of the ethical conditions is that authorization for such sterilization be obtained from the court.

This creates a dilemma in Canada, because the Supreme Court of Canada has judged that the courts do not have inherent parental, or *parens patriae*, jurisdiction to authorize such sterilizations, even in cases where contraceptive sterilization would be ethically justifiable under the conditions discussed above. The Court established that only provincial legislation can create this power, and that legislation will have to satisfy the criteria set by the *Canadian Charter of Rights and Freedoms*.

Of course, the Supreme Court of Canada can change its own decisions (Dickens, 1987). However, until it does, it is extremely unlikely that lower courts in Canada would give approval or authorization for contraceptive non-consensual sterilization, without clear authority from provincial legislation.

It would be ethically irresponsible, and perilous for the welfare of intellectually handicapped persons, to advocate that parents, physicians, and guardians should now, as it were, "take the law into their own hands," when they are convinced that an intellectually handicapped person in their charge requires contraceptive sterilization for his or her best interests. This could well lead to abuse. Their recourse is to encourage their provincial legislature to give courts the power they lack, under their inherent jurisdiction, to approve contraceptive sterilization.

An ethically responsible approach would be to marshal evidence to show that the Supreme Court decision in the case of Eve is causing hardship and suffering for intellectually disabled persons, who would benefit from contraceptive sterilization to achieve their life plans. A provincial legislature, persuaded by such evidence, might take the available political initiative to give its provincial courts the power the Supreme Court found they lack under their inherent jurisdiction. If such legislation met *Charter* standards, it would be upheld by the Supreme Court as lawful and constitutional, as not violating rights to liberty, security and nondiscrimination.

The issue of contraceptive sterilization of intellectually disabled persons demonstrates the tension that can exist between clinical ethics and law; between clinical ethics and public policy. Clinical ethics is governed by concern for individual patients, and the goal of this particular patient now is the norm of clinical ethics. But law and public policy are rightly concerned with the common good, and a generalization of acts, such as contraceptive sterilization of intellectually disabled persons, that could be justified in an individual case, could lead to a spate of intolerable abuse. The resolution of such tensions and dilemmas, as discussed earlier in Chapter 2, may necessitate the experimental use of a public policy for a time, and until accumulating experience and evidence make it clear that a change in policy is required.

REFERENCES

B (a minor) (1987), 2 *All England Reports* 212.

Bayles M. "Sterilization of the Retarded: The Legal Precedents." *Hastings Center Report* 1978; 8/3:37-41.

D (a minor) (1976), *All England Reports* (Family Division) 327.

Dickens B. "No Contraceptive Sterilization of the Mentally Retarded: The Dawn of Eve." *Canadian Medical Association Journal* 1987;137:65-67.

E. (P.E.I.) (1979), 10 *Reports of Family Law* (2d) 317.

Eve (P.E.I.) (1981), 115 *Dominion Law Reports* (3d) 283.

Eve v. Mrs. E. (1986), 2 *Supreme Court Reports* 5.

Gaylin W. "Sterilizing the Retarded Child." *Hastings Center Report* 1976;6:15.

Gillon R. "On Sterilizing Severely Mentally Handicapped People." *Journal of Medical Ethics* 1987;13:59-61.

Law Reform Commission of Canada *Sterilization.* Working Paper #24. Ottawa: The Minister of Supply and Services, 1979.

Neville R. "Sterilization of the Retarded: The Philosophical Arguments." *Hastings Center Report* 1978;8/3:33-37.

Perelman C. *Justice, Law, and Argument.* Dordrecht, Holland: D. Reidel Publishing Company, 1980.

Thompson T. "Sterilization of the Retarded: The Behavioral Perspective." *Hastings Center Report* 1978;8/3:29-32.

Walters L. "Sterilizing the Retarded Child." *Hastings Center Report* 1976;6:13-14.

P A R T 3

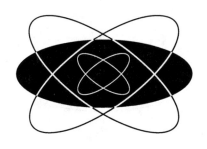

WHEN HUMAN HEALTH AND LIFE ARE THREATENED

10

WHEN A NEW EPIDEMIC OCCURS: THE ETHICS OF HIV INFECTION AND AIDS

The worldwide epidemic of HIV (human immunodeficiency virus) infection and AIDS (acquired immunodeficiency syndrome) is now into its second decade. Scientists have been hot on the track of this virus, actually a retrovirus as we shall explain below, for ten years. Because of spectacular advances in molecular biology and genetics, which were made possible by the discovery of recombinant-DNA technology in the early 1970s (see Chapter 18), scientists in the 1980s were equipped to probe the genetic structure of this retrovirus, and to seek out sites in this structure where the virus could be attacked. Much of the scientific work of the last eight years has concentrated on the design and testing of drugs to cripple the virus or, at least, to slow down its destructive effects on the human immune system. However, as of the end of 1992, there is no vaccine to prevent HIV infection, and there is no cure for AIDS, which is the advanced stage of HIV disease.

The virus (retrovirus) leading to AIDS works slowly, and ten years, accordingly, is a short time in this epidemic. The magnitude of HIV's human destruction builds cumulatively and, with the exception of the highly publicized AIDS-related deaths of famous persons, somewhat unobtrusively over decades. In this respect, and also in other ways, as we shall discuss later, the epidemic of HIV and AIDS differs from some of the great contagious plagues, such as the bubonic plague, called the Black Death, when thousands upon thousands of people died within a relatively short time in Europe, in the year 1347. In another bubonic plague that hit London in 1665, at least 68,000 people, and probably many more, died between May and December of that year.

Though the initial scientific and medical bafflement regarding this new epidemic, and also much of the initial panic and hysteria of the early 1980s, have passed into history, the HIV epidemic is still challenging individual citizens, health care professionals, and governments in countries throughout the world to confront phobias, paranoia, and prejudice; to declare whether they stand for or against the values of civilization; for or against inhumanity and indifference in the battle against this infection, and in the care of the afflicted.

Mounting an effective response to short-lived emergencies requires the fast mobilization of great amounts of energy and resources. It is, however, so much more difficult to maintain such a response over decades, when the epidemic to be mastered grows inexorably and slowly.

SCIENTIFIC AND MEDICAL BACKGROUND

Sometimes children are born with genetic defects that prevent them from developing a normal immune system. Their bodies cannot fight off infections, and they die rapidly from multiple infections unless they are kept in a totally sterile enclosure, like a bubble tent or a spaceman type of suit. This kind of immune deficiency is said to be congenital, because children are born with the condition.

AIDS stands for *acquired* immune deficiency syndrome. We are talking about an immune deficiency that people acquire after being infected with a special virus, called the human immunodeficiency virus, or HIV. This virus causes a breakdown in the body's system of defence against infections. As the HIV-infected immune system deteriorates, HIV-infected persons begin to show symptoms of various kinds of infections. These are called *opportunistic infections*, because a weakening of the body's immune defences offers an opportunity for widely prevalent microorganisms, such as viruses and bacteria, to take command and cause infections, resulting in severe illness and death. When the immune system is functioning efficiently, these widely present microorganisms are kept in check and do not cause illness and death.

AIDS, then, is not one single disease. It is a syndrome, meaning a collection of symptoms and signs, indicating various kinds of infections and diseases. AIDS is the advanced stage in the progression of HIV disease.

HIV Infection

There is widespread scientific agreement, despite some continuing controversy, that the human immunodeficiency virus, or HIV, is the principal cause of the deterioration of the immune system, a deterioration resulting in AIDS and death for most HIV-infected persons.

Viruses are among the smallest and simplest forms of life known to biological science. Though there are many kinds of viruses, they all share the characteristic of being unable to reproduce themselves without using the biological mechanisms of the cells they infect.

The HIV is a special kind of virus, and belongs to the family of viruses called *retroviruses*, so named because they reverse the normal flow of genetic information. Genes on the chromosomes in cells are made of DNA and they can only be expressed, or get to do what they are supposed to do, by being transcribed into messenger RNA that serves as the basis for the production of proteins, one of the principal functions of genes. In retroviruses, a reverse process has to take place before the virus can be reproduced in the body. The genes of a retrovirus are coded in RNA, not in DNA. Once this RNA is converted into retroviral DNA, the retrovirus can enter into the DNA of the cell it infects and thereby reproduce new retroviruses, in this case, new HIV, every time the infected cell divides and reproduces itself. Once the retrovirus HIV enters the DNA of its target cells, infection is permanent (Haseltine, 1988).

HIV preferentially infects one of the most important set of cells in the human immune system, a set of white blood cells called lymphocytes. HIV preferentially, though not exclusively, infects a subset of these lymphocytes, called the helper T cells, the command centre of the body's defence system against viruses, bacteria, and other kinds of infectious microorganisms. As HIV infection progresses, these helper T cells die and the body is increasingly defenceless against a host of infections that define the advanced stage of HIV disease we call AIDS.

The Detection of HIV Infection

There is no simple, widely usable test available that can directly find the human immunodeficiency virus in the body. Detection of HIV in the body is indirect, and based on the fact that the immune system produces antibodies against invading microorganisms like HIV. Since 1985, tests exist to detect the presence in blood samples of antibodies to HIV. The most widely used such test is called ELISA, which stands for enzyme-linked immunosorbent assay. Because HIV-antibody tests are performed on a component of blood, called serum, persons who test positive are said to be HIV-seropositive, if the positive ELISA test results are confirmed by one of several more sophisticated and reliable tests. Such confirmation, as we shall discuss later, is one of the ethical conditions for acceptable uses of the HIV-antibody test.

Confirmation of ELISA results is necessary, because tests for antibodies to HIV can produce false-positive results. A number of factors linked to biochemistry and to the way such tests are performed can make the test show up positive, even when the HIV is not in the body of a person whose blood has been tested. This will happen more frequently when the test is used for populations within which the HIV is not very prevalent.

It is also important to emphasize that failure of the ELISA test to detect HIV antibodies in blood samples can occur, even when people have HIV in their bodies. This is because the body does not produce antibodies to HIV immediately. It usually takes anywhere from four to six weeks, sometimes even months, before antibodies to HIV are produced. During this time, a person who has been infected with HIV, and who can infect others, will test negatively on HIV-antibody tests.

The Transmission of HIV Infection

HIV has to enter the body's bloodstream to cause HIV infection and HIV disease. This can happen through vaginal and anal sexual intercourse, and as a result of other exchanges of semen or vaginal secretions, especially if these secretions contact skin or membranes that have open wounds. Intravenous drug use, via needles contaminated with HIV-infected blood, is another primary mode of transmitting HIV infection. Blood transfusions of HIV-infected blood, and reception of plasma products from such blood, such as factor VIII used in the treatment of hemophiliacs, also can transmit, and, indeed, have transmitted HIV infection. However, the risk of HIV infection from blood transfusions and plasma products, such as factor VIII, is now very low in all countries using both strict blood donor screening programmes and special heat treatment of plasma products. HIV infection can also be transmitted from mother to child during pregnancy or delivery, and possibly also through breast-feeding.

HIV infection is not very contagious. People do not acquire HIV infection simply by using cups, telephones, drinking fountains, locker rooms, and toilets that have been touched or used by HIV-infected persons. HIV infection is not spread or acquired by touching, holding, or carrying an HIV-infected person. Some have feared they could acquire infection from handling the same books or papers as an infected student, or from using the same word processor or other office equipment previously touched by an HIV-infected co-worker. These fears have no basis in fact. They should not be cultivated or supported in any fashion. These fears should, rather, be exposed as unjustified and inappropriate as often as they appear.

The Diagnosis of AIDS

People can be HIV-infected for long periods of time, before their bodies begin to show symptoms that justify the diagnosis of AIDS. People are said to be *asymptomatic* if they are infected with HIV, but do not yet show the symptoms of HIV disease. After infection with HIV, some people initially show very few symptoms, or none at all; others suffer from fever, fatigue and general aches and pains. Still others suffer from swollen glands in the neck, armpits, and groin. These symptoms are called *lymphadenopathy*, because they indicate a pathology, or diseased condition, of the lymph glands.

These early symptoms usually last only for a relatively short time. Many HIV-infected people, after the passing of these symptoms, feel healthy and strong, and are able to carry on with all life's normal activities during the asymptomatic phase of HIV disease. However, as HIV disease progresses, and as increasing numbers of helper T cells (T_4 lymphocytes, also called CD_4 cells because they carry the CD_4 receptor molecule on their surface) die, HIV-infected persons begin to show increasing symptoms of life-threatening infections. They suffer weight loss or diarrhea, and show symptoms of rare lung infections and rare cancers that eventually prove to be fatal. The opportunistic infections increase as the immune system deteriorates, and these infections can attack the lung, the brain, the gastrointestinal system and, for all practical purposes, every organ system of the body.

There is no cure for AIDS, though skilful use of drugs now available can usually offer those with advanced HIV disease a longer span of life than was the case when AIDS was first identified, in the early 1980s. It is uncertain whether everyone infected with HIV will eventually move through the continuum of HIV disease up to the stage of AIDS. Most people with HIV infection, according to current knowledge, do follow this progression. Moreover, very few persons diagnosed as having advanced HIV disease and AIDS live much beyond three or four years after the diagnosis. As of early 1993, AIDS, on average, is uniformly fatal over a span of three to four years after diagnosis.

THE HISTORY OF THE HIV EPIDEMIC: MILESTONES

An epidemic is an outbreak of a communicable disease that spreads to affect large numbers of people. When the disease extends to many people in various parts of the world it is sometimes called a pandemic, from Greek words suggesting that people all over the world, not only people in one particular region or country, court a risk of contracting the disease.

Early Indications of the Epidemic

In 1981, the Centers for Disease Control (CDC) in Atlanta, Georgia, began to receive reports of rare infections and cancers in young men; infections such as a peculiar sort of pneumonia called pneumocystis carinii (a primitive microorganism) pneumonia (PCP); and cancers such as Kaposi's sarcoma, a tumor leading to the development of purple-coloured patches and bumps on the skin, and also affecting various organs in the body. Prior to 1981, these conditions were noticed only rarely, and then only in people who had been submitted to known causes of immune system weakening, such as rare genetic diseases, immuno-suppressive drug treatments in connection with organ transplantation, or cancer chemotherapy.

At first, these rare opportunistic conditions were found only, or almost only, in homosexual men, and the unexplained condition came to be known temporarily and popularly by a number of names, such as "the gay plague," "gay cancer," and "GRID (gay-related immune disease)." This last term recognized the common denominator (disruption of the immune system) among the various opportunistic infections and conditions that, from 1982 and thereafter, came to be diagnosed, not only in homosexual men, but in bisexual men also, and in hemophiliacs, intravenous drug users, and sexual partners of these persons.

The Syndrome, the Virus, the Test, and AZT

By the end of 1982, AIDS came to be the officially recognized name for the collection of infections and symptoms resulting from a new, and as yet unexplained, deterioration of the body's immune defenses. Cases of AIDS increased rapidly in the U.S., Canada, and many of the European countries. Careful observation and analysis of the reported cases supported the conclusion that an agent, a microorganism of some sort, transmitted from one person to another by contact with infected blood and in sexual relations, was causing this immunological breakdown. The work of laboratories directed by Professor Luc Montagnier at the Pasteur Institute in Paris, and by Dr. Robert Gallo at the National Cancer Institute in Bethesda, Maryland, led to the identification in 1983 and 1984 of a virus, a retrovirus, as the cause of AIDS. That virus came to be known as HIV, the human immunodeficiency virus. By 1985, a blood test, the ELISA test, was developed to detect anti-HIV antibodies in the blood. This test, along with other stronger confirmatory tests, came to be widely used to screen blood, and to identify people who are carriers of HIV infection. By the end of 1986, clinical studies demonstrated that treatment with an agent called azidothymidine (AZT), also called zidovudine (ZDV), would prolong the survival of persons with AIDS. Since 1986, numerous additional studies have shown that early treatment with AZT or other antiretroviral agents also slows down the progression of HIV infection to the AIDS stage of HIV disease.

The Origin of HIV Infection

The precise origin of HIV infection is unknown. Earlier rumors that HIV originated intentionally, as a new infectious organism constructed in laboratories for developing biological weapons, can be quite easily discounted. HIV-antibody tests of stored blood samples, carried out after AIDS came to be recognized as a new syndrome, indicate that there were cases of HIV-induced AIDS going back to the late 1960s, a time when the techniques of molecular biology required to create an HIV-like virus did not exist. The more recently mentioned idea that HIV infection entered the human population from a virus used to construct the polio vaccine in the 1950s has been examined and found to be both without evidence and unlikely. The human immunodeficiency virus probably did evolve in Africa, and may have been present in human populations there for many decades, without causing AIDS. The virus could also have caused AIDS-like diseases and deaths that were never recognized as such, against the heavy background of other lethal infectious diseases present in those populations (Anderson, 1992, 59).

The Spread of HIV Infection and AIDS

Cases of AIDS have now been reported in nearly every country of the world. As of January 1993, 7,282 cases of AIDS had been reported to Health and Welfare Canada, over the period 1979-1992 (December). Among these 7,282 cases, there have been 4,685 deaths. However, Dr. Donald Sutherland, chief of HIV-AIDS epidemiology at the Laboratory Centre for Disease Control in Ottawa, believes that the real number of AIDS cases in Canada is greater than the number of reported cases. Taking account of cases not reported, and of late reporting, Dr. Sutherland estimates that the cumulative number of AIDS cases in Canada may be as high as 11,000 by the end of 1992 (Mickleburgh, 1992, A-4). As of March 1992, Mexico had 9,562 reported cases of AIDS, and the United States had 242,146 reported cases of AIDS as of October, 1992 (Laboratory Centre for Disease Control, 1993, 1).

The reported number of AIDS cases is only the tip of the iceberg of HIV infection in any one country, and also in the world at large. If Dr. Sutherland's estimate that 1 in 670 Canadians is HIV-infected is correct, then there would be something over 40,000 HIV-infected Canadian citizens and residents, as of 1992. The recently published *AIDS in the World - A Global Report* estimates that nearly 13 million people worldwide have been infected with HIV. In over 2.5 million of these people, HIV disease has progressed to AIDS, and over 90% of those with AIDS (about 2.5 million persons) have died. The spread of HIV infection worldwide has not stopped, and estimates are that nearly 7 million more people around the world will become HIV-infected by 1995. On a conservative estimate, these numbers will reach 38 million HIV-infected by the turn of the century. Some believe 110 million is a more realistic projection of the numbers of people who will have become HIV-infected by the year 2000 (Mann, 1992, 4-5). HIV infection and HIV disease have, without doubt, attained pandemic proportions over the last decade. The pandemic will not rapidly go into demise and disappearance, because HIV is now endemic in the human population.

ETHICS AND THE EPIDEMIC: AN OVERVIEW

Though the HIV epidemic exhibits very distinct biological characteristics, in comparison to epidemics of earlier centuries, this epidemic's social effects, some have said, are unparalleled in history (Society Services Committee, 1987). Along with the suffering and death it has wrought, this epidemic has also functioned like a social electron-scanning microscope, amplifying and revealing deep deficiencies in science, medicine, and systems of health care. It has also amplified and expressed widespread and latent ignorance, as well as complacency regarding the infectious and potentially lethal microorganisms with which human beings must coexist in the biosphere. People generally thought, prior to the outbreak of HIV infection, that science and medicine had lethal infectious diseases largely under control. The outbreak of this epidemic shook that confidence. It also revealed that HIV infection, linked from the outset to people living on the margins of social respectability, was awakening phobias, prejudices, paranoias, and discrimination of new and unique intensity.

Response to the HIV epidemic is calling upon, and calling forth, a society's basic values. These values are the terms in which a society defines and exhibits its identity, what it stands for, and what it stands against. These values are a foundation for policies, laws, regulations; for setting priorities and supporting projects; and for decisions about the just distribution of increasingly limited resources.

The central moral and social issues of how society should relate to individuals, of how the spread of HIV infection can be prevented without trampling upon the rights, or neglecting the needs, of those already infected recur over and over again, in an extraordinarily wide range of specific and difficult ethical issues relating to HIV infection and HIV disease. These issues involve uncertainties and conflicts of many sorts, including conflicts of perception, assumptions, and beliefs (ethos); and conflicts of values and responsibilities (morality and professional ethics).

People have confronted these issues repeatedly over the last decade, and continue to do so, as they seek consensus on questions about:

- HIV-antibody testing, and the need to protect HIV-infected persons against discrimination;

- nominal or anonymous reporting of positive HIV test results and of diagnoses of AIDS to public health authorities;

- whether, how, and by whom contact tracing and partner notification should be undertaken;

- HIV screening, whether it be for promoting behavioural change, for clinical purposes, for safety, for epidemiological research and surveillance studies, or for the imposition of constraints on travel, immigration, employment, or insurance;

- the role of information, education, counselling, and behaviour modification in preventing the transmission of HIV infection;
- confidentiality, versus the need to warn;
- the need clinically to evaluate new treatments, versus the desire and demand of HIV-infected persons for rapid access to potentially beneficial new drugs;
- the duty to treat, versus the risks in treating HIV-infected people;
- the right of HIV-infected health care professionals to pursue their careers, versus their responsibility to protect patients against HIV infection;
- the myriad of recurrent dilemmas, with emphasis on euthanasia, that can occur in the care of persons in the final stages of HIV disease.

THE NATURAL HISTORY OF HIV ETHICS

Values have dates, and so do issues in HIV ethics. The term "natural history" is used in medical circles to cover the progression of a disease, particularly when treatments are not available to alter the course of a disease progression.

We borrow that term to indicate that there is also a progression, though not inevitably progress, in our perception, analysis, and resolution of ethical and social issues related to HIV infection and HIV disease.

Some issues have been resolved; others have been resolved, but opened again. Some issues, on the other hand, are still subject to controversy, and have never been resolved. Other issues are new or still just emerging.

An Issue as Resolved

An issue is considered to be *resolved* when sufficient consensus has been achieved to end dispute on a matter requiring decision, policy, and action. One of several conflicting positions gains a sufficient measure of public support to become the basis for public ethics, policy, or law.

Anonymous HIV seroprevalence studies offer an example of an issue that has been resolved. Four to five years ago, there was considerable controversy about the ethical justifiability of using leftover blood samples to conduct studies, to determine how far HIV infection had spread in given subpopulations in a society. For example, proposals were put forward for studies that would use blood samples routinely taken from newborn babies, to determine anonymously how far HIV infection had spread into the population of childbearing women. For at least twelve months after birth, a baby cannot produce antibodies of its own against HIV. So the presence of HIV antibodies in the baby's blood would reveal that its mother was HIV-infected. For a time, thoughtful people were adopting quite opposed positions on the matter of whether it was ethical to conduct tests on anonymous leftover samples of blood without mothers' consent. Gradually, and after much discussion, differing perceptions came into closer alignment and, finally, the issue was resolved in favour of allowing such epidemiological studies, under carefully specified conditions (Roy, 1990; Federal Center for AIDS, 1990).

An Issue as Unresolved

An issue is *unresolved* if controversy continues, and societal consensus cannot be achieved about which of two or more conflicting courses of action should be ethically or legally supported. Such is the case with euthanasia and assisted euthanasia for persons with AIDS. Such also is the case regarding what means may justifiably be taken to protect patients against HIV transmission, when a surgeon, for example, or a dentist, is HIV-infected.

An Issue as Reopened

A *resolved* issue may be *reopened*. The consensus and support required to resolve an issue may not be universal. Opposition to the proposed resolution may be silent and unorganized, at the time a resolution is adopted. In such circumstances, the consensus may be only apparently universal, and the resolution of the issue may be only temporary. Such is the case with HIV-antibody testing of health care professionals, and of patients. Consensus, apparently, had been achieved, and the apparently widely accepted policy, during the period 1980 to 1990, was against any routine, systematic, or mandatory HIV-antibody testing of patients or health care professionals. This issue, as we shall see, now seems to be returning to the centre of public discourse, in this second decade of the epidemic. Some health care professionals are, for their own protection against HIV infection, arguing that patients, particularly those requiring invasive procedures, should be routinely tested for HIV antibodies; others are demanding that health care professionals be periodically tested, to protect patients against receiving HIV infection from doctors, dentists, nurses, and others entrusted with their care.

An Issue as New

Controversies take time *to mature*. A dispute may begin, for example, with disagreement between two surgeons in a surgical specialty unit about the justification of a surgeon's refusal to do elective surgery, or about the justifiability of an HIV-infected surgeon's continuing to practise surgery. The dispute gradually grows into an issue, as more and more people, and various institutions, are drawn into the discussion, and the dispute becomes a public controversy. While this process is going on, an issue is *maturing*. During this process, perceptions, for instance, about risk, come into clearer focus. Facts and reasons are marshalled and organized to build arguments. Positions and counterpositions crystallize and become rallying points of public controversy. When this point is reached, we have a *new* issue in the domain of HIV disease.

An Issue as Emerging

An issue is only *emerging*, when controversy is still at an embryonic stage of development. People then have spontaneous feelings for or against a course of action. At this stage, the facts involved in the dispute usually have not been precisely determined. Perceptions are out of focus, arguments have not been organized, positions have not hardened. A public controversy may or may not arise out of the initial malaise, and the early sense that things here are not quite right. People do not yet really know "what is at stake," when an issue is only just emerging. Are important values being threatened, or not, by a possible new course of action? What values will a new course of action support and enhance? Once clarity is achieved on the answers to these questions, a potential controversy may rapidly fade away, or mature into a new ethical or legal issue.

At the beginning of the HIV epidemic in 1981 and 1982, persons tended to die quite rapidly after they reached the stage of HIV disease that later came to be known as AIDS. Many lived barely six months to a year after the start of treatment for their infections. Since the introduction of several new treatments against the virus itself, such as AZT and ddI (dideoxyinosine, a drug acting against retroviruses), and with more effective treatments available for a number of infections that HIV-infected people acquire as their immune systems weaken, people tend, on average, to live three or more years after a diagnosis of AIDS, particularly when they are tested early after HIV infection, and begin to receive treatment early in the course of HIV disease. These persons live longer, and their care becomes more expensive as new drugs are developed. A new version of the just distribution of limited resources is an example of an emerging issue, in the 1990s. Some hospitals, saddled with serious budgetary constraints, refuse to allocate money for some of the expensive new drug treatments for AIDS. Can we ethically tolerate the emergence of two classes of AIDS patients: those who live longer because they can pay for the drugs, and those without personal means who will die earlier than need be?

The Focus of This Chapter

This chapter will concentrate on selected unresolved, as well as on new and emerging, ethical issues in the domain of HIV infection and AIDS. A selection is necessary, because a chapter cannot cover the same ground as a book, and books have already been needed to discuss HIV ethics comprehensively (Reamer, 1991). Our selection is based on two criteria: centrality of the issue to the well-being of HIV-infected persons, and intensity of the controversy generated by the issue.

THE ETHICS OF PERCEPTION AND ATTITUDE

The attitudes towards HIV-infected persons, and towards persons with AIDS, that should be adopted and promoted, both individually and publicly, are an ethical issue, an example of conflicts on the level of ethos.

Individuals and groups can control and modify perceptions and choose attitudes based on disgust and fear, or upon compassion and solidarity. There is a danger that prejudice and panic may shape behaviour and policies, regarding HIV-infected persons and persons with AIDS. Some may transfer their fear of the syndrome and of death, or their repugnance against homosexual behaviour and drug abuse, to the human beings who face the sufferings of isolation and loneliness, guilt and hopelessness, gradual loss of strength and function, and eventually death. The primary ethical challenge is on the level of perception. To see persons as greater than their infection, disability, and disease, and as possessing a worth and dignity incalculably superior to forms of behaviour many may scorn, is the core of the challenge. The ethical tragedy is when the infection and the syndrome become the identity of the affected person, in his or her own eyes, and in the eyes of others.

Health care professionals, and others who counsel seropositive persons and who treat and care for AIDS patients, perhaps particularly those who aspire to offer palliative care to terminally ill AIDS patients, should ponder what some persons with AIDS have said to those who proffer help: "You cannot really say that you accept me as a human being while you reject the sexuality that constitutes a central dimension of my own personal identity and being." We should all ponder, though many may not be prepared to accept, that sexuality is not reprehensible because it is homosexual, rather than heterosexual. It is perhaps, rather, the case that sexual activity, whether it be homosexual or heterosexual, is immoral when it expresses the trivialization of human beings, or their domination and betrayal, rather than supporting presence, fidelity, and liberation.

Many persons with AIDS are demonstrating that death is not the greatest pain. That pain is, rather, to be found in the abandonment of suffering people, by those of us who are complacent in the conviction of our moral superiority to those whose behaviours we reject, and complacent also in the conviction of our social superiority to those who, because of their colour, poverty, or life-style, we consider marginal, unimportant, and undeserving of our care.

One physician has observed that AIDS, this dreadful disease, "is not only killing young people in the prime of life and destroying their familial and social relationships, it also is damaging the bond between the caregiver and the patient with AIDS as well." (Rogers, 1988) The professional and personal bond between caregivers and HIV-seropositive persons at all stages of their infection needs to be fostered, for at least three reasons:

- that bond is essential for effective counselling and education;
- that bond is an integral part of the healing process, "healing" being a comprehensive mind-body event, and possible even when medical "cures" are not available;
- that bond may be an AIDS patient's only, or most important, mooring of support as the disease advances to its terminal stages.

Appropriate professional attitudes towards patients, though as important as knowledge and technical skills in the education of doctors, nurses, and other caregivers, cannot be commanded or legislated into existence. In this regard, there is no substitute for "teaching by example." It is, however, extremely difficult to demonstrate humane and sensitive attitudes towards patients, if the members of a treatment team work in an environment that tends to foster their own dehumanization at work. Time is needed with others on a treatment team, to explore together the fears, suspicion, and negative feelings that can be so destructive of a healing relationship with patients, whatever the disease they may have.

There is some evidence that AIDS is drawing forth quite powerful phobias and negative attitudes towards HIV-seropositive persons, and towards those who are symptomatic. A study of the attitudes of randomly selected physicians in three large cities of the United States found "that the AIDS diagnosis carries emotional charge and elicits judgmental, negative evaluations about the patient even by health care providers. Attitudes of this kind indicate that many physicians experience discomfort interacting with AIDS patients which can interfere with the development of a positive, constructive, and open doctor-AIDS patient relationship." (Kelly, 1987, 791) These negative attitudes were associated strongly with the physicians' idea that persons with AIDS are responsible for their illness. Some physicians believe, for this reason, that AIDS patients are less deserving than other patients, and should occupy lower places on waiting lists for scarce and expensive diagnostic and therapeutic procedures. "Why all the fuss? They're going to die anyway!" This reaction of one physician, though not representative of physicians' or caregivers' attitudes generally, does underscore the point that destructive attitudes can destroy the quality of life, and even the lives, of HIV-infected persons.

Attitudes towards HIV-infected persons, and the willingness of professionals to care for them are also influenced by the professionals' perception of the risk they face of becoming HIV-infected. A study of physicians in three geographical regions of North America (Ohio, Chicago, Ontario) found that physicians' perception of risk affects their behaviour. Physicians who perceived the risk of becoming infected in treating HIV-infected persons as high were more likely than others to adopt the position that surgeons have the right to refuse to treat patients who refuse to undergo HIV-antibody testing (Taylor, 1990, 499).

ETHICS, LAW, AND DISCRIMINATION

The failure to make intellectually relevant distinctions leads to unjust discrimination against human beings. The guiding ethical rule should be: judge each person on the basis of his or her unique qualities, competence, abilities, and unique reserves of physical and psychic strength. Unjust discrimination begins when people are lumped together and treated as members of a class, while their unique distinguishing characteristics are ignored, and count for little or nothing in deliberations that affect their lives.

The term *discriminate*, however, is usually not used in the positive sense of making intellectually relevant distinctions (that is, of being a person of "discrimination"). Discrimination usually means making adverse distinctions against persons. It means distinguishing someone or some group unfavourably from others, in an arbitrary way. People are unjustly discriminated against when the adverse treatment they receive, when the goods, services, and opportunities from which they are excluded, are out of proportion with the characteristics that do differentiate them from others. Minor differences, and differences unrelated to specific goods, services and opportunities, do not justify excluding persons from benefits enjoyed by others with whom those discriminated against share major similarities.

The Québec *Charter of Human Rights and Freedoms*, a comprehensive bill of rights, defines discrimination in the following terms:

> Every person has a right to full and equal recognition and exercise of his human rights and freedoms, without distinction, exclusion or preference based on race, colour, sex, pregnancy, sexual orientation, civil status, age except as provided by law, religion, political convictions, language, ethnic or national origin, social condition, a handicap or the use of any means to palliate a handicap.
>
> Discrimination exists where such a distinction, exclusion or preference has the effect of nullifying or impairing such right. (*Charter of Human Rights and Freedoms*, s.10)

Discrimination, in this *Charter*, is a distinction or exclusion that restricts or bars a person's right of access to goods, services, facilities, employment, and other benefits for which citizens should enjoy equal opportunity. The grounds for such adverse distinction are specified, and include adverse distinction on the basis of handicap (Tarnopolsky, 1985, 274). Provincial human rights codes generally prohibit discrimination on the basis of handicap or disability, though the language used varies considerably (MacKinnon, 1988, 380; Ritter, 1987, 70).

The question arises as to whether AIDS, HIV seropositivity, perceived HIV infection, sexual orientation, or perceived sexual orientation are included as grounds upon which discrimination should be considered unlawful.

The Yukon, Québec, Manitoba, and Ontario prohibit discrimination based on a person's sexual orientation. Ontario's and Québec's legislation also prohibit discrimination based upon a perception of handicap. AIDS, presumably, would qualify as a handicap or disability protected by provincial antidiscrimination legislation. However, it is not clear that discrimination against an asymptomatic HIV-seropositive person is unlawful everywhere in Canada. For this reason, the Royal Society Working Group on AIDS has recommended that all human rights legislation in Canada be amended to prohibit discrimination based on evidence of HIV infection, perceived infection, sexual orientation, or perceived sexual orientation (Royal Society of Canada, 1988, 11). This direct, explicit approach is perhaps more promising than semantic attempts to protect persons against unreasonable discrimination, by trying to cover them with the term *handicap*, when they are in no fashion disabled or impaired. But the U.S. Supreme Court, in the *Arline* case, held that a person suffers discrimination if he or she is disabled due to others' prejudiced responses or prejudiced denials of opportunity; that is, an otherwise able person becomes disabled because of how others treat him or her, and so many suffer discrimination on grounds of disability (*School Board of Nassau County*, 1987).

THE ETHICS OF PREVENTION

Public health authorities have a moral and legal mandate to prevent the spread of contagious and potentially lethal infections and diseases. That is beyond dispute, and is based on the assumption that the good of the community may, *under certain conditions*, justifiably compel individuals to accept or suffer constraints on their liberties. On these assumptions, there is nothing *inherently* unethical in the bestowal upon, and the exercise by, health authorities of power to compel such procedures as testing, reporting, contact tracing, immunization, treatment, and even isolation and quarantine.

However, the commanding values, beliefs, and perceptions of a community, at any given period in its history, will greatly affect how the balance is struck between the individual's interest in liberty and privacy and the public's interest in health safety. Moreover, societies will differ, and any given society may, at different periods in its own history, hold quite different views on the ethical and legal conditions that have to be met to justify the use of coercive measures against individuals, to protect public health. Some of the measures previously tolerated in Canada to control venereal diseases (Cassel, 1987) are no longer consonant with our current views and values, nor are they necessary or effective in the control of HIV infection and AIDS today. Historically, public health measures were applied under the state's policing powers, rather that health care powers, hence the use of coercion, rather than free and informed consent.

A Voluntarist Policy

After ten years of experience with HIV infection and AIDS, people around the world have come to realize that the current biological, medical, and social characteristics of the HIV epidemic demand a voluntarist, rather than a coercive, model of public health intervention, to reach the goal of maximally containing the spread of this infection. The reasons supporting a voluntarist, rather than a coercive, policy are many, and have been discussed in numerous publications.

A voluntarist policy of prevention would emphasize public information and education, counselling to support HIV-infected persons, voluntary HIV-antibody testing, anonymous reporting to public authorities of HIV test results and of AIDS diagnoses (that is, for epidemiological determination of prevalence levels in a community, rather than for mandatory management of infected individuals), the protection of the privacy of HIV-infected persons and of persons with AIDS.

A voluntarist ethic should be pursued in all efforts to stem the spread of the HIV epidemic, to develop treatments for AIDS, and to care for those with HIV disease. The use of coercion or force threatens the fabric of our society, designed as it is on a pattern of liberties, rights, and freely assumed responsibilities. Mandatory requirements may be justified, but they do require justification. Arbitrary, discriminatory, or falsely based restrictions on rights and liberties are intolerable in an open and democratic society.

Contact Tracing and Partner Notification

Identification and notification of sex partners of persons carrying venereal disease have, for many years, been standard elements in the public health strategy to control sexually transmitted diseases such as syphilis and gonorrhea. The goal of this strategy has been to break the chain of transmission, through early treatment of the infected persons and their sexual contacts. Though there is no cure yet available for HIV disease, and no vaccine that can prevent infection, identification and notification of sexual and needle-sharing contacts of HIV-infected persons can allow these contacts to seek testing, to be counselled, to modify their behaviour and reduce further transmission of the virus, and to begin an early course of medical care and treatment.

The goals — what can be done for contact persons, and what they can do for themselves once they know of the risk they have faced — are important and realistic, both for the welfare of individuals and for the protection of the common good. These goals justify contact tracing and partner notification in principle.

The key ethical question is about method. There are *three general models* of how identification and notification of partners can be achieved. *Active contact tracing* seeks out as many contacts of an infected person as possible. Public health officials are centrally involved. They solicit the names of a patient's contacts, locate them, and warn them about their exposure to HIV, but without deliberately or explicitly revealing the infected person's name. *Limited contact tracing* applies the same approach as active contact tracing, but on a restricted and specifically targeted subpopulation, such as unsuspecting heterosexual contacts, women of childbearing age, or blood-product recipients. *Voluntary contact tracing* and partner notification are much less invasive of privacy than is active contact tracing. In the voluntary process, the infected person undertakes to notify his or her contacts personally and to refer the contacts for testing and counselling (Levine, 1988).

The voluntary contact tracing and partner notification model has two variants. The *patient referral process* has infected persons informing their own partners of the HIV risk to which they have been exposed. Public health officials or physicians may instruct and aid them in this process. With the *provider referral process*, infected persons provide names, telephone numbers, or addresses of their known sexual or needle-sharing partners, and public health officials, or a physician, or a specially trained nurse does the work of contacting and notifying the partners (Centers for Disease Control, 1988).

It would be difficult ethically to justify any model of contact tracing and partner notification that would jeopardize the goals of a voluntarist public health care policy, in the matter of HIV infection. Systematic active contact tracing models that pressure HIV-infected persons to reveal the names of their partners, that infiltrate strangers into the spheres of personal and sexual privacy of HIV-infected persons and their partners, and that store highly sensitive, as well as potentially damaging, information, particularly when stored in ways that permit identification of individuals by name, do seriously threaten both a voluntarist policy and the collaboration of HIV-infected persons with partner notification programmes. Voluntary contact tracing and partner notification, properly organized and implemented by sensitive and well-trained persons, are a practicable approach to controlling the spread of HIV infection. This approach is also consistent with human rights, and with the human dignity of HIV-infected persons and their sexual partners.

Mandatory Testing of Tissue Donors: An Exception to the Voluntarist Ethic

Mandatory testing for HIV infection implies an element of coercion. A person may refuse to be tested, but at the price of being excluded from some activity, or of foregoing some benefit or privilege. Prospective donors of blood, semen, ova, organs, and other tissues for transplantation constitute the widely recognized category of necessary exceptions to a voluntarist policy of HIV-antibody testing. Testing of donors should be mandatory. Restrictions on the liberty of donating blood, or organs, or tissues are justified by the need to protect recipients from potentially lethal infections.

The Ethical Response to Unreasonable Demands for Mandatory Testing for HIV Infection

Mandatory HIV-antibody testing has been proposed for a wide range of groups in society, including those planning marriage, pregnant women, patients scheduled for surgery, persons admitted to hospitals, surgeons and health care personnel, homosexuals, prostitutes, intravenous drug users, insurance applicants, school children, teachers, prisoners, employees for various occupations, recruits or volunteers for military service, and immigrants.

An ethical position requires the comprehensive consideration and balancing of all relevant factors. Balanced consideration of all relevant factors relating to HIV infection and AIDS leads to the following conclusion: mandatory HIV-antibody testing programmes, with the exception of mandatory testing of donors of human blood and tissue, are unnecessary, impracticable, and likely to be injurious both to individuals and to society. Mandatory policies will discourage cooperation of people with health authorities, will heighten fear and hysteria, and will force the epidemic spread of HIV infection underground. The ability to control the spread of that infection will be lost, and everyone will suffer the consequences.

The Ethics of Safer Sex

Sex is at the heart of the human drama of HIV infection and AIDS. The HIV pandemic presses us to rethink the question of the ethics of sex, but not only in the way some people would like to think.

Some believe that those who acquire HIV infection from sexual activity are responsible for their own actions, and for the terrible consequences they have to pay. Some narrow their focus on homosexual persons, and believe these persons should never engage in sexual activity. They would believe that *heterosexual eros* is the only sexual way to realize *agape*, that increasingly unselfish love that wills the full flowering of another human being.

However, the ethics based on this view of sex falls far short of the tolerance and understanding that human solidarity requires. That solidarity does not expect, nor does it demand, that a human being renounce being bodily and intimately cherished for a lifetime, because his or her desire is for a human being of the same sex.

The ethics of homosexual relations, as is equally true of heterosexual relations, is based on humanity's commands: do not trivialize, enslave, or betray another human being! Do not give death when you love! These are the terms of the human drama, when it is acted out in sex.

However, it is essential to realize that sexual relations can and do transmit the human immunodeficiency virus, and with that virus follows HIV disease, AIDS, and death. So, sexual relations are the place where the spread of this virus can also be prevented and stopped. How?

Primarily, by not having unprotected sexual relations with an HIV-infected person. It is very difficult, however, to know who is HIV-infected and who is not. Evidently, people who are in a long-standing sexual relationship, and who are completely faithful sexually to each other, run a very low risk of transmitting the virus or of becoming infected themselves. Of course, sexual fidelity is not a hallmark of our culture. Couples and marriages break up frequently. New sexual relationships are then started. Moreover, many people have more than one sexual partner in any given year.

It is for this reason that those who preach safer sex advise the use of condoms. Use of condoms has helped to reduce the spread of venereal disease, and they can help to prevent the spread of HIV infection. Condoms, of course, are not fail-safe. There are perhaps many who believe that sexual relations outside of marriage are morally reprehensible. Some of these people also affirm that it is, therefore, morally irresponsible to counsel the use of condoms. That would be equivalent, they say, to condoning immoral activity.

There is quite another way of thinking about this issue. We should be doing everything we can to promote the survival of people who do not accept, or cannot live up to, the moral ideals others proclaim to be of the highest importance. Collaboration with public health authorities in promoting every reasonable measure to prevent the spread of HIV disease, AIDS, and death is ethically just as important as proclaiming moral ideals that many will never espouse or cannot achieve.

HIV ETHICS IN HEALTH CARE INSTITUTIONS

If values have dates, as was said earlier in this chapter, ethical conflicts have their arenas. The workplace and the school were arenas for some of the most acrimonious ethical conflicts of the 1980s. The issues confronted there have now been largely resolved.

As to the workplace, general consensus has been achieved on the following points. First, HIV-infected employees and employees with AIDS should be allowed to work as long as they are able to do so, and they should be treated like any other employees with life-threatening diseases, in respect to medical coverage, disability leave, and life insurance. Second, employers should not routinely screen current employees or job applicants for HIV infection. Any exception to this rule in individual cases would have to be justified in terms of bona fide occupational requirement, and must respect informed voluntary consent and confidentiality requirements.

As to the school, people now generally recognize and accept that barring HIV-infected children (infected usually from blood transfusions or *in utero*) from school serves no valid purpose. Segregation of HIV-infected school children from their peers would fail the proportionality test. Such isolation would cause the HIV-infected child harm totally out of proportion to the insignificant risk such a child would pose to other school children or to teachers. Refusal to accept HIV-infected children in the school would be discriminatory and unreasonable. Moreover, HIV-antibody testing of children, for purposes of deciding about their attendance at school, is totally unwarranted.

Nothing stands still for very long in the world of HIV infection and AIDS, and ethical controversy has now, early in the 1990s, shifted from the workplace and school to hospitals and health care institutions. Some physicians and surgeons have refused to treat HIV-infected persons, and are requesting that patients be tested for antibodies to HIV before undergoing invasive procedures like surgery. There is widespread and unresolved controversy as to whether HIV-infected surgeons and dentists should be allowed to continue to practise their professions. HIV-antibody testing is again at the centre of controversy, when the idea is put forth that all health care workers, especially those who perform surgery and other invasive procedures, should be periodically tested. The issue of how limited health care resources should be distributed is returning to the centre of ethical controversy over HIV disease in the 1990s. Are budgetary decisions justified, if they force doctors to treat AIDS patients according to standards that are now no longer optimal?

When Physicians Refuse to Treat

There have been a number of reports of the reluctance of health care professionals, including dentists, physicians, and surgeons, to treat HIV-infected persons and persons with AIDS. The motivation for this reluctance is multiple. Some refuse treatment because they fear acquiring HIV infection and passing it on to their families. They fear for their careers and the stability and security of their family lives, if they become infected. Some physicians have refused or are reluctant to treat HIV-infected persons, because they fear that the presence in their practices of persons with AIDS will scare away other patients. There are also some physicians who are totally ill at ease with homosexuals and intravenous (IV) drug users, and their refusal to treat such persons is phobia-motivated. Caring adequately for AIDS patients is also a fairly complex business, requiring the use of novel drugs, and combinations of drugs, often with unknown or unfamiliar side effects, for the treatment of the multiple opportunistic infections characteristic of advanced HIV disease. Some doctors simply do not want all the bother, particularly when death is seen as the inevitable result of all their efforts (Zuger, 1991; Levine R.J., 1991).

Now there is controversy about both the basis and the extent of a physician's duty to treat persons with HIV disease. Those who support a physician's right to refuse to treat certain patients emphasize the contractual nature of the doctor-patient relationship, and see a doctor's rights as parallel to those of a patient (Reed, 1987). Those who reject a doctor's refusal to treat as unethical insist on what could be called the covenant character of the professional relationship between a physician and a sick person in need of care (May, 1983). That insistence encompasses the notion that medical ethics imposes, on those who freely choose the medical profession, obligations that are greater and more demanding than the obligations of citizens in other walks of life (Brennan, 1991). This is an essential and distinguishing mark of a profession. Still others find that the reasoning in support of this view is weak and faulty, and that a legal statute specifically defining a doctor's duty to treat persons with AIDS may be necessary to resolve ethical uncertainty (Tegtmeier, 1990).

There is a quite general recognition that doctors do possess the liberty to enter or not to enter into contract with people requesting their care. Doctors are not obligated to accept each and every person requesting their services. However, that liberty is not absolute. In emergencies, doctors are not free to refuse treatment. Moreover, in some provinces, discrimination against persons on the basis of disability or, for instance, their sexual orientation, is illegal. Indeed, if a recent amendment to the *Code of Medical Ethics* of the Professional Corporation of Physicians is adopted and implemented, doctors in Québec will not be at liberty to refuse to treat persons on the basis of their HIV seropositivity, or on the basis of their having AIDS.

Five years ago, the American College of Physicians and the Infectious Diseases Society of America emphasized that physicians, other health care professionals, and hospitals are under ethical obligation to provide competent and humane care to patients with AIDS, with other conditions related to HIV disease, and to HIV-infected persons with other medical problems not directly related to HIV disease. The denial of appropriate care to these patients and refusal to treat them was deemed to be unethical (Health and Public Policy Committee, 1988, 462).

Physicians, surgeons, dentists, and other health care professionals should realize that HIV infection is widespread in our society, and can remain latent and asymptomatic for years. This means that the burden of HIV disease and AIDS will increase over the coming years. Moreover, as continuing medical advances will offer increasingly prolonged life expectancy to those with HIV infection, HIV disease will become a more prevalent chronic condition in our society, and in societies throughout the world. Doctors, surgeons, and others should realize that contact with HIV-infected persons is an integral part of the reality they will have to accept, if they want to practise a health care profession over the next decades.

If we are ever to gain control of the HIV epidemic, and if we are to be in a position to offer competent and sensitive care to those with HIV disease, we need a solid, well-organized system of health care that we can trust and upon which we can rely, particularly in times of crisis. Acceptance of the thesis that physicians are at ethical liberty to refuse treatment for those in serious need will contribute to the breakdown of the system of care, upon which the entire community depends.

When a Surgeon Is HIV-Infected

The general common-sense view is that a single HIV-infected health care worker who does invasive procedures, such as a surgeon does, can infect many more patients than an HIV-infected patient can infect health care workers (Brennan, 1991; Gostin, 1989). Whether HIV-infected surgeons should continue to practise surgery, and how this question should be decided and by whom are foci of an emerging ethical issue in the 1990s.

We direct attention briefly to the question about an HIV-infected surgeon continuing his or her practice. There is currently no consensus on this issue, and recommendations are often evasive rather than definite.

Some recommendations, however, are very definite indeed. The American Medical Association has said that physicians who know they carry an infectious disease should desist from any activity that poses even a minimal risk of transmitting the disease to patients (Council, 1988). The same Association has even counselled HIV-seropositive health care providers to warn patients or cease practising (Altman, 1991, A-3). Others have denied that HIV-infected physicians should report their HIV status to their patients (Brennan, 1991; Altman, 1991, A-1).

There seems to be no justification for drastic, radical approaches, such as demanding that an HIV-infected surgeon immediately cease all practise of surgery. The general idea is: let the decision match the risk.

The first essential consideration is that HIV-infected physicians and surgeons, and their patients, can be best helped by creating a non-draconian, confidential, and sympathetic environment that encourages them to seek help (Adler, 1987).

The second essential consideration is that HIV-infected physicians, particularly those whose specialty requires that they perform invasive procedures, should seek specialist advice on the extent to which they should limit their professional practices, in order to protect their patients. HIV-infected physicians and surgeons should not continue their practices solely on the basis of their own assessments of the risk they pose to patients (Walter, 1987).

A third essential consideration is that restricting HIV-infected surgeons only from practising certain particularly high-risk procedures, not from practising surgery altogether, may offer patients sufficient protection. For example, HIV-infected surgeons at the University of Minnesota Hospital are required to avoid performing surgery that requires blind, by-feel manipulation of sharp instruments (Rhame, 1990).

A fourth essential consideration directs attention to the care that should be provided for physicians, surgeons, and others who have contracted HIV infection — some would emphasize — while professionally helping the sick. These professionals should never be abandoned. Every effort should be made to prepare proper alternative career opportunities and fitting financial security for them, when the moment does arrive when they can no longer practise the specialty for which they were trained.

HIV-Antibody Testing in Hospitals

The basic ethical principles, set down over the last decade, governing HIV testing have not changed, and there is no sound reason to change them now. HIV testing should be voluntary. This means that HIV testing should not be done without patients' informed *consent*. This means that patients should be informed about the reasons for the test, and the implications of negative and positive HIV-antibody test results. ELISA tests have to be *confirmed*. Patients should know what this means, and should understand the significance of false-positive and false-negative antibody tests. They should realize that every reasonable effort will be made to confirm the antibody tests, so that patients can trust the results that are finally given to them by their physicians. Patients should be told that the results of their HIV tests will be kept *confidential*, and that the health care personnel who need to know about the patients' HIV status, to offer proper treatment and care, are bound by the professional and legal obligation of protecting confidentiality. Pre- and post-test *counselling* are also essential ethical conditions for HIV testing. Post-test counselling may involve the need of psychological and emotional support and, when results are positive, will necessarily involve extensive discussions about coming medical events, about the course of HIV disease, about treatment options, and about responsible behaviour to avoid transmitting HIV infection to lovers and loved ones.

Physicians have a profound responsibility to educate themselves about the meaning, appropriate use, and potential adverse consequences of the HIV-antibody test, before ordering a single test. The impact of test results on the patient, and the impact on the patient's life if positive results become known to others, are potentially devastating. This is still the case in the early 1990s. It is, therefore, wrong and misguided to view HIV testing as "routine," and as no longer requiring the safeguards of confidentiality, counselling, and consent (Sherer, 1988).

Some hospitals and health care professionals, it seems, tolerate, if they do not advocate, clandestine or coercive HIV-antibody testing of patients who have been the source of blood involved in needle stick, or other kinds of accidental injuries to health care workers. Testing of a patient's blood without his or her knowledge is clandestine. Testing of a patient's blood despite his or her refusal is coercive. Such testing, of course, can be both clandestine and coercive.

Health care workers who have been exposed, by accidental injury, to potentially HIV-infected blood will, understandably, want to know as soon as possible if they have become HIV-infected. These workers, typically doctors or nurses, will have to wait months for their own immune systems to produce antibodies to HIV, if the virus has indeed entered their blood systems via accidental injuries. The period of waiting can be terribly stressful, and may well require changes in their normal ways of living a sexual life.

One should not minimize the reassurance health care workers can gain from knowing the HIV status of the patients to whose blood the workers have been accidentally exposed. However, the realistic limits to this reassurance also have to be recognized. If, for example, a patient's test is negative, but the health professional's test is positive, shortly after the accidental exposure or subsequently, the health professional may suffer suspicion and stigmatization, rather than sympathy. Moreover, a patient's negative HIV-antibody test result may be due to the patient being in the incubation period, that period of time between becoming HIV-infected and producing antibodies to the virus. This period can vary considerably. So a patient's negative test result cannot give a health professional complete reassurance. If, on the other hand, a patient's test result is positive, this does not mean that the health care professional, who has been exposed to the patient's blood, has necessarily become infected with HIV.

The degree of reassurance a health care professional can obtain from knowing the HIV status of the source-patient involved in an accidental exposure of the professional to blood, is an argument for the reasonableness of asking source-patients to consent to HIV testing. It is not an argument, however, that can justify clandestine or coercive, nonvoluntary testing of these patients.

Ethics and Limited Resources in HIV Disease

Patients at various stages of HIV disease should not be singled out as a special focus for questions about the justifiability of acceding to wishes and needs for costly drug treatments of opportunistic infections, for intensive care, and for life-prolonging procedures. Sick people come to hospitals and to doctors for counsel, care, relief, and cure, for prolongation of meaningful life if cure is not possible, and for sensitive support when death is inevitable. These expectations are reasonable, and fidelity in responding to them should be a cardinal principle of institutional and professional ethics. This principle sets a basic right of patients, and a corresponding fundamental duty of hospitals and doctors, above any utilitarian and discriminatory calculus that would tolerate a sacrifice of the duration or quality of life of some patients, for the greater good of society, of other patients, or of patients tomorrow.

This position will come under challenge over the coming decade, particularly as persons with HIV disease live longer and the cumulative costs of their treatment escalate. Some people are already claiming that persons with HIV disease and AIDS are being given preferential treatment in the distribution of limited resources, when compared with patients with other kinds of life-threatening diseases requiring prolonged and costly treatment.

Claims and counterclaims of this sort need to be settled by appeal to objective studies about how limited health care resources are, in fact, being allocated to various groups of patients. But once the studies are completed, the difficult societal choice will remain. Are we prepared, or not, to accept and endorse the sacrifices all will have to make to guarantee that no one in our society will have to suffer diminished quality and length of life, because he or she could not afford to pay for treatments that are available on the shelves of our pharmacies and hospitals?

THE ETHICS OF CONFIDENTIALITY

Persons with HIV infection have been seriously harmed by stigmatization and discrimination, following upon disclosure of their HIV seropositivity by persons, other than their physicians, who had become privy to this information. Protection of confidentiality is a personal, not only a professional, ethical responsibility.

Nevertheless, we direct attention in this section primarily to physicians, in discussing the ethics of confidentiality in connection with HIV infection. Physicians, perhaps more frequently than other health care professionals, may find themselves drawn in one direction by their obligation to keep secret information patients have entrusted to them, and drawn in the opposite direction by their sense of a need to warn other persons who are endangered by their patients' behaviour.

There are few acceptable exceptions to a physician's duty to keep confidential the information he or she has received about a person's body, life, and secrets, in the course of diagnosis and treatment. Patients' trust in physician confidentiality is essential for treatment and healing and, given the stigma and discrimination associated with seropositivity and AIDS, is equally important for effective surveillance of this epidemic and the prevention of the spread of HIV infection.

However, when a physician's patient is sexually irresponsible or blinded by psychological denial, and places the health and lives of others in danger, is a physician justified in disclosing confidential information? Some physicians have the strongest reservations against doing this. But when the physician is the only one, other than the recalcitrant patient, who possesses the knowledge needed to protect others from an unsuspected danger of an almost certain personal disaster, is he or she then justified in doing so?

A Real-Life Story

A 24-year-old woman went to her physician for an examination of symptoms related to her hay fever. She asked her physician if he would be willing to examine her husband also, because her husband was feeling chronically tired. The woman also wanted a general checkup, because she wanted to have a child soon.

The 31-year-old husband was investigated for the fatigue he was experiencing, and he was found to have mild to moderate immunodeficiency on laboratory testing. He had generalized lymphadenopathy (swollen lymph glands in the neck, armpits, and groin), and was found to be HIV-antibody positive.

The following additional facts describe the issue of confidentiality:

* The husband admitted to the doctor that he had lived a promiscuous gay life before marriage, and that he continued, even after marriage, to have occasional gay sexual relations.
* The physician told the husband he must not have unprotected sexual intercourse with his wife, and that he should not try to get her pregnant. The doctor stressed that unprotected sexual intercourse would endanger the life of the wife, and of any child they might conceive.
* The physician realized three months later, after a conversation with the wife, that her husband had told her nothing about his HIV infection, and also was continuing to have unprotected intercourse with his wife. The wife, not knowing about her husband's HIV infection, was very eager to get pregnant.
* The physician warned the husband to tell his wife the truth about his HIV infection, and to stop having unprotected sexual intercourse with her. The husband refused to accept the warning.

Ethical Considerations

Would the physician in this case be justified in breaking confidentiality, and warning the wife about her husband's HIV infection?

The professional obligation to protect confidentiality is strong, but is not absolute. There are both ethical and legal limits to this obligation (Dickens, 1988). The Canadian Medical Association's *Code of Ethics* recognizes two instances when physicians must or may disclose information about their patients to third parties: when the law demands or when the patient authorizes such disclosure. A resolution passed at the Association's annual meeting in Prince Edward Island, in the summer of 1987, added another circumstance similar to that already recognized in the *Code of Medical Ethics* of the Professional Corporation of Physicians of Québec. Protection of the health or life of others may be an ethical justification for breaking confidentiality. The text of the Québec *Code* states:

> The physician must keep in confidence what he has learned in the practice of his profession. However, he may divulge those facts he knows personally, when the patient so authorizes him, when the law permits, when there are imperative and justifiable motives relating to the health of his patient or of the community or in the case of a commanding higher objective. (Professional Corporation of Physicians of Québec, 1978, 6)

The health and life of a spouse or partner, endangered by the sexual irresponsibility of an HIV-infected person, is *a commanding higher objective* that would justify a physician's breaking confidentiality to warn such third parties.

However, breaking confidentiality to warn the spouse or partner of an HIV-infected person should be an action of last resort. A physician should sensitively educate an HIV-infected person, realizing that people may need time to grow in strength before they can face and carry the full impact and consequences of this terrible infection. We should never underestimate the costs an HIV-infected person may have to pay, in living up to the demands of moral responsibility. The social, familial, emotional, and financial costs of honesty and responsibility can be very high, indeed. People have lost their jobs, their apartments, their reputations, or have been excluded from school and university because professionals, colleagues, or even friends have been indiscreet. The other side of this story, of course, is that the price an unsuspecting spouse may have to pay for not being warned could quite well be HIV infection, AIDS, and death.

HIV RESEARCH ETHICS

Clinical trials of new treatments, when run according to the methodology outlined in Chapter 13, tend to be formal, rigid, and slow. These trials take a long time to complete, too long for many persons with advanced HIV disease ever to benefit from the clinical trial results. So, quite understandably, both persons with HIV disease and a number of scientists have increasingly and vigorously challenged research designs that would, in their view, sacrifice the needs of persons with HIV disease for the sake of respecting overly fastidious and purist ideals of clinical trials methodology.

The pressing need to develop rapidly new, safe, and effective antiretroviral treatments and treatments for opportunistic infections has been increasingly accompanied by pressure from HIV-infected persons and community groups to change the strategy of controlled clinical trials. Why? So that increasing numbers of HIV-infected persons and persons with AIDS can have a better chance of obtaining more rapid access to promising new drugs that are available only in trials, while they remain scientifically unproven.

Pressure for changes in the way clinical trials for treatments of HIV disease are run has led to intense ethical and scientific controversy. As frequently happens in such controversies, two important values are at stake, and the controversy is rooted in uncertainty about the possibility of simultaneously honouring both values.

If a promising but unvalidated new drug is available only to persons with HIV disease who participate in a clinical trial, many HIV-infected persons and persons with AIDS will never get the drug, because they will not be able to enter the clinical trial. This may happen for a number of reasons: either there are not enough clinical trials of the new drug to enroll all HIV-infected persons who would want to participate; or overly restrictive inclusion criteria will eliminate a number of persons who would want to participate; or HIV-infected persons do not want to face the lottery of randomization, and the chance of being assigned to receive either standard therapy or placebo, rather than the new drug.

On the other hand, if a promising new drug, not yet evaluated for safety and efficacy, is made widely available to persons with HIV disease, a methodically sound clinical trial of the new drug may never get off the ground, for want of a sufficient number of HIV-infected persons prepared to enter a randomized trial.

Moreover, if a promising but unvalidated new drug is made widely available outside the context of a clinical trial, many HIV-infected persons receiving the drug run the risk of being seriously harmed, if this new drug is, in fact, either unsafe or inefficacious. Of course, we will never really come to know this if a properly organized clinical trial is never conducted.

Though we cannot discuss the tactical details in this chapter, considerable progress has been made, over the last several years, in arriving at a strategy to bypass this apparently unresolvable ethical-scientific dilemma. One of the most important moves towards a successful strategy has been an ever-increasing collaboration between HIV-infected persons, persons with AIDS, clinical researchers, and clinical trials methodologists, in the design of trials for new drugs and treatments (Levine C., 1991; Byar, 1990; Merigan, 1990).

A GLOBAL ETHICS FOR THE GLOBAL IMPACT OF THE HIV PANDEMIC?

A global ethics for AIDS, hunger, poverty, disease, and homelessness around the world will, as emphasized in Chapter 14, require an epochal change in consciousness, an epochal change in our perception of the boundaries of the community to which we belong, and within which the principles of justice govern our actions. If humanity, understood here as global solidarity among human beings, is the required measure of a global ethics for the HIV pandemic, then our

Northern ethics, to borrow Hans Jonas's statement about philosophy, is sadly unprepared for its planetary challenge (Jonas, 1974, 80).

The rich, developed, and privileged peoples of the Northern zones of this planet, operate on the principle of justice at home and charity abroad — providing the charity is not too costly, and not demanding of too many sacrifices. For all it is worth, the maxim, "Think globally, act locally," can be invoked to support complacent and inoperative ideals. Ethics, as discussed in Chapter 2, is dependent upon an ethos, a guiding vision or belief about the kind of community towards which human beings should aspire. And what vision of community determines how we interpret the global requirements of justice today? What is the vision of community that currently determines how power is shared, how resources are exploited, how capital is amassed, how goods, food, medicines, and services are shared between the affluent nations of the North and the many nations and countries struggling for development?

It is very difficult to detect, in the operative concept of community now governing the behaviour of the affluent countries of the North, any real presence of the idea that everyone in the world has a claim on everyone else, simply because we are all human beings. A global ethics for the HIV pandemic, though, needs the ethos of global solidarity, the realization that people geographically distant and culturally different from us are bound to us by the demands of global justice. Those demands create global responsibilities, requiring that each person act globally and not only think globally.

Is this not utopian? How can each person act globally to counter and diminish the intense burden of suffering from HIV disease, carried disproportionately by peoples now deprived of resources, medicines, and services in so many parts of the world? Jon Gates's proposal offers only one example, a perhaps highly controversial example, of what a global ethics for the HIV pandemic might require of those who commit themselves to an ethos of human solidarity.

Jon Gates, who died early in December 1992 of an AIDS-related illness, was formerly coordinator of the Inter-Agency Coalition on AIDS and Development, a branch of the Canadian Council on International Cooperation. In his keynote address at an annual meeting of the Canadian AIDS Society in Halifax, Nova Scotia, in May 1992, Mr. Gates proposed that people call on governments and multinational organizations to delay release of any new vaccine or cure for AIDS, when and if such should become available, until three conditions could be fulfilled. These conditions are:

- that the drug or vaccine be affordable worldwide;
- that it be accessible worldwide;
- that it be available worldwide.

The idea behind this proposal is "that we will not allow the lifeboat to leave until we are assured that everyone will be on board." (Gates, 1992)

The chapters of this book document the process of working out what clinical ethics, research ethics, and public policy ethics require, as each new issue arises in bioethics. No one yet is very skilled in specifying the requirements of global ethics. Is Jon Gates showing us an example of what a global ethics, in this case for AIDS, might require of us all?

REFERENCES

Adler M.W. "Patient Safety and Doctors with HIV Infection." *British Medical Journal* 1987;295:1297-1298.

Altman L.K. "AIDS-Infected Doctors and Dentists Are Urged to Warn Patients or Quit." *New York Times* January 18, 1991:A-3.

Altman L.K. "New York Won't Tell Doctors with AIDS to Inform Patients." *New York Times* January 19, 1991:A-1.

Anderson R.M. and **May R.M.** "Understanding the AIDS Pandemic." *Scientific American* 1992;266:58-66.

Brennan T.A. "Transmission of the Human Immunodeficiency Virus in the Health Care Setting — Time for Action." *The New England Journal of Medicine* 1991;324:1504-1509.

Byar D.P. et al. "Design Considerations for AIDS Trials." *The New England Journal of Medicine* 1990;323:1343-1348.

Cassel J. *The Secret Plague. Venereal Disease in Canada 1838-1939.* Toronto: University of Toronto Press, 1987.

Charter of Human Rights and Freedoms, R.S.Q., c. C-12.

Council on Ethical and Judicial Affairs "Ethical Issues Involved in the Growing AIDS Crisis." *Journal of the American Medical Association* 1988;259:1360-1361.

Dickens B.M. "Legal Limits of AIDS Confidentiality." *Journal of the American Medical Association* 1988;259:3449-3451.

Federal Center for AIDS, Working Group on Anonymous Unlinked HIV Seroprevalence "Guidelines on Ethical and Legal Considerations in Anonymous Unlinked HIV Seroprevalence Research." *Canadian Medical Association Journal* 1990;143(7):625-627.

Gates J. "A Call to Fight AIDS around the World." *The Globe and Mail* (Toronto) December 15, 1992:A-17.

Gostin L. "HIV-Infected Physicians and the Practice of Seriously Invasive Procedures." *Hastings Center Report* 1989;19:32-39.

Haseltine W.A. and **Wong-Staal F.** "The Molecular Biology of the AIDS Virus." *Scientific American* 1988;259:52-62.

Health and Public Policy Committee, American College of Physicians and Infectious Diseases Society of America "The Acquired Immunodeficiency Syndrome (AIDS) and Infection with the Human Immunodeficiency Virus (HIV)." *Annals of Internal Medicine* 1988;108:460-469.

Jonas H. *Philosophical Essays. From Ancient Creed to Technological Man.* Englewood Cliffs, New Jersey: Prentice Hall Inc., 1974.

Kelly J.A. et al. "Stigmatization of AIDS Patients by Physicians." *American Journal of Public Health* 1987;77:789-791.

Laboratory Centre for Disease Control *Quarterly AIDS Update, January 1993.* Ottawa: Health and Welfare Canada, Health Protection Branch, Division of HIV/AIDS Epidemiology, Bureau of Communicable Disease Epidemiology.

Centers for Disease Control, Leads from the MMWR "Partner Notification for Preventing Human Immunodeficiency Virus (HIV Infection) - Colorado, Idaho, South Carolina, Virginia." *Journal of the American Medical Association* 1988;260:613-615.

Levine C., Dubler N.N. and **Levine R.J.** "Building a New Consensus: Ethical Principles and Policies for Clinical Research on HIV/AIDS." *IRB: A Review of Human Subjects Research* 1991;13/1-2:1-17.

Levine M.L. "Contact Tracing for HIV Infection: A Plea for Privacy." *Columbia Human Rights Law Review* 1988;20:157-201.

Levine R.J. "AIDS and the Physician-Patient Relationship." In: F.G. Reamer, ed. *AIDS & Ethics.* New York: Columbia University Press, 1991:188-214.

MacKinnon M. and **Krever H.** "Legal and Social Aspects of AIDS in Canada." In: The Royal Society of Canada. *AIDS. A Perspective for Canadians. Background Papers.* Ottawa: The Royal Society of Canada, 1988:347-404.

Mann J., Tarantola D.J.M. and **Netter T.W.**, eds. *AIDS in the World — A Global Report.* Cambridge, MA: Harvard University Press, 1992.

May W.F. *The Physician's Covenant.* Philadelphia: The Westminster Press, 1983.

Merigan T.C. "You 'Can' Teach an Old Dog New Tricks. How AIDS Trials Are Pioneering New Strategies." *The New England Journal of Medicine* 1990;323:1341-1343.

Mickleburgh R. "Canada's Estimates of AIDS Cases Low." *The Globe and Mail* (Toronto) October 1, 1992:A-1, A-4.

Professional Corporation of Physicians of Québec *Code of Medical Ethics.* 2nd Edition. 1978.

Reamer F.G., ed. *AIDS & Ethics.* New York: Columbia University Press, 1991.

Reed R.R. and **Evans D.** "The Deprofessionalization of Medicine: Causes, Effects, and Responses." *Journal of the American Medical Association* 1987;258:3279-3282.

Rhame F.S. "The HIV-Infected Surgeon." *Journal of the American Medical Association* 1990;264:507-508.

Ritter D.B. and **Turner R.** "AIDS: Employer Concerns and Options." *Labor Law Journal* 1987;38:67-83.

Rogers D.E. "Caring for the Patient with AIDS." *Journal of the American Medical Association* 1988;259:1368.

Roy D.J. "Anonymous HIV Seroprevalence Studies: Ethical Conditions." In: C.M. Laberge and B.M. Knoppers, eds. *Genetic Screening. From Newborns to DNA Typing.* Amsterdam, New York, Oxford: Excerpta Medica, Elsevier Science Publishers, 1990:95-103.

Royal Society of Canada *AIDS. A Perspective for Canadians. Summary Report and Recommendations.* Ottawa: The Royal Society of Canada, 1988.

School Board of Nassau County, Florida v. Arline (1987), 107 Supreme Court 1123 .

Sherer R. "Physician Use of the HIV-Antibody Test. The Need for Consent, Counseling, Confidentiality, and Caution." *Journal of the American Medical Association* 1988;259:264-265.

Society Services Committee, House of Commons, U.K. *Problems Associated with AIDS.* Vol. I: *Report together with the Proceedings of the Committee.* London: Her Majesty's Stationery Office, 1987:X-XIII.

Tarnopolsky W.S. "Equality and Discrimination." In: R.S. Abella and M.L. Rothman, eds. *Justice Beyond Orwell.* Montréal: Yvon Blais, 1985, 267-283.

Taylor K.M. et al. "Physicians' Perception of Personal Risk of HIV Infection and AIDS through Occupational Exposure." *Canadian Medical Association Journal* 1990;143(6):493-500.

Tegtmeier J.W. "Ethics and AIDS: A Summary of the Law and a Critical Analysis of the Individual Physician's Ethical Duty to Treat." *American Journal of Law and Medicine* 1990;16/1,2:249-265.

Walter Sir John, quoted in: Anon. "GMC Warns Doctors Infected with HIV or Suffering from AIDS." *British Medical Journal* 1987;295:1500.

Zuger A. "AIDS and the Obligations of Health Care Professionals." In: F.G. Reamer, ed. *AIDS & Ethics.* New York: Columbia University Press, 1991:215-239.

11

WHEN PEOPLE ARE DIAGNOSED AS MENTALLY ILL: ETHICS, LAW, AND PSYCHIATRY

MENTAL ILLNESS AND PSYCHIATRY: SCANNING FIVE DECADES

Dr. Heinz Lehmann, one of Canada's leading psychiatrists and now professor emeritus of the department of psychiatry at McGill University's Faculty of Medicine, left his native Germany in 1937 to begin work in psychiatry at the Douglas Hospital, then called Verdun Protestant Hospital, in Verdun, Québec, near Montréal. In an interview conducted by Michel Dongois, Dr. Lehmann recently reviewed the major turning points and some of the problematic aspects of psychiatry over five decades (1937-1992). We allow Dr. Lehmann to guide us into this chapter, since he highlights some of the issues on which we shall focus attention in our discussion of ethical and legal issues in the care of persons diagnosed as mentally ill (Lehmann, 1992).

Milestones in Psychiatry

Psychiatry has undergone major changes in this century, as have also the understanding of mental illness and the treatment of mental disorders. Dr. Lehmann points to four milestones.

First, Sigmund Freud's development of psychoanalysis and his notion of the unconscious represented a revolutionary attempt to uncover the biographical roots of mental illness; an attempt to make sense of madness, to discover its meanings. Psychoanalysis has emphasized the process of communication and close interaction between therapist and mentally ill persons, in the search for healing. While philosophers such as Paul Ricoeur have explored the role of meaning in this healing process (Ricoeur, 1965), biologically-oriented psychiatrists prefer to emphasize that Freud himself was also a neurologist, and he never abandoned the belief that the underlying and complete explanation of mental disorder would come from biology (Fink, 1978, 14).

Second, biologically-oriented psychiatry has made significant advances over the last five decades, in uncovering the biological, neurological, and genetic roots of some mental disorders. Psychologically-oriented approaches to the treatment of mental illness utilize methods such as psychoanalysis and various types of psychotherapy (for example, individual, group, and family therapy). It has been argued, for example, by P.W. Medewar, that these therapeutic preoccupations with the human psyche, with the mind, with language, and with personal relationships distracted attention away from, and impeded the discovery of, the true (that is, the biological) causes of mental disorder (Grenell, 1976, xiii). Some mental disorders undoubtedly *do* have a direct biological cause, such as an infection in the case of syphilis-induced general paresis (paralysis), or vitamin B deficiency in the case of pellagra-induced severe psychosis. Only a biological intervention can prevent *these* and similar kinds of mental disorders from occurring. Dr. Lehmann refers to the severe mental disorder resulting from untreated advanced syphilis. Ten percent of patients suffered from this mental disorder when Dr. Lehmann first started work at the Douglas Hospital, and since the discovery of antibiotics for the treatment of syphilis, he has not seen a case of syphilis-induced psychosis in thirty years (Lehmann, 1992).

Third, the revolution in psychopharmacology in the 1950s produced antipsychotic, antidepressant, and anxiety-controlling drugs that greatly increased psychiatrists' effectiveness in managing disturbing symptoms, in relieving mental suffering, and in modifying bizarre behaviours.

Dr. Lehmann's *fourth* milestone in the care of the mentally ill, namely the movement for deinstitutionalization and for integration of the mentally ill into the community, can be located in the late 1950s and early 1960s, close in time to the psychopharmacology milestone, and the post-World War II renewed emphasis on psychotherapy. That renewed emphasis was partly the result of a shift in understanding and in treating the mental trauma soldiers suffered in battle. During World War I (1914-1918) that trauma was called "shell shock" and it was treated with electroshock therapy, on the assumption that the trauma resulted from disturbances in the brain caused by the pounding noise of exploding shells. During World War II (1939-1945) this mental trauma came to be called "battle fatigue." It was treated with rest and psychotherapy, on the quite different assumption that battle-related mental trauma resulted from psychological, rather than from physical, disturbances; from perturbations of the psyche or mind, and not from direct perturbations of the brain (Lehmann, 1992).

This shifting back and forth between biological and psychological approaches to the understanding and treatment of mental illness occurs again in Dr. Lehmann's review, when he considers some of the problematical aspects of psychiatry over the last fifty years. We use the term *pitfalls* in grouping together and expanding upon the points Dr. Lehmann has raised.

The Pitfalls of Psychiatry

In the early days of psychiatry, little was known about the biological, neurological, and genetic causes of mental disorders, and emphasis was placed on psychological and social approaches to the diagnosis and treatment of mental illness. The differentiation of psychiatry into two broad diagnostic and therapeutic approaches to mental illness — the biological and the psychosocial approaches — was, in and of itself, a positive development. However, the increasing dissociation and polarization of these approaches in the 1990s is, according to Dr. Lehmann, provoking the disintegration of psychiatry. The ideal situation would be the integration of the two approaches. Dr. Lehmann refers to the attitude of some psychiatrists who see little sense in spending much time talking to their patients, because these psychiatrists see the real cause of mental illness as located in the genes or in the brains, not in the minds, of those who come, or who are sent to psychiatry for help. This is the *polarization pitfall*.

A *second* pitfall, the *pitfall of superficiality*, centres on the diagnostic use of existing classifications of mental disorders.

There are two main classifications, widely used throughout the world, of the many and diverse conditions covered by the broad term *mental illness*: the American Psychiatric Association's *Diagnostic and Statistical Manual of Mental Disorders*, now into its third revised edition (1987), and usually referred to as DSM-III-R; and the World Health Organization's *International Classification of Diseases*, now into its tenth edition (1992), and known in abbreviation as ICD-10.

These classifications, results of the much-needed and laudable effort to put some order into the diagnostic process in psychiatry, also serve to reduce the likelihood of psychiatric misdiagnosis, and all of its associated tragic consequences (Reich, 1991, 104). Yet, Dr. Lehmann has pointed out the *superficiality pitfall* that awaits injudicious use of classifications such as the DSM-III-R. Routine mechanical use of these categories and criteria, accompanied by only a minimum of clinical thought and attention to the full particularity of patients (see Chapter 5 on the doctor-patient relationship), can deteriorate to the labelling of people and to the therapeutically futile squeezing of people into diagnostic boxes, too narrow and too shallow to encompass and explain the unique and full story of their suffering. Dr. Lehmann's term for this approach to sick people is *dehumanization* (Lehmann, 1992).

Use of the DSM-III-R need not result in dehumanizing, "recipe-style" psychiatry. In fact, the manual contains several cautionary statements to guard against this: statements to the effect that a DSM-III-R diagnosis is only one step towards a comprehensive psychiatric evaluation; that use of DSM-III-R categories and criteria requires specialized clinical training; that indiscriminate application of the manual's diagnostic criteria to non-Western ethnic groups and cultures can result in the false branding of mentally healthy people and of culturally-specific normal behaviours as pathological (American Psychiatric Association, 1987, xxvi).

Superficiality in diagnosis, however, remains a potential pitfall of a purely descriptive diagnostic scheme. The same symptoms could have quite different causes, but the causes of most of the mental disorders classified in the DSM-III-R are unknown. The DSM-III-R has adopted an *atheoretical* approach to unknown aetiology or causation: *atheoretical* meaning that the manual remains neutral regarding the many competing causation theories of mental disorders, and does not discuss these theories. This atheoretical stance may have been pragmatically wise. Psychiatrists, though, can hardly avoid the pitfall of superficiality if they stop at the level of symptoms in their evaluation and treatment of patients, and fail to probe to the roots of their patients' mental suffering.

The *third* pitfall is that of *psychiatric misdiagnosis*, which is quite different, as we shall discuss later in the chapter, from the honest mistakes that can occur at any time in clinical practice. Psychiatric diagnosis is a socially powerful instrument. It can serve social and political purposes, not just the goals of therapy and care. When emphasis in the use of psychiatry is placed, not on genuinely needed mental therapy, but rather on finding a solution for a vexing social problem, psychiatric diagnosis can slide into misdiagnosis, and degrade to an instrument of psychiatric abuse. People may then be confined to institutions and deprived of their rights, liberties, and opportunities for healthy personal development when, in fact, they are not mentally ill at all. They may become mentally ill, however, as a result of such injustice and such an abuse of psychiatry.

One need not look to the widely acknowledged abuses of psychiatry in the former Soviet Union for examples (Bloch, 1991; Bloch, 1984; Podrabinck, 1980). Kenneth Donaldson, a man who survived fifteen years of unjustified confinement because of misdiagnosed illness, and whose case reached the Supreme Court of the United States, has already told his own story (Donaldson, 1976). Dr. Lehmann's interview refers to the "Duplessis orphans," those illegitimate and homeless children in the province of Québec who were institutionalized under the guise of mental disorder while Maurice Duplessis was Premier of Québec (1944-1959). The story of one of these children, Alice Quinton, institutionalized from 1945 to 1961, has just recently been published (Gill, 1991). Dr.

Lehmann asserts that psychiatry owes these children an apology, but he asks how to apologize. Society owes these children an apology too, an apology for the misuse it made of psychiatry, but the form that social apology should take is still to be determined, most probably in the courts.

Deinstitutionalization, a movement marred by many failures, illustrates the *social and political pitfall* of psychiatry, the *fourth* and last of the pitfalls to be mentioned here. Money was involved in some of the failures of this well-intentioned movement, and money still is, when these failures are repeated. Dr. Lehmann observes that deinstitutionalization was politically attractive, because it costs society less to release people from mental hospitals into the community than to pay for hospital-bed occupancy and all the attendant care. Some people who should have stayed in hospital were released. Others, who were ready to live outside the mental hospital, but who were still mentally fragile and vulnerable, were released but never really integrated into the community. Many left the back wards of mental institutions, only to land in the back alleys of the cities, neglected and largely helpless (Bazelon, 1976, xi). The "revolving door" phenomenon ensued: out of the hospital one week, back the next, and so on and so forth. Integration into the community after deinstitutionalization would have required — as it still requires — the wise use of resources to build bridges between the hospital and the community, and to organize systems of support to shelter successfully treated, but still vulnerable, people. However, these bridges and systems were, by and large, never constructed, and deinstitutionalization increased the misery of many patients and of their families and friends (Klerman, 1977; Bassuk, 1978).

The Future of Psychiatry

Some of the current speculation on the future of psychiatry concentrates on the inner dynamics of its evolution as a discipline. Some emphasize the need to establish closer collaboration between neurology and psychiatry; and the need, as well, to submit psychiatric diagnosis and treatment to more rigorously controlled clinical trials (Detre, 1987). Others highlight the likelihood that psychiatric diagnosis and treatment will become more precise and refined as psychiatry becomes more solidly anchored as a medical specialty (Michels, 1990). Moreover, few would doubt that closer links will be established between psychiatry, molecular biology, and genetics over the next decade. The search for the hereditary factors and gene defects involved in some of the mental disorders has already been underway for several years (Pardes, 1989; McGuffin, 1992).

Dr. Lehmann has considered the future of psychiatry from the quite different perspective of two critically important social revolutions. If these revolutions take place, they will, in his view, profoundly affect psychiatry because of the effect they will have on the incidence of mental illness. The first revolution would centre on the rearing of children. Dr. Lehmann estimates that the incidence of mental illness could be reduced by as much as 20% or 30% if adults, particularly parents, spent more time with children, and entered more sensitively into the world of children's fears, anxieties, symbols, concerns, and dreams. It is within trusting and solid relationships with parents and adults that children can acquire the strength and sense of personal identity and self-worth needed to hold together, when they later confront life's crises as adolescents and adults. The second revolution would centre on the closing years of life, and would involve a social transformation of values, a shift of emphasis on what should be most highly esteemed by everyone in society, and by the elderly themselves, as people age. Old people have very little place in a society that esteems only the activities, goals, and values of youth and middle age. People can easily fall apart when the new identity into which they must grow, after passing through their central years of social status, power, and productivity, does not really exist as a *persona* in the social drama. The Latin word, *persona*, and the related Greek word, *prosopon*, referred to the mask an actor wore to indicate his or her role and existence in the play. When the elderly can find no role, no place for themselves, and no esteem in the social drama, they can succumb to the experience of facelessness, and withdraw into the off-stage darkness of depression, loneliness, and a premature desire for death.

The Focus and Objectives of the Chapter

The concept of mental illness, and its psychiatric diagnosis, are socially powerful: they permit, and even command, departures from the ethos that normally governs clinical practice and clinical ethics. That ethos is based on autonomy, emphasizes respect for the will of the patient, dictates the norm of informed and voluntary consent, and safeguards privacy and confidentiality, a condition for patients' trust in doctors. However, when people are diagnosed as mentally ill, they are often deprived of their liberties, and confined to institutions against their will. Treatment may be forced upon them, for their own good or for the good and protection of others. Moreover, even if that treatment is sometimes safe and effective, at other times it is not. If patients are judged, usually by psychiatrists, to be dangerous to others, their personal and medical secrets may be in danger of being divulged to third parties and to authorities. The protection of confidentiality in psychiatry poses particularly complex ethical and legal issues (Dickens, 1986).

We choose, then, in this chapter to concentrate on those aspects of mental illness and psychiatry that most prominently exemplify a departure from the traditional ethos of clinical practice and from clinical ethics. Some would say this departure is necessary and inevitable, given the nature of mental illness, for such illness alienates persons from their own true selves, and diminishes, when it does not outright suppress, their freedom and capacity to function at work, in the family, and in society generally. The goal and function of psychiatry, in this view, are to liberate people from the mental disorders in which they are imprisoned (Hollender, 1978). Others, most notably Dr. Thomas Szasz, have stated that the concept of mental illness itself is largely a social construction without objective foundations; that the concept is erroneous and misleading; that the interlocking assumptions, social arrangements, and coercive treatment practices based on this concept constitute an immoral ideology of intolerance (Szasz, 1970, xv; Szasz, 1974). The goal and function of ethics, in this view, and even in the view of persons who are not as extremely critical of psychiatry as is Dr. Szasz, are to scrutinize the ways psychiatric power is used (and abused) when it primarily serves not to liberate people, but to control them (Robitscher, 1980).

The chapter, then, focuses attention on the ethical issues that are most prominent in the space where psychiatry is in tension between liberating people and controlling them. We focus on that tension and its related ethical issues, as they appear in the definition and classifications of mental illness, in psychiatric diagnosis and prognosis, and in coerced commitment and treatment of people diagnosed as mentally ill. We then close the chapter with a brief reflection on the limits of ethics in "impossible" situations. A detailed study of the many and varied issues in *clinical ethics* and *research ethics*, insofar as these fields of bioethics relate to psychiatry, would exceed the space available for a chapter. Moreover, excellent discussions of many of these issues have already been published (Bloch and Chodoff, 1991; Committee on Medical Education, 1990; Lakin, 1988; Dickens, 1981; Gaylin, 1975). Canada offers an historical and controversial reference point for the ethics of psychiatric research, a reference point centring on the work of Dr. Ewen Cameron at the Allan Memorial Hospital in Montréal in the 1950s and 1960s. That story is complex, courts cases have occurred, and commentaries are still being written (Collins, 1988).

MENTAL ILLNESS AND DISEASE: ETHICALLY NEUTRAL CONCEPTS?

We now return to the statement made above, that there is a strong link in psychiatry between theory and practice, and between theory and ethics, as well. The theory of mental illness and its related diagnostic theory shape what psychiatrists see, and what they do when mentally distressed people come, or are sent to them for help (Reich, 1991). The basic assumptions that psychiatrists make when they diagnose mental disorders in people largely determine how these people will be treated. Among the most important of these basic assumptions are the concepts of mental illness and disease, through which psychiatrists perceive, and in terms of which they classify, the behaviours and patients before them. Some of the deepest and still unresolved conflicts in psychiatry occur at this level of basic assumptions and perceptions. This is the level of ethos, as explained in Chapter 2. So our concern with the concepts of mental illness and disease links semantics (the theory of how words relate to reality), hermeneutics (the theory of interpretation), and the logic of medicine in laying the ethical foundations of psychiatry (Fulford, 1991, 77). Our purpose here is not to develop and explain these links, for that of itself would require at least a chapter-length discussion, but rather to describe how the concepts of mental illness and disease are not ethically neutral, either in their content or in their consequences.

Disease and Illness: Two Different Concepts

First, the *distinction between illness and disease* is itself ethically loaded, because this distinction, depending on how it is understood, can shift patients in their full particularity either to the periphery or to the centre of medical and psychiatric practice. If, as explained in Chapter 2, the patient, body and biography, is the norm of clinical ethics, ethical problems will abound if the healing process targets the body, and for all practical purposes, leaves the mind and personal history of the patient out of account. In the field of psychiatry, *disease*, defined in the factual terms of the basic sciences — for example, microbiology (for infections), neurology, neurochemistry, molecular biology, genetics, and so forth — is the starting and end point of the diagnostic and therapeutic process. This assumption (one might even say the still *reigning* assumption) tends to give pre-eminence to doctors' perceptions of what is wrong, and to marginalize (or even quite fatally ignore) patients' perceptions of how, where, and why they are suffering, of how and why they are ill. *Illness*, as defined in terms of patients' perceptions, not *disease*, as defined in terms of scientific perceptions, is the starting point and the end point of sick people's search for healing (Fulford, 1991, 86).

Disease versus Illness

When the concepts of illness and disease, as described above, are not only distinguished, but are actually *polarized* in the therapeutic encounter, doctors' goals and priorities may then push the goals and priorities of sick people far out onto the penumbra of inattention and lack of concern. Some may think, *so what!* What really matters is that sick people are cared for, or at least given the best medical treatment available. That should be the common goal of both doctors and patients, so where is the problem? The problem appears and intensifies when "illness" remains, and even worsens, after "disease" has been treated with every approach available. A woman afflicted with a very severe form of cancer, now under control at least temporarily, was quite horribly disfigured both by the cancer and its treatments, and persistently complained of intense pain. This was the central and high point of her suffering at a given moment in her hospitalization. The doctors tried every possible combination of analgesics (pain-control medication), varying both the dosages and frequency of administration. Nothing worked, and the woman continued complaining and, so the doctors thought, continued harassing them. Some, in frustration, withdrew from her care. Their focus had been on her body as the source of her pain. They totally ignored the woman's intense suffering over the loss of her once-remarkable beauty; over being abandoned by her husband, who had left her during her illness for another, younger woman. That suffering deep in her mind, and her personal history, got lost in the penumbra of the doctors' inattention. That suffering (illness), unattended to, translated itself into the woman's complaints of intense pain, the only reality her doctors seemed capable of perceiving and treating.

Values, Functions, and Intentions

This case story of controlled cancer, and uncontrolled pain and suffering, illustrates two additional features that distinguish the concept of illness, as contrasted with the reigning scientific concept of disease. Values, value perceptions, and value judgments — perceptions and judgments about what is of greatest and most central importance to a sick person — are integral components in the concept of illness. According to the reigning reductionistic assumption, this evaluation dimension, and with it ethics, are supposed to have little or no place either in the concept of disease or in its diagnosis and treatment.

Moreover, whereas the *concept of disease* emphasizes failure of organic functions, such as those of the immune system or of such vital organs as the heart, liver, lungs, and brain, the concept of illness focuses on sick persons' sense of loss of control; on their sense of helplessness; and on their experience of incapacitation. These central experiences in illness primarily express failures of personal intention and of personally intended action, rather than failure of organic function (Fulford, 1991, 89-91).

Both these elements in the concept of illness, namely, values and the inability to realize one's cherished intentions, are evident in the above case story of the woman with cancer. Regaining her lost beauty and the lost love of her husband were beyond her control. Moreover, she could not integrate these losses into her life all by herself, and her complaints of intense pain failed totally to draw her doctors' attention, and their care, to the prime source of her suffering.

This failure of intention and of intended action is often most dramatically evident in the various forms of mental illness, both the less and the most severe. The story of Mr. X illustrates this failure of intention, when mental illness is not severe. When his wife did not answer his telephone call one evening, while he was hundreds of miles away from home on a business trip, Mr. X wanted to resist his irrational, jealous compulsion to drive back to check if his wife were cheating on him. He just could not resist, he *had* to interrupt his business trip and drive home, although he knew with his every memory that his wife was faithful.

The severely deluded Mr. Nouville, in Dr. S. Baur's stories about madness and enchantment from the back ward, complains that his thoughts just will not stay down where they belong, so he feels he is going to throw up (Baur, 1991, 120).

Disease or Illness? Which Predominates in Psychiatry?

Some assume that the concept of illness, with its emphasis on values and on the patient's point of view, predominates in psychiatry over the mere scientific, factual, and organic function-oriented disease concept. That concept may well predominate in the practice of some psychiatrists. Perhaps it should predominate wherever psychiatry is practised, particularly where medically controllable infections and lesions are not the cause of mental disorder. However, the concept of illness, with its central focus on the full particularity of the patient, often does not direct psychiatric practice, and the patients' own views about themselves and their suffering are often ignored.

Dr. Baur, for example, admits that, for years, she never thought of asking severely delusioned patients what was wrong. She believed that the diagnostic labels in the patients' hospital charts contained the explanation of what had gone wrong, as well as the indications of the therapeutic ways to set things right (Baur, 1991, 87). She and her colleagues worked with the concept of disease, rather than with the concept of illness. The disease concept implies that mental disorders are rooted in a genetic predisposition that comes to expression in an abnormality of the brain's chemistry, so chemicals or drugs are needed to restore normal functioning of the brain. Sometimes drugs do bring mentally ill people back, even completely back, to normal thinking and behaviour. Unfortunately, as Dr. Baur observes, drugs do little more than subdue the feelings of a sizeable minority of the mentally ill, particularly those very severely mentally ill persons who often remain confined to hospital for the rest of their lives. These people are sedated and controlled. Rarely are they listened to carefully, or ever asked about themselves, their needs, desires, fears. The disease concept reveals its flaws on these back wards.

What is its key flaw? This concept, and the medical model of mental illness it underpins, simply exclude, in Dr. Baur's view, too much of the patient. Only parts of the patient are attended to, and these are reassembled by a multidisciplinary team into a facsimile of the real patient. "The spirit that animates the real person gets lost." (Baur, 1991, 106)

Dr. Baur's conviction and conclusion, formed over years of work on the back wards, is that treatment must begin with the patient's own story, with the patients' perceptions of how and why they are suffering. On this view, the essence of healing, if not of cure, is the moving experience of being listened to, of being believed, and of being understood (Baur, 1991, 106). How can healing begin, when patients, caught in the total difference between their own explanations of their suffering and their doctors' explanations, conclude, as did Mr. Bartlett, "Because our accounts don't agree, I don't exist."? (Baur, 1991, 96)

Can Mental Illness, Mental Disease, or Mental Disorder Be Defined?

The DSM-III-R is only one of the latest efforts, and surely not the last, to standardize and sharpen the descriptions, categories, and criteria used by psychiatrists in diagnosing mental illnesses or mental disorders. The DSM-III-R admits that there is no definition available that adequately specifies precise boundaries for the concept of "mental disorder." Significantly, the term *mental disorder*, and not *mental illness*, is the central concept of the DSM-III-R. Mental disorder is closely linked to failure of functioning, to dysfunction. This emphasis associates psychiatry more closely to medicine, while increasing the distance between psychiatry, psychoanalysis and psychotherapeutic theories deemed by many to be less scientific than medicine. Dr. Robert L. Spitzer, the driving force behind DSM-III (1979) and DSM-III-R (1987) has been quoted as stating that he and the DSM Task Force came to believe that mental disorders were merely a subset of medical disorders (Robitscher, 1980, 178).

However, there is little agreement among psychiatrists themselves about how "medical" psychiatry should be. Some mental disorders, as already noted, are expressions of organic disease, and require a medical approach for their prevention and treatment. The psychoses, with or without organic cause, would generally be accepted by psychiatrists as exemplifying true disease. Yet there has been, and there will continue to be, considerable disagreement about the "disease" status of, and about the appropriateness of medical hegemony over, many of the other conditions included in the DSM-III-R classification of mental disorders.

Psychiatrists, if Jonas Robitscher is correct, do not agree on the definition of mental illness, on its scope, and on the proper role of psychiatrists, when expanding definitions of mental illness shift psychiatric intervention away from therapy and towards control of people. Some psychiatrists would restrict the mental-disease concept to the organic and other kinds of severe mental disorder; others, such as those adopting a community mental health or social approach, would extend the definition of mental illness or disease as widely as possible (Robitscher, 1980, 159).

Besides these trends to link psychiatry closely with, or to extend it beyond, medicine, other forces have exerted an accordion effect on the understanding of mental illness, since the beginning of systematic attempts reliably to classify its many behavioural and personality phenomena. Homosexuality, for example, was once considered to be a crime. Social pressures to free persons engaging in homosexual activity from criminal punishment, led to the classification of homosexuality as a mental disease or disorder. A similar process, applied to a number of other behaviours, expanded the concept and the categories of mental disorder. In DSM-II, which took effect in 1968, homosexuality was classified as a disease, and placed in the category *personality disorders and certain other non-psychotic mental disorders*. For years, psychiatrists agreed on the disease status and pathological character of homosexuality. Then, social attitudes changed and so did the psychiatric classification of homosexuality. In 1973, the trustees of the American Psychiatric Association, under pressure from homosexuals who saw discrimination in their being labelled as having a mental disorder, voted to strike homosexuality from the DSM-II classification of mental disorders. In the DSM-III-R, homosexuality remains excluded from any category of mental disorder, but "persistent and marked distress about one's sexual orientation" is listed under the category *sexual disorder not otherwise specified* (American Psychiatric Association, 1987, 296).

There is, indeed, no existing definition establishing precise and clear boundaries to the concept of mental illness (disease or disorder). Social, economic, political, and legal considerations have influenced, at times strongly, decisions about which conditions are to be included and excluded (or removed after previous inclusion) from the official classifications of the mental disorders. The social, economic, political, and legal influences are not likely to abate. This situation sets the stage for a consideration of the ethical and legal concerns raised by psychiatric diagnosis and psychiatric prediction.

PSYCHIATRIC DIAGNOSIS: ETHICAL CONCERNS

The inherent ethic underlying the search for a precise diagnosis is that doctors should *know what they are doing*, before they intervene into the bodies, brains, genes, minds, and lives of sick, vulnerable, and threatened human beings. "Know what they are doing" comprises three kinds of knowledge: knowledge of what is wrong with persons who are ill (diagnosis); knowledge of how those wrongs can be safely and effectively corrected or controlled (treatment); knowledge of the impact of treatment or nontreatment on the wrong or disorder underlying the illness (prognosis).

The logic of medicine (Murphy, 1976) links these three kinds of knowledge and these three moments of the therapeutic and healing process. Treatment, of course, is the central, critical moment. This is true even if only comfort, or relief of symptoms and pain, or arresting of a disease progression, and not a definitive cure, define the limits of what available treatments, at any particular moment, can achieve. Both diagnosis and prognosis guide the choice of treatments.

Without a differential diagnosis — a diagnosis that distinguishes as precisely as possible one condition from another, or from several others, that may be wreaking different kinds of havoc in a sick person — treatment can be little more than haphazard and experimental. In a sense, the roles of diagnosis and treatment may be reversed in such a situation: treatments may be tried as probes to find the disease process that is at work. The general idea would be: "You could be suffering from C_1, C_2, C_3 or a combination of two or three of these conditions. So we will try treatments T_1, T_2, or T_3, observe the changes, and see if we can determine (diagnose) what is wrong with you." Sometimes, as Victor Adebimpe, a psychiatrist, puts it, "you have no way of knowing whether your diagnosis is better than anyone else's ... until you see if the treatment works." J. Robitscher adds that treatment success would, of itself alone, not be a scientific validation of the diagnosis (Robitscher, 1980, 181).

A judicious, that is, a patient-benefiting rather than a patient-harming, choice of treatment is no less dependent upon prognosis and prediction. Diagnosis is not an end unto itself, but serves to direct and channel the predictive process, namely, the ability to foresee how specific treatments will or will not alter the natural course and progression of a disease. The prime purpose of clinical research (see Chapter 13) is to ground the predictive process on the best available evidence. Even if the best possible differential diagnosis is available for a given patient, the logic of medicine in this particular case may well come to nought, if doctors cannot reliably predict whether and how their treatments will change the course of the disease. Moreover, the treatments may be more damaging than the disease itself.

Against the background of this classical logic of therapy, we attempt, both in this section and in the next, to highlight the particular ethical and legal concerns raised by the uses of diagnosis and prediction in psychiatry. In this section, we are particularly concerned with:

- the reliability and validity of psychiatric diagnosis;
- the possible dehumanizing effects of psychiatric labelling;
- the possibility and consequences of misdiagnosis, when psychiatry is used primarily to control, rather than to heal people.

The Reliability and Validity of Psychiatric Diagnosis

The *reliability* of psychiatric diagnosis rises and falls in tandem with the degree of uniformity or discordance in psychiatrists' perceptions and evaluations of symptoms. Reliability is high, when psychiatrists agree on what mental disorder is present when a person manifests a given array of symptoms. Reliability of diagnosis is low, when psychiatrists attribute quite different mental disorders to the same person or people who manifest the same symptoms. High diagnostic reliability is an indication, but not a guarantee, that the diagnosis is correct and can be trusted as a basis for treatment decisions. High reliability is not a guarantee of diagnostic validity, because psychiatrists could agree on what disorder is indicated by a set of symptoms, and they could all be wrong (Townsend, 1981, 33).

Many psychiatrists, before Freud and right to the present day, have held a firm hope, if not the expectation, that psychiatric diagnosis will gradually acquire the same degree of reliability as other diagnoses in medicine, particularly if progress continues in identifying the biological causes of mental illness. Others believe this expectation is illusory. The symptoms in terms of which the mental disorders are currently distinguished and classified, in all likelihood, will never be completely reducible to, or completely explained by, genetic, neurological, or organic disorders. Forms of mental illness and mental suffering that have no one-to-one cause-effect link to bodily disease will continue to plague human beings, as long as the human psyche continues to function as it does now. If this view of things is correct, and we believe it is, then the attribution of mental illness to people will always be more susceptible to doubt, and to disagreement among psychiatrists, than is the diagnosis of bodily disease. For this reason, mental illness, as W. Fulford has emphasized, is an ethically tricky concept, and diagnosis in psychiatry will long continue to be ethically more problematical than in medicine and surgery (Fulford, 1991, 94).

As long as there are only a few, if any, unambiguous objective tests against which psychiatric diagnoses can be checked, there will be confusion and uncertainty about how people, who are possibly mentally ill, possibly not, are to be treated when psychiatrists disagree on diagnosis. As J.M. Townsend has observed, mental illnesses consist of symptoms, and if psychiatrists disagree on the interpretation of symptoms, even the presence of a mental disorder is questionable (Townsend, 1981, 29). And psychiatrists do disagree, not only on their interpretation of symptoms, but — and this is ethically much more significant — also in their very perception of the presence or absence of symptoms that characterize the various mental disorders. In one study, some psychiatrists perceived certain symptoms in a woman and diagnosed one or another disorder; other psychiatrists observed other symptoms in the same woman and diagnosed a totally different disorder. The study involved both American and British psychiatrists, and although one third of the American psychiatrists diagnosed schizophrenia in the woman, not one of the British psychiatrists did. These differences did not derive from the American and British use of different diagnostic terms for the same symptoms, but from their very divergent perceptions of symptoms in the same person (Townsend, 1981, 28; Katz, 1969).

Psychiatric diagnosis depends upon psychiatrists' perceptions, and their patients' perceptions, of symptoms. However, the paradox of mental illness is that some persons who are seriously mentally ill complain of no symptoms whatsoever, and deny any suggestion that their behaviour is symptomatic of mental illness. Others, who have no detectable serious mental disorder, complain unendingly of an array of symptoms (Robitscher, 1980, 148). Moreover, the symptoms upon which psychiatric diagnosis is based, unlike the persistent and localized symptoms of most physical diseases, are linked to rapidly changing and evanescent behaviours; here one moment, gone the next; of one profile today, another tomorrow (Koran, 1975, 1065). Over thirty years ago, Karl Menninger observed a feature that still characterizes psychiatric diagnosis today, namely, that a psychiatric diagnosis is continuous and changing, not punctual and definitive: "... no sooner has a description been entered upon a case record than it begins to be out of date."(Menninger, 1959, 234).

Although the reliability of psychiatric diagnoses has improved since the successive updatings and revisions of the classifications of the mental disorders, that reliability still varies considerably across the various categories of these disorders. A leading view, over ten years ago, was that psychiatric diagnoses are only reliable in acute, classical (disorders that have been recognized through the centuries), and extreme cases (Robitscher, 1980, 166). The more recent view is similar. Psychiatrists are more likely to agree when diagnosing mental illnesses marked by easily recognizable and describable symptoms, such as the psychoses, of which there are many types. Where criteria are less precise, as is the case for many of the mental disorders listed in DSM-III-R, reliability of diagnosis is variably low (Reich, 1991, 106). Psychiatric diagnosis, even after standards and criteria have been carefully formulated, will remain a subjective activity (Loring, 1988, 19).

If the relative unreliability of psychiatric diagnosis sets in motion a train of ethical concerns, regarding the safety and efficacy of psychiatric treatment, that train gathers speed when psychiatry enters the space where its powers are used more for the control of patients than for their therapeutic care. Moreover, the reliability of psychiatric diagnosis and treatment becomes even more ethically significant when, as we shall note below, there is question of involuntary commitment and involuntary treatment of mentally ill persons. Even if we assume, for the moment, that involuntary treatment may be justified in some circumstances, it is surely never ethically justifiable to give the wrong treatments to the wrong people.

Psychiatric Labelling: The Risks of Dehumanization

Dr. Lehmann used the term *dehumanization* to characterize a diagnostic process that would confine people to diagnostic boxes that are too narrow and too shallow to encompass the unique history of their suffering (see above).

A second, and related, aspect of dehumanization relates to the tendency to reduce mentally ill persons themselves to their particular mental disorder. They are then no longer seen and related to in terms of *who* they are, but rather, in terms of the mental disorder they *have*. The DSM-III-R warns against the misconception that the classification of the mental disorders is a classification of people. It is not. Dehumanization and the distortion of therapy and care will occur when patients' unique personalities and personal histories are lost to view, and all are seen and treated exclusively from the point of view of the symptoms they happen to share. People *are* classified, though, when they are spoken of, and perceived exclusively as, that "schizophrenic," that "manic-depressive," that "alcoholic," that "psychotic." Dehumanization occurs when the adjective indicating the mental disorder becomes a noun, and that noun comes to substitute for the person. This can also happen to people afflicted with physical diseases. But because mental illness so typically displays distortions of thought, emotion, and behaviour, the tendency is stronger to behave towards mentally ill persons as though these distortions are the whole person.

In Chapter 5, we noted that *humanity* is one of the four marks of a genuine doctor-patient, professional-patient relationship, and that *humanity* emphasizes the unique, particular, and incomparable nature of each human being. In this light, a profoundly wounding dehumanization of people occurs, when they are persistently misdiagnosed and correspondingly mistreated. Some children afflicted with *distonia musculorum deformans*, an inherited progressive disease, notable for the pain and crippling effects it causes, spent months and years under basically useless psychiatric treatment because they were persistently misdiagnosed as having a mental disorder. The children needed surgery, not any of the variants of psychotherapy, and as long as they did not get that surgery, the disease progressed, compounded all along by family shame, anxiety, guilt, and the disintegration of family life (Siegler, 1974, 173; Cooper, 1973).

If it is difficult to know who is right when psychiatrists disagree on a diagnosis, then how, in the absence of unambiguous, objective tests, can psychiatrists ever come to admit that their diagnoses have possibly been wrong? Dr. W. Reich has emphasized that one of the most enraging features of a psychiatric diagnosis is its tendency to become a self-confirming hypothesis (Reich, 1991, 123). For years, Kenneth Donaldson's pleas and plaints that his confinement in a mental institution was totally unwarranted were, for his doctors, nothing more than further proof of his paranoia (Bazelon, 1976, xii). If psychiatric diagnoses tend to be irreversible (Neisser, 1973), the stigmatizing psychiatric labels that stick to people, as a result of diagnosis, tend to be permanent. It is profoundly dehumanizing to be seen by others, and thereby to be induced to see oneself, as definitively incapable of change, of improvement, and of ever regaining normalcy. Psychiatrists aggravate their dehumanizing tendencies when they describe patients they believe not to need further treatment as being "in remission," rather than cured.

The opprobrium attaching to mental illness is still both deep and extensive. If "once labelled," in fact, turns out to be "always labelled," the resulting stigmatization can become easily compounded by a lifelong threat, or even the actual lifelong experience, of discrimination (Robitscher, 1980, 230-242).

The Occasions and Consequences of Psychiatric Misdiagnosis

Our focus of attention here is on misapplications of the classifications of mental disorders. Dr. W. Reich distinguishes *purposeful* and *nonpurposeful misdiagnoses* from *mistakes in diagnosis*. *Mistakes in diagnosis* typically result from lack of adequate information about the patient, or from insufficient education and training of the psychiatrist. *Misdiagnoses*, in contrast, derive primarily from the fact that psychiatrists, unlike doctors in other fields of medicine, have a wide scope of freedom and discretion in their use of diagnostic labels; discretion, as J. Robitscher has observed, "to apply them at one time and not another, or for one purpose and not another." (Robitscher, 1980, 165)

Purposeful misdiagnoses involve the intentional misapplication of a mental disorder to a person, for objectives that are neither medical nor therapeutic. The person himself or herself may demand or request such a misdiagnosis to escape a worse fate; for example, lengthy imprisonment after a criminal act, or professional disbarment after an act of fraud or gross negligence. *Nonpurposeful misdiagnoses*, in contrast, are more subtle. They are not overtly intentional, and do not occur in the full light of awareness. They result, rather, from nonmedical needs, pressures, and compromises that can contaminate the diagnostic process, particularly when psychiatry is called upon to solve problems that are primarily social, not medical in nature. Nonpurposeful misdiagnoses, in W. Reich's view, should be the central focus of ethical concern, because they are more frequent, much more insidious, much more part of the fabric of psychiatry itself, and much more difficult to identify and prevent than are purposeful misdiagnoses (Reich, 1991, 102-103).

Nonpurposeful misdiagnoses, though more likely to occur when diagnostic reliability is low, really derive most prominently from the fact that the psychiatric diagnostic process can be used, and is used, not for medical objectives, but to solve or to shelve vexing and complex human and social problems. Psychiatric diagnoses (misdiagnoses) can be used as a means for an array of ends, identified by W. Reich as to mitigate or excuse from guilt; to reassure; to transform social deviance into medical illness; to exclude and dehumanize; to discredit and punish (Reich, 1991, 114-126). When psychiatric diagnosis is diverted from the goals of healing people towards the goals of controlling people, misdiagnosis can occur and provoke great damage to individuals. These damages can range from involuntary commitment to noxious environments; to involuntary and possibly injurious treatments; to loss of civil liberties, opportunities, and privileges; and to potentially lifelong stigmatization and discrimination.

Because psychiatric diagnosis is socially so powerful an instrument, and because society relies on psychiatry to manage and control people who are disturbing, the psychiatric diagnostic process requires continuous vigilant and careful scrutiny. The abuse of psychiatric diagnosis, and of psychiatry itself, is a pervasive ethical concern, a concern, however, that should be seen as arising much less from the corruptibility of the profession of psychiatry itself than from the fears, biases, vulnerabilities, and possibly the reigning ideologies of the moment, in which everyone has a share (Reich, 1991, 127). This may occur, for example, when psychiatrists overdiagnose mental dysfunction in women who are angry and frustrated over the discrimination they experience, regarding education, employment, advancement, and equal treatment.

PREDICTIONS OF DANGEROUSNESS IN THE PSYCHIATRIC TREATMENT AND CONTROL OF PEOPLE

Complex ethical and legal issues, highly resistant to easy solution, arise where psychiatry is caught in the tension between *treating* people who, because they are a danger to themselves, *have a need* to be put away, and *controlling* people who, because of their perceived dangerousness to others, are seen as *needing* to be put away (Reich, 1991, 121).

A diagnosis of mental illness may well be disadvantageous for a person's reputation, work, status in the community, and ability to conduct his or her own affairs. Nevertheless, of itself alone, a diagnosis of mental illness does not usually result in massive invasions of a mentally ill person's privacy, in deprivations of liberty, or in enforced commitment or involuntary treatment. It is for such extensive deprivations of liberty and invasive control of people's lives that predictions of dangerousness are both legally required and socially most frequently used. Part 24 of the *Criminal Code*, for instance, requires psychiatric assessments of offenders who, once found to be dangerous offenders, become liable to indeterminate detention.

Generally speaking, people cannot be sent to prison or detained there for purely preventive purposes, or for the protection of others, if they have committed no crime. Frequently enough, however, the diagnosis of mental illness is linked to a prediction of a person's dangerousness to others, as a basis for his or her involuntary commitment to a mental institution for periods of indeterminate duration.

In this section, we *first* examine the ethical and legal issues associated with the use of psychiatric predictions of dangerousness to justify involuntary commitment, and treatment of persons for their own good. *Second*, we consider controversial consequences of using a psychiatric diagnosis of mental illness to shift a person from the criminal-justice system to the psychiatric-care system. *Third*, we discuss the troubling situations that can occur, when predictions of danger-ousness are used to justify preventive detention of people in mental institutions for the protection of others from harm.

When People Are Seen as a Danger to Themselves

The majority of people who are involuntarily committed to mental institutions, or who voluntarily admit themselves to psychiatric wards of general hospitals, need comprehensive psychiatric evaluation, asylum, or a protected environ-ment, and treatment, whether it be medication or psychotherapy, or a sequen-tial combination of both (Robitscher, 1980, 191). These needs are usually temporary, even if often recurrent, for those who voluntarily admit themselves to psychiatric care. For those who are involuntarily committed to mental hos-pitals, the needs may be long-term or even lifelong. We limit our attention in this chapter to involuntary commitment.

J. Robitscher has emphasized that there is no perfect balance attainable between protection of people from harming themselves and protection of their liberties (Robitscher, 1980, 196). If psychiatrists emphasize protection of patients' liberties, some patients will harm or kill themselves. If protection of the health, physical integrity, and life of patients is emphasized, some patients will be unjustifiably deprived of liberty, perhaps for a very long time. The critical point in either case is the difficulty of making reliable predictions of long-term future dangerousness. How long may patients be justifiably kept in protective custody in a mental institution, to prevent them from harming themselves?

The Peter Mayock case illustrates this ethical dilemma. Six months after he was released from the Connecticut State Hospital in Norwich, Mr. Mayock, fol-lowing his literal interpretation of the Sermon on the Mount (Matthew, 5:29-30), gouged out his right eye. He was recommitted to hospital and, after a period of treatment, was released on a psychiatrist's recommendation that Mr. Mayock was ready for unconditional liberty. Three days after his release from hospital Mr. Mayock, again following his interpretation of the Sermon on the Mount, cut off his right hand. Mr. Mayock was recommitted to hospital and, twenty-one years later, tried to obtain his release, rightly claiming he had never injured himself during those many years of hospitalization, and that continuing commitment to the hospital was no longer necessary.

Was the fact that Mr. Mayock had never attempted again to harm himself, during his twenty-one years in the protected environment of the mental hos-pital, a sufficient basis to conclude that he was no longer a danger to himself? The psychiatrists' uncertainty increased considerably when Mr. Mayock admit-ted, in response to their questions, that he would cut off his foot if he ever came to the conclusion that the Sermon on the Mount was commanding him to do so. Was the possibility, or the unmeasurable probability, that Mr. Mayock would one day "receive such a divine command" a sufficient basis to keep him in mental hospital for another future indeterminate period, perhaps for the rest of his life? The courts thought yes; one dissenting judge thought no (Robitscher, 1980, 196-197).

This tension between protecting patients from themselves and honouring their rights to liberty is particularly taut when the suspicion is strong that patients will remain suicidal for long periods of time. While psychiatrists are at risk of being sued, if they fail to adopt reasonable measures to protect patients from harming or killing themselves, the reasonable measures to be taken while a patient is in hospital have already been quite clearly specified (Peterson, 1990, 102-104). Although these measures do frequently succeed in preventing patients from killing themselves while they are in hospital, the prevention is often little more than a delay. Many people under psychiatric care do succeed in killing themselves. Some psychiatrists are reluctant to discharge patients from hospital when they fear, but cannot reliably predict, that these patients will again try to kill themselves when they are out of the hospital's protective environment. The ethical issue here, and the crux of the matter, as Mr. Mayock wrote, is whether people who now demonstrate reasonable behaviour can be confined to hospital, because of what others presume they may do to themselves in the future (Robitscher, 1980, 198). This issue is even more complex when suicide is the presumed likely future behaviour. Though the majority of suicide attempts and completed suicides are linked to treatable depressions, and to mental conditions that should be treated, the possibility of rational suicide remains an open and controversial question. Moreover, suicide is not just a psychiatric and medical issue, but a profoundly existential and ethical issue about the meaning of life, and about whether there is a human obligation to live at all. The philosophical controversy is of long duration, and has not yet been closed (Heyd, 1991, 243, 248-252).

Crime and Punishment or Mental Illness and Indefinite Commitment?

Psychiatric diagnoses of mental disorder, combined with predictions of dangerousness, have at times been, and they may at times continue to be, an excessive measure to protect the public against potential acts of relatively low damage or danger. In some circumstances, it is reasonable to ask whether sentencing and punishment would not be a wiser and ethically more justifiable way of handling some disordered behaviours than is shifting or deviating delinquent people from the system of justice to the system of mental care.

Mr. Maurice Millard's story, dating back to 1962 and recounted by J. Robitscher, exemplifies this issue. After Mr. Millard had been charged with indecent exposure and masturbation in public, he was first diagnosed by two psychiatrists as a sexual psychopath (a label no longer used), and subsequently diagnosed in hospital as afflicted with a personality disorder. While the maximum punishment for these public sexual acts would have been a ninety-day imprisonment term or a $300 US fine or both, Mr. Millard, six years later, was still trying to obtain his release from the mental hospital. After one court agreed with psychiatrists' opinions that Mr. Millard was a continuing danger to others, Judge Bazelon of the Court of Appeals focused attention on the gravity of the danger Mr. Millard posed to others. Judge Bazelon found that there was no proportion between the harm Mr. Millard would cause others, were he again to expose himself indecently, and the harm Mr. Millard would suffer from continuing and indeterminate loss of his liberty (Robitscher, 1980, 193-194).

Dangerousness: Does Involuntary Commitment Entail Involuntary Treatment?

Involuntary commitment of people to mental institutions becomes particularly controversial, both legally and ethically, when there are no safe and effective treatments for the disorders afflicting the people committed, or when those committed refuse the treatments that may be available.

The right to treatment has been emphasized since the 1960s, when Dr. Birnbaum introduced the term (Birnbaum, 1960). The enduring ethical issue arises from an inadequate allocation of resources, which so often disallows mental health professionals from fulfilling their responsibilities, and disbars mentally ill persons from receiving much more than custodial care or chemical sedation (Miller, 1991, 275).

The right and the ability of persons, diagnosed as mentally ill, to refuse treatment is at the centre of continuing ethical and legal controversy. Though mentally ill persons have a generally recognized right to refuse psychiatric treatments, overriding such refusals has been justified, in the past, in three situations: when there is an emergency; when treatment of mentally ill persons is required for the protection of others; and when treatment is refused because the mentally ill person's reasoning is disturbed precisely by the mental disorder for which treatment is indicated (Miller, 1991, 276). The last of these three situations has been the target of extensive commentary, and there are many sides to the issue (Gutheil, 1980; Appelbaum, 1980; Ford, 1980; Lasagna, 1982).

There is the psychiatrists' side of the issue, which is linked to their frustration at being forced to be little more than hospital jailers for patients who need treatment and refuse it. So the tendency of psychiatrists may be to set very low thresholds for declaring patients to be incompetent to consent to treatment, so as to be able to obtain substituted consent. Moreover, authorization to impose treatment may be easier to obtain, if the psychiatrist can allege that the person refusing hospitalization and treatment poses a danger to others (Miller, 1991, 278). In support of psychiatrists' pressure for involuntary treatment is the truth that some patients refuse treatment because they are denying their illness, and that these patients are often later happy to have been treated. However, there is another side to this issue, the patients' side. Some patients may be refusing treatment because of their earlier painful experiences with the side effects of some of the medications they have received in the past. Their present refusal, despite their mental illness, may consequently be quite highly informed, particularly when it is based on experience deriving from their own personal history of treatment (Miller, 1991, 271-272).

Proposals to do away with involuntary hospitalization of persons who will refuse treatment, and to concentrate limited psychiatric resources on the care of the many who voluntarily seek treatment, court the risk of provoking abandonment of the severely mentally ill. They are, first of all, most in need of care and, secondly, most likely neither to seek treatment nor to accept it voluntarily (Miller, 1991, 270). More recent proposals would make incompetency to consent to treatment a necessary condition for involuntary hospitalization. This would reduce the number of people who are committed against their wills, who refuse treatment, and for whom psychiatrists can offer nothing more than custodial care. According to this model, incompetence to consent to treatment, when combined with the existence of a severe mental disorder, availability of treatment, and likelihood of deterioration without treatment, would constitute a sufficient basis for involuntary commitment and involuntary treatment (Brouillette, 1991, 288). While *competent* mentally ill patients are likely to be protected against the imposition of treatment in Canada, there is no solid trend in Canada yet evident to support the right of *incompetent* mentally ill persons to refuse psychiatric treatment (Verdun-Jones, 1988, 60).

Dangerousness: Involuntary Commitment for the Protection of Others?

Media stories have appeared almost weekly, over the last several years, about women who were first threatened, and then murdered, by their lovers or husbands. Shocked, many have asked, "Why were these men allowed to roam about free in the community? Why were they not locked up? Why were these women not protected?" These tragic stories of violence and murder, and the questions they provoke, lead us into the thicket of complex ethical and legal issues raised by the combination of a social need to predict dangerousness, the uncertainty of these predictions, and the social use of psychiatry both to identify and to control potentially dangerous persons.

Because of the frailty and unreliability of psychiatrists' predictions of dangerousness, particularly of their predictions of long-term future dangerousness, some have suggested that psychiatrists, ideally, should refuse to make such predictions. However, if psychiatrists cannot realistically and pragmatically be expected totally to refuse to make predictions of dangerousness, these predictions should at least be tightly controlled (Rogers, 1991, 83).

Dangerousness is the strongest criterion upon which persons may currently be involuntarily committed to mental institutions. Because people may not be detained in prison for acts of violence they may possibly commit, but have not yet committed, psychiatrists may find themselves burdened with the social responsibility of preventing dangerous conduct. They may well not be able to do so, when those potentially dangerous persons, committed involuntarily to mental institutions, are afflicted with disorders for which there *is* no effective treatment. Should such persons then be held in mental institutions indefinitely? (Brouillette, 1991, 285) This situation and its question bring us to our closing reflection on the "impossible situations" with which psychiatrists, *faute de mieux* in society, are often confronted.

PSYCHIATRY AND LABYRINTHINE ETHICS

Although the diagnosis, "borderline personality disorder," is extraordinarily heterogeneous, many of the persons who have this disorder are self-damaging, disruptive, hostile, impulsive, demanding, unreasonable, and depressed. They can burn out one psychiatrist and clinical team after another, and some persons with particularly aggressive borderline personalities can disrupt a number of health care institutions in a city within a short period of time. They frequently bounce from one mental institution to another, often resist every treatment proposed, and terrorize hospital staff. Others, confined to hospital for lengthy periods of time, frustrate every therapeutic effort psychiatrists can imagine trying. Some persons with borderline personality disorder will refuse treatment when competent to do so, then deteriorate, to the point of incompetency, then receive court-ordered imposed treatment, then improve, only to refuse treatment again, deteriorate again, and the eternal cycle starts all over again.

Persons afflicted with extreme versions of borderline personality disorder reduce us, as one psychiatrist has characterized their impact, "to our final common human denominator" (Stone, 1990, 267). These persons also frequently lead psychiatrists, clinical staff, social workers, and other health care professionals into situations one can only describe as "impossible." The situations are often labyrinthine, for there is no exit, no solution that works, no place where these persons and those caring for them can find stability and a measure of peace. Every attempt to find a solution to the multiple problems of people with borderline personalities typically leads to multiple additional problems. One treatment plan after another ends in failure and frustration.

We coin the term *labyrinthine ethics* to capture the fact that psychiatrists, judges, and clinical staff are often reduced, in their dealings with people with borderline personalities, to a choice between the lesser of two or more evils. The ideal solution constantly recedes over the horizon. In the most tragic circumstances, the repeated cycles of frustrated treatment plans, and the experience of wandering through a maze without exit, ends only with the death of the patient.

There is no immediate psychiatric solution to the suffering of some patients with borderline personality. Their suffering is tragic, all the more so because it is often rooted far back in the past, rooted in the early rejection and abuse these people have experienced. The future solution, if there will ever be one, directs us towards the social revolution sketched at the beginning of this chapter, a social revolution in how we care for and raise children. That revolution is not the responsibility of psychiatrists as such. It is the responsibility of us all.

REFERENCES

American Psychiatric Association *DSM-III-R. Diagnostic and Statistical Manual of Mental Disorders*. 3rd Edition - Revised. Washington, D.C.: The American Psychiatric Association, 1987.

Appelbaum P.S. and **Gutheil T.G.** "The Boston State Hospital Case: 'Involuntary Mind Control,' the Constitution, and the 'Right to Rot'." *American Journal of Psychiatry* 1980;137:720-723.

Bassuk E.L. and **Gerson S.** "Deinstitutionalization and Mental Health Services." *Scientific American* 1978;238:46-53.

Baur S. *The Dinosaur Man. Tales of Madness and Enchantment from the Back Ward.* New York: Edward Burlingame Books, 1991.

Bazelon D.L. "Foreword." In: K. Donaldson. *Insanity Inside Out.* New York: Crown Publishers, 1976, viii-xii.

Birnbaum M. "The Right to Treatment." *American Bar Association Journal* 1960;46:499-505.

Bloch S. and **Chodoff P.**, eds. *Psychiatric Ethics.* 2nd Edition. Oxford, New York: Oxford University Press, 1991.

Bloch S. and **Reddaway P.** *Soviet Psychiatric Abuse. The Shadow over World Psychiatry.* London: Gollancz, 1984.

Bloch S. "The Political Misuse of Psychiatry in the Soviet Union." In: S. Bloch and P. Chodoff, eds. *Psychiatric Ethics.* 2nd Edition. Oxford, New York: Oxford University Press, 1991, 493-515.

Brouillette M.J. and **Paris J.** "The Dangerousness Criterion for Civil Commitment: The Problem and a Possible Solution." *Canadian Journal of Psychiatry* 1991;36:285-289.

Collins A. *In the Sleep Room. The Story of CIA Brainwashing Experiments in Canada.* Toronto: Lester and Orpen Dennys, 1988.

Committee on Medical Education, Group for the Advancement of Psychiatry *A Casebook in Psychiatric Ethics.* New York: Brunner/Mazel, 1990.

Cooper I.S. *The Victim Is Always the Same.* New York: Harper & Row, 1973.

Detre T. "The Future of Psychiatry." *American Journal of Psychiatry* 1987;144:621-625.

Dickens B.M. "Ethical Issues in Psychiatric Research." *International Journal of Law and Psychiatry* 1981;4:271-292.

Dickens B.M. "Legal Issues in Medical Management of Violent and Threatening Patients." *Canadian Journal of Psychiatry* 1986;31:772-780.

Donaldson K. *Insanity Inside Out.* New York: Crown Publishers, 1976.

Fink P.J. "Psychiatric Must Remain a Medical Specialty." In: J.P. Brady and H.K.H. Brodie, eds. *Controversy in Psychiatry.* Toronto: W.B. Saunders, 1978, 13-27.

Ford M.D. "The Psychiatrist's Double Bind: The Right to Refuse Medication." *American Journal of Psychiatry* 1980;137:332-339.

Fulford W. "The Concept of Disease." In: S. Bloch and P. Chodoff, eds. *Psychiatric Ethics.* 2nd Edition. Oxford, New York: Oxford University Press, 1991, 77-99.

Gaylin W.M. et al. *Operating on the Mind. The Psychosurgery Conflict.* New York: Basic Books, 1975.

Gill P. *Les enfants de Duplessis.* Montréal: Éditions Libre Expression, 1991.

Grenell R.G. and **Gabay S.**, eds. *Biological Foundations of Psychiatry.* Vol. 1. New York: Raven Press, 1976.

Gutheil T.G. "In Search of True Freedom: Drug Refusal, Involuntary Medication, and 'Rotting with your Rights On'." *American Journal of Psychiatry* 1980;137:327-328.

Heyd D. and **Bloch S.** "The Ethics of Suicide." In: S. Bloch and P. Chodoff, eds. *Psychiatric Ethics.* 2nd Edition. Oxford, New York: Oxford University Press, 1991, 243-264.

Hollender M.H. "Should Psychiatric Patients Ever Be Hospitalized Involuntarily? Under some Circumstances - Yes." In: J.P. Brady and H.K.H. Brodie, eds. *Controversy in Psychiatry.* Toronto: W.B. Saunders, 1978, 955-964.

Katz M., Cole J. and **Lowery H.** "Studies of the Diagnostic Process." *American Journal of Psychiatry* 1969;125:937-947.

Klerman G.L. "Better But Not Well: Social and Ethical Issues in the Deinstitutionalization of the Mentally Ill." *Schizophrenia Bulletin* 1977;3:617-631.

Koran L. "Controversy in Medicine and Psychiatry." *American Journal of Psychiatry* 1975;132:1064-1066.

Lakin M. *Ethical Issues in the Psychotherapies.* Oxford, New York: Oxford University Press, 1988.

Lasagna L. "The Boston State Hospital Case (Rogers v. Okin): A Legal, Ethical, and Medical Morass." *Perspectives in Biology and Medicine* 1982;25:382-403.

Lehmann H. "Utiliser le DSM-III en clinique, c'est une tragédie!" Interview by M. Dongois. *L'Actualité médicale* 1992;13/43:14.

Loring M. and **Powell B.** "Gender, Race, and DSM-III: A Study of the Objectivity of Psychiatric Diagnostic Behaviour." *Journal of Health and Social Behaviour* 1988;29:1-22.

McGuffin P. and **Thapar A.** "The Genetics of Personality Disorder." *British Journal of Psychiatry* 1992;160:12-23.

Menninger K. "The Psychiatric Diagnosis." *Bulletin of the Menninger Clinic* 1959;23:226-240.

Michels R. and **Markowitz J.C.** "The Future of Psychiatry." *The Journal of Medicine and Philosophy* 1990;15:5-19.

Miller R. "The Ethics of Involuntary Commitment to Mental Health Treatment." In: S. Bloch and P. Chodoff, eds. *Psychiatric Ethics.* 2nd Edition. Oxford, New York: Oxford University Press, 1991, 265-289.

Murphy E.A. *The Logic of Medicine.* Baltimore: The Johns Hopkins University Press, 1976.

Neisser U. "Letter. Reversibility of Psychiatric Diagnosis." *Science* 1973;180:1116.

Pardes H. et al. "Genetics and Psychiatry: Past Discoveries, Current Dilemmas, and Future Directions." *American Journal of Psychiatry* 1989;146:435-443.

Peterson L.G. and **Bongar B.** "Training Physicians in the Clinical Evaluation of the Suicidal Patient." In: M.S. Hale, ed. *Methods in Teaching Consultation - Liaison Psychiatry. Advances in Psychosomatic Medicine* 1990;20:89-108.

Podrabinck A. *Punitive Medicine.* Ann Arbor: Karoma, 1980.

Reich W. "Psychiatric Diagnosis as an Ethical Problem." In: S. Bloch and P. Chodoff, eds. *Psychiatric Ethics.* 2nd Edition. Oxford, New York: Oxford University Press, 1991, 101-133.

Ricoeur P. *De l'interprétation. Essai sur Freud.* Paris: Éditions du Seuil, 1965.

Robitscher J. *The Powers of Psychiatry.* Boston: Houghton Mifflin, 1980.

Rogers R. and **Lynett E.** "The Role of Canadian Psychiatry in Dangerous Offender Testimony." *Canadian Journal of Psychiatry* 1991;36:79-84.

Siegler M. and **Osmond H.** *Models of Madness, Models of Medicine.* New York: MacMillan, 1974.

Stone M.H. "Treatment of Borderline Patients: A Pragmatic Approach." *Psychiatric Clinics of North America* 1990;13:265-285.

Szasz T.S. *The Manufacture of Madness. A Comparative Study of the Inquisition and the Mental Health Movement.* New York: Harper & Row, 1970.

Szasz T.S. *The Myth of Mental Illness. Foundations of a Theory of Personal Conduct.* Revised Edition. New York: Harper & Row, 1974.

Townsend J.M. "Psychiatric Diagnosis: Scientific Classification and Social Control." In: M. Dongier and E.D. Wittkower, eds. *Divergent Views in Psychiatry.* Hagerstown, Maryland: Harper & Row, 1981, 23-45.

Verdun-Jones S.N. "The Right to Refuse Treatment: Recent Developments in Canadian Jurisprudence." *International Journal of Law and Psychiatry* 1988;11:51-60.

12

WHEN PATIENTS ARE OLD: THE ETHICAL DILEMMAS OF CARING FOR THE ELDERLY

Canadians are ambivalent about aging. On the one hand, most of us would like to live to a "ripe old age," and we regard premature death as a tragedy. On the other hand, we do not accord elderly persons much respect. When asked, they tell us that they often feel useless or burdensome, in a world devoted to the cult of youthfulness. Nowhere is this conflict of attitudes towards the elderly more manifest than in the health care system.

In this chapter, we will focus on the bioethical issues that arise in the care of the elderly. This group is defined rather arbitrarily, according to age — 65 and over in countries such as Canada. Persons who have reached this age are also known as golden agers, senior citizens, or simply the aged. Most of them are healthy most of the time, but they are still more likely than any other age group to become, and remain, ill. And of course, their death rate far exceeds that of younger people.

The chapter will proceed as follows: first we will look at the demographic characteristics of the elderly population of Canada, in order to see why they are attracting so much attention from health care planners. Next, we shall consider the phenomenon of ageism, which accounts for much of the discrimination elderly people experience. The central part of the chapter will deal with the ethical issues in the care of the elderly, in each of the three

fields of bioethics: public, clinical, and research. We will close with an examination of the duties and responsibilities of those who provide health care to the
elderly.

THE ELDERLY IN CANADA

In recent years, the elderly population has been singled out for close scrutiny by
government planners and health economists. The reasons for this not-always-
welcome attention are easy to identify: the numbers of elderly people are growing rapidly; many of them cannot care for themselves and require the services of
others; the supply of family members as caregivers is diminishing, and the cost
of alternative arrangements is becoming prohibitive. These three factors are the
source of many of the ethical issues in the care of the elderly. Let us examine
each of them in some detail.

Numbers

The rapid increase in both the absolute number and the percentage of the elderly, in countries such as Canada, is evident in the following statistics:

- Between 1931 and 1981, life expectancy in Canada increased from 60 to
  71.9 years for men, and from 62.1 to 79 years for women.
- In 1981, the elderly (65 and over) constituted 9.7% of the Canadian population. This will increase to between 12.8% and 14% in 2001, 15% and
  18.4% in 2016, and 18.9% and 26.6% in 2031. The actual ratio will depend
  on the number of births and young immigrants.
- The percentage of the very old (over 80) is rising faster than the elderly as a
  group. In 1981, those over 80 constituted 2% of the entire population. This
  will increase to approximately 4% in 2001, and 6% in 2021.
- In 1981, there were 15.6 elderly people for every 100 Canadians between
  18 and 65. By 2031, this ratio could be as high as 51 out of 100 (McDaniel,
  1986, 36-39, 101-114).

Health Status

The extra years of life expectancy that have been gained during the past fifty
years are not an unmixed blessing. The older we get, the more likely we are to
become ill. Advances in medical technology often serve to keep the elderly alive,
but in a permanently incapacitated condition. As a result, medical costs for this
group of patients, especially hospital care, are very high in proportion to their
numbers. In 1981, the elderly 9.7% of the population accounted for approximately 40% of total Canadian health care expenditures, including 48% of occu-

pancy in general and specialized hospitals, 33% in psychiatric hospitals, and 72% in long-term care facilities. Almost one third of those aged 85 or over are permanently institutionalized (Canadian Medical Association, 1987, 4).

Family Situation

In addition to the rapid growth in their numbers, the elderly are undergoing other changes that have significant implications for their health care. Many of these changes involve their family situations. For example:

- The difference of seven years in life expectancy between men and women, combined with the earlier age of women at marriage, results in a high proportion of widows among the elderly, especially the very old.

- The increased divorce rate since 1969, when the Canadian law was relaxed, has added to the number of single, elderly persons who lack a spouse to care for them, when they fall ill.

- The drastic reduction in the birth rate during the past thirty years will mean a significant decline in the number of children to care for their elderly parents in the future. This situation is exacerbated, because many children no longer live close to their parents, and most women work outside the home and can no longer provide continuous care for needy parents.

- The frequency of divorce and remarriage among young and middle-aged adults contributes to the separation of the elderly from their grandchildren.

- Many elderly immigrants do not speak English or French fluently and, as a result, have difficulty gaining access to public services.

Almost 10% of elderly people in Canada currently live in institutions, a figure that is considerably higher than Great Britain (5%), the U.S.A. (5.3%), or Australia (5.9%) (Horne, 1987, 72). It is likely that this rate will increase over the next decades, unless a new source of caregivers for the elderly is found to replace the depleted ranks of spouses and children.

Taken together, these demographic, medical, and social facts about the elderly in Canada point to an impending crisis in their health care. Certain aspects of this crisis will be dealt with more fully in later chapters, especially 14 and 16. Here, we will focus on the special problems that the elderly encounter from society in general, and the health care system in particular.

RESPECT FOR THE ELDERLY

How do we see the elderly? As a "crabbit old woman"? This was the key phrase in a poem left by an old lady, after she died in the geriatric ward of Ashludie Hospital, near Dundee, Scotland. She addressed her poem to nurses, asking, with the opening line, what they saw when they looked at her. A crabbit old woman, withdrawn, passive, slovenly, and uncommunicative? She then asked them to open their eyes, because, if that was what they saw, they were not looking at her. She proceeded to tell them who she was: still a small child, a young girl of sixteen, a bride, a mother, a lonely woman whose children had left home, a grieving woman whose husband had died. As an old woman, from whom grace and vigour had departed, she was still all of these persons she once had been. She vigorously assured them that, in her old carcass, a young girl still dwelt.

How do we view the aged? Will we ever see, in an old woman or an old man, all of the persons they once were and still are? How can we do so, if we are blinded by what Butler has called the myths of aging, unproductivity, disengagement, inflexibility, senility, and serenity? (Butler, 1975, 6-11) These myths are perception filters, through which pass, indeed, a great number of truths about the aged. What they filter out, however, is an older person's unique individuality. When we miss seeing that, we are close to discrimination and mind-crippling bias.

Bias, a reduction of affirmations and decisions to unexamined perceptions, is how we come to diverge systematically from the truth. Bias is the bane of scientific research, and every effort is made to reduce its devastating effects on our search for reliable medical knowledge. Bias can also cause us to diverge systematically, and tragically, from that which is right and demanded by the primordial canons of humanity. This is the threat of the bias of ageism.

It is now widely recognized that disrespect for persons on the basis of their race (racism) or sex (sexism) is wrong, and should not be tolerated. In recent years, ageism has joined racism and sexism on the list of attitudes that offend against current norms of human rights. Ageism can be defined as unjustified discrimination against elderly people, on the grounds of their age. Its manifestations range from laws and regulations about compulsory retirement, through attitudinal problems such as paternalism in medical and nursing care, to extreme forms of physical and mental abuse of elderly people.

In Canada, compulsory retirement has been opposed by elderly persons and their advocates, because it is based on the assumption that, at the age of 65, people are no longer capable of earning their living. In 1979, a Special Senate Committee on Retirement Age Policies produced a report entitled *Retirement Without Tears*, which recommended that mandatory retirement be abolished. The *Canadian Charter of Rights and Freedoms* (1982) forbids discrimination on the basis of age (section 15[1]), although the following subsection qualifies this provision as not precluding "any program or activity that has as its object the amelioration of conditions of disadvantaged individuals or groups ..." Proponents of mandatory retirement have argued before the courts that unemployed youth are disadvantaged by the refusal of 65-year-old persons to yield their jobs. Some provinces, such as Manitoba and Québec, have already acted to abolish mandatory retirement at age 65. Others, including Ontario, have retained it, and have been supported in their action by the Supreme Court of Canada, which has observed that, although age discrimination in principle contradicts the Charter, compulsory retirement is reasonable and demonstrably justified in our society (section 1). Despite these legal decisions, there is a strong ethical argument against forcing people to give up their employment, on the sole basis of having reached a certain age.

A more insidious expression of ageism is the widespread paternalism that elderly people encounter in health care professionals, public officials, and society in general. Advanced age is often regarded as a debilitating disease, which reduces elderly people to the status of small children or mental incompetents, incapable of making rational decisions about their health and welfare. Even less severe manifestations of this attitude, such as addressing elderly (usually female) patients as "dear" or by their first names, can be an affront to their human dignity.

Physical and mental abuse of elderly people is now recognized as a growing social problem. Such abuse is perpetrated in the course of violent criminal activity, where elderly people are seen as "easy" victims (Brillon, 1987). It also occurs in domestic settings, with family members or nursing home staff as the aggressors. As is the case with spouse and child abuse, society is only beginning to realize the extent of this problem and to find ways of dealing with it.

Ageism is, to a considerable extent, intertwined with sexism, since a large majority of elderly people are women. They are often the victims of considerable economic disadvantage, as well as bearing the brunt of the other manifestations of ageism described above (Gee, 1987). Overcoming these injustices will require special attention to the social and health care needs of elderly women by the health care professions, government agencies, and voluntary organizations.

PUBLIC ETHICS

In Chapter 14 below, we will examine in depth one of the major problems in public bioethics, the allocation of scarce health care resources. Here, we will discuss this problem as it relates to the care of elderly persons. The rapidly growing size of this group in Canada and in many other countries, and their disproportionate use of health care resources, have led some to question whether elderly people are receiving more than their fair share of these resources. Positions on this issue range from the rejection of old age as a criterion for treatment (Canadian Medical Association, 1991, 72), all the way to the encouragement of suicide by elderly people before they require any expensive care (Battin, 1987). A wide spectrum of intermediate positions would consider advanced age to be one factor among many in the determination of appropriate medical treatment.

In proposing one of these intermediate positions, Daniel Callahan distinguishes between age as a medical or technical criterion, and age as a person- or patient-centred criterion. He rejects the former, on the grounds that age is not, by itself, a justifiable reason for withholding or withdrawing treatment. Some 80-year-olds can be restored to good health by surgery that would not benefit a 60-year-old who has other complications. However, as an important element in the biography of a patient, age can and should be considered as one factor, among others, in the determination of appropriate treatment. By this he means that elderly people have already lived a pretty full life, and even if they successfully undergo major medical interventions, they are still drawing near to the end of their time on Earth. Callahan concludes that medicine should give up its relentless drive to extend the life of the elderly, for example by organ transplantation, and turn its attention instead to the relief of their suffering, and improvements in their physical and mental quality of life (Callahan, 1987).

Callahan's position has been widely criticized as being unfair to elderly people, since he would deny them access to medical treatments that are available to other, younger patients (Kapp, 1991, 80-82). His response to this charge is that the present allocation of health care resources to extending the lives of the elderly is unfair to younger generations, who need these resources to provide such basic necessities as education, employment, and preventive health care.

The suggestion that elderly people are in competition with other age groups for health resources is considered by Norman Daniels to be both inaccurate and unhelpful for resolving the debate about the allocation of health care resources among generations. He agrees that the elderly use far more of these resources *per capita* than do others, but it is important to realize that all of these elderly patients were once young, and most were in much less need of health care. According to Daniels, we should consider the resources used by the elderly as their own, derived from earlier savings, rather than as transfers from their younger contemporaries. In this respect, health resources are similar to pension funds. Daniels agrees with Callahan that expenditures on elderly patients may have to be limited, but the principle underlying such limits is that the savings that younger people accumulate are generally not sufficient to pay for all possible medical interventions, when they reach old age (Daniels, 1988).

In the Canadian health care system, there is, at present, no explicit rationing by age. Elderly patients have the same right to needed medical services as any other patients, and in most provinces they have easier access to these services, especially prescription drugs, because of special benefit programmes provided by government. However, there are signs that such programmes are being targeted by governments, as they try to restrain health care spending. It remains to be seen whether these cutbacks will be justified strictly by economic criteria, or whether there will be a place for ethical arguments, such as those advanced by Callahan and Daniels.

CLINICAL ETHICS

Because of their propensity to ill health, often of a life-threatening nature, elderly persons frequently present ethical dilemmas to caregivers, whether health care professionals or family members. The most common ethical problems in the care of the elderly are obtaining informed consent for treatment or non-treatment, and determining the most appropriate treatment to be offered.

Informed Consent and Competency

Elderly people have the same moral and legal right to make decisions about their health care as any other competent adults. They are, however, more subject to medical problems that can impair their competency to make such decisions. Accordingly, the doctrine of informed consent, which was discussed in Chapter 5, requires a certain adaptation to the situation of the elderly (Thomasma, 1984).

In cases of elderly persons' total and permanent incompetency, such as individuals suffering from advanced dementia, caregivers must determine appropriate treatment according to: (1) the patient's expressed wishes while competent; (2) the best interests of the patient; and (3) the instructions of "significant others," such as family members or friends. In cases of conflict, it may be advisable to have recourse to a dispute-settling mechanism, such as an ethics committee.

A more difficult task is dealing with cases of doubtful or intermittent competency. Many elderly persons experience temporary confusion and loss of memory. At such times, it is difficult for them to make decisions about their medical care. One national organization of Canadian doctors, the Royal College of Physicians and Surgeons of Canada, has advised its members to employ the following procedure in such cases:

> If the patients' competence is uncertain, the physicians should attempt to minimize the uncertainty by seeking medical consultation before trying to secure informed consent. If the patients' decisions or refusals to decide seem unreasonable and are likely to result in serious harm to them, the physicians should consult with the families, colleagues, and hospital authorities about the advisability of acting against, or in the absence of the patients' expressed wishes, at least until their competence is no longer in doubt (Royal College of Physicians, 1988).

These guidelines can be used by other caregivers — nurses, social workers, family members — as well. They, just as much as doctors, have an obligation to respect the elderly person's decision, no matter how unreasonable it appears, as long as it is not likely to cause serious harm. There are often considerable burdens involved in respecting patient autonomy, since many patients choose to do things that make life difficult for their caregivers. There is a strong temptation at these times to treat the person as incompetent, in order to solve such behavioural problems. However, such an approach is generally unethical, and other solutions should be sought.

Since competency is a prerequisite for the exercise of informed consent, it follows that caregivers should strive to preserve competency whenever it is threatened. In particular, they should avoid administering medication that diminishes competency, unless absolutely necessary.

In many health care institutions, caregivers frequently employ restraints to prevent patients from acting in what they (the caregivers) consider to be a dangerous or bothersome fashion. Restraints may be chemical, such as sedative drugs, or mechanical, such as bedrails or restrictive jackets. When patients object to these restraints, they are considered to be incompetent to make their own decisions. While this may be true in some cases, in many others the declaration of incompetency is clearly an excuse to impose the caregiver's will on a powerless patient.

Whether or not the patient is incompetent, the use of restraints requires strong justification. Not only are they against the patient's will, but they can be extremely dangerous, causing emotional distress, bedsores, and even death by strangulation. Moreover, they may not even be very effective. For example, the incidence of falls among home-bound, unrestrained, elderly patients is not greater than among institutionalized, restrained, elderly patients (Moss, 1991, 23). The greater expense of employing personnel to care for patients who may be dangerous to themselves or to others should not be the only factor in deciding whether or not to use restraints.

In their article on this topic, Moss and La Puma make the following recommendations:

- Mechanical restraints should not be used routinely, in either the acute or long-term care settings.
- Restraint use should be governed by the doctrine of informed consent. If patients are unable to consent, proxy consent should be obtained. Only in cases of violent assault, or for the immediate protection of staff, is informed consent unnecessary.
- When restraints appear to be warranted, the least restrictive means should be used.
- Underlying disturbances of gait, mobility, behaviour, and cognition should be identified, and alternative therapies to decrease the risk of falling should be considered in restrained patients.
- Restraints are generally not indicated when patients are near the end of life, or when the goals of therapy are to promote patient comfort (Moss, 1991, 24).

Since incompetency, like death, can strike at any time, elderly people (and, for that matter, people of any age) are well advised to prepare advance directives to ensure that their wishes will be known to caregivers and proxies, if and when they are unable to make their own decisions about medical treatment. The question of advance directives is discussed in greater detail in Chapter 16 below.

Appropriate Treatment

As we saw when we dealt with the issue of allocation of resources, earlier in this chapter, the definition of "appropriate" treatment for elderly patients is a matter of considerable debate. Some argue that, although the elderly may have different requirements for medical and surgical care than other age groups, the principle of respect for them as persons means that their age should not be a decisive consideration in deciding whether or not to provide treatment. Like all other patients, elderly people may decline any such treatment for whatever reasons they find compelling, but they should have access to all appropriate and needed medical services. Others believe that expensive, life-prolonging treatments are inappropriate for the elderly, and should not be available to them.

The following types of medical treatment pose special difficulties for elderly patients: surgery, resuscitation, infection control, and nutrition and hydration. The choice to offer or withdraw these treatments is further complicated in the case of patients who are incompetent.

Surgery

Several years ago, a woman in her late sixties suffered a stroke that left her conscious, but paralysed from the neck down and unable to communicate. Several weeks after this stroke, she was losing weight dramatically and her doctor, after consultation with specialists, decided that a gastrostomy would be necessary to assure this woman would receive adequate nutrition. A gastrostomy is an operation permitting introduction of nutrients directly into the stomach. The alternative was tubal feeding, but the woman's doctor feared this could lead to pneumonia, if food particles were aspirated into the lungs.

This gastrostomy proposal seemed to be quite straightforward and ethically uncomplicated. However, the woman's sons were asked to give permission for the operation, and for resuscitation should their mother suffer a cardiac arrest in connection with the operation. They refused, because their mother had already suffered heart attacks, they had witnessed what she had gone through during resuscitation, and they said she would never agree to go through resuscitation procedures again, especially now, when she would be "brought back" only to remain totally paralyzed for the rest of her life. The sons preferred to see their mother run the risk of aspiration pneumonia than face the risks of surgery, possible cardiac arrest, and resuscitation.

In this situation, the doctor's view of surgery as the best approach to assure adequate nutrition conflicted with the sons' view of what was an unacceptable risk for their mother.

Ethical conflicts of an intense kind can occur when patients themselves, or their families, refuse surgery that is necessary to preserve life. One example will illustrate these ethical issues. Gangrene had set into the foot and lower leg of a man in his mid-seventies, as a result of very poor blood circulation due to several underlying diseases. Amputation of the leg from below the knee would definitely prolong the man's life for a number of years. The surgeon, however, found it difficult to hold a continuous coherent conversation with the man. Sometimes the patient was lucid, at others not, and it was far from clear that he understood what was at stake. But the young surgeon, heavily indoctrinated on the need for informed consent, kept pushing the issue, until the old man broke down crying one day, while his brother was there during the surgeon's attempt to obtain informed consent.

The surgeon eventually gave up pressuring the patient, and asked the brother to authorize the amputation. The brother refused, explaining that his brother had always been proud of his independence, and would rather die than be a cripple. The doctor retorted that we do not let people die from gangrene in the twentieth century, and that perhaps the brother was more worried about having to care for the patient after surgery than really concerned about the patient's best interests.

Situations such as these illustrate some of the ethical conflicts that can arise, when caregivers perceive a need for surgery for the elderly. It is, however, perhaps ethically more tragic when there is no conflict and people, whether health care personnel or family members, simply assume that the elderly are too old for an operation. This attitude is generally contrary to the best interests of the elderly, and to the record of surgical success in operations on the elderly.

People should not be refused life-prolonging or life-enhancing surgery, simply because they are old. Some elderly people, 65 years of age and older, may have healthier and stronger arteries and vital organs than persons in their forties and fifties. The criterion of physiologic, as contrasted with chronologic, age acts as a corrective to the already mentioned myth of "ageism," and to the unfair discrimination against the elderly that that myth can stimulate. Decisions to withhold surgery from the aged are justified when the operations would be futile, or when older people themselves, after being adequately informed, refuse to be operated upon. And the elderly may have many valid reasons for refusing surgery. When older people are unable to express their own wishes, close family members should generally be trusted and heeded when they either authorize or refuse surgery for their elderly relative. The exception to this, of course, arises when relatives do not understand what is at stake, or are in a conflict of interests. It would also be ethically quite unacceptable to refuse surgery to the eldery, because of a calculation that their best interests are too expensive, and in conflict with the greater interests of society as a whole.

Resuscitation

Cardiopulmonary resuscitation (CPR) is a normal treatment for the sudden cessation of heart and lung functioning. Once these functions have been restored, they can be sustained artificially with the help of medical devices, such as respirators, until the organs are well enough to work on their own. Unfortunately, for the vast majority of elderly people, this return to good health never occurs, and they remain permanently dependent on the machines, if they survive at all.

Given these poor results of CPR for elderly patients, it is often asked whether it would be better not to attempt resuscitation in the first place. Many hospitals and nursing homes have developed "do not resuscitate" policies, which give competent patients the opportunity to refuse such treatment in advance (see Chapter 16 below, for a discussion of such policies). However, for those who have not indicated their desires, and for incompetent patients who are unable to do so, these policies often require that CPR be given, even when there is little chance of success.

On the basis of current medical knowledge about the expected results of CPR for the elderly (Schiedermayer, 1988, 2096), one can argue that it would be wrong to make universal rules, either denying or requiring such treatment. To refuse CPR to all patients over a certain age, whether or not they are incompetent, could be considered an example of ageism, as defined above. However, it would be both a cause of useless suffering to patients and a waste of medical resources to resuscitate all elderly patients who undergo cardiac arrest. The ethical challenge is to identify those patients who are likely to benefit from this procedure, and who would be likely to want it if they could make their wishes known.

Infection Control

The second type of medical treatment that frequently poses ethical problems in the care of the elderly is the use of antibiotics to control infections. Many elderly patients are very susceptible to pneumonia and other infectious diseases. Before antibiotics were widely available, pneumonia was known as the "old person's friend," because it brought about a quick and easy end to an often-painful decline in health. Now, however, antibiotics are administered routinely to combat infections, and patients are usually cured of that particular condition. Unfortunately, the quality of life that remains is often very low, and the question arises whether it is in the patients' best interests to prevent death by such means.

Physicians are often reluctant to forego the use of antibiotics to combat life-threatening infections, since they consider themselves obligated to use all ordinary means to preserve life. However, there are good reasons for considering antibiotics in the same class of medical treatments as CPR, when dealing with elderly persons with severe disabilities, especially those who are permanently unconscious or demented. As with resuscitation, respect for these patients requires that two extreme positions be avoided: (a) incompetent elderly persons should not be given antibiotics, because their lives are of very little value; and (b) antibiotics must be given in every case where there is a chance of prolonging life. The difficult process of deciding when such life-preserving measures should be administered will be discussed in greater detail in Chapter 16.

Nutrition and Hydration

Eating and drinking are not generally thought to be forms of medical treatment. However, when a person can no longer perform these functions spontaneously, there are several ways in which nutrition and hydration can be given artificially, for example, intravenously or through a nasogastric tube. These measures are often sufficient to keep a person alive indefinitely. When such patients are permanently unconscious or demented, however, the question arises whether it would be better for them if these procedures were terminated, and they were allowed to die. The problem is especially urgent when patients of uncertain competency attempt to remove their feeding tubes, and caregivers have to decide whether the tubes should be reinserted against the patients' apparent wishes.

As with resuscitation and antibiotics, respect for these patients requires that two extreme positions be avoided: (a) incompetent elderly persons should not be nourished artificially, because their lives are of very little value; and (b) they must be kept alive by all available means, even if this means going against their own wishes. In place of such rigid rules, which leave no room for consideration of differing circumstances in particular cases, several groups have proposed guidelines for deciding when artificial nourishment should or should not be administered. The Committee on Ethics of the American Nurses Association has proposed the following exceptions to the general requirement to provide such nourishment:

- when patients would clearly be more harmed by receiving than by the withholding of food and fluids;
- when competent patients refuse treatment, including food and water, for "good reasons";
- when the provision of food and fluid is considered "futile," "severely

burdensome" to the patient, sustains life only long enough for the patient to die of other more painful causes, or inflicts suffering or harm that is not outweighed by an important long-term benefit (Fry, 1988, 148).

These guidelines are very general, but they do provide some help to care-givers in making decisions for incompetent patients on this important matter.

RESEARCH ETHICS

The participation of elderly persons in medical research poses numerous ethical problems. There is a great need for such research, since some diseases (e.g., Alzheimer's) affect primarily the elderly, and they react to many drugs differently than do younger patients. At the same time, such research is hindered both by the reluctance of elderly persons to participate and by their special requirements for protection from the loss of privacy and the risks associated with research.

Although some elderly persons enjoy the attention they receive as research subjects, many others refuse to participate. Their reasons include not liking needles, not feeling well, not wanting to bother, and a distrust of medical research. Follow-up is hindered by lack of transportation, and their reluctance to go outside in bad weather or to leave homes or apartments vacant for visits to the research site.

Even when elderly persons express interest in taking part in research, their ability to give informed consent can be compromised by the following factors:

- dependency on the health care system — they may feel that their level of care will be diminished if they do not take part in research studies;
- reluctance to offend authorities — medical researchers, who may also be their primary physicians, are seen by the elderly as powerful and caring persons, who are owed gratitude and respect, not questioning or refusal;
- low educational attainments and/or intellectual decline — based on a comparison with U.S. figures (Taub, 1986, 8), it would seem that less than 50% of elderly Canadians completed high school;
- diminished ability to understand and evaluate degrees of risk — the elderly may consider death in familiar surroundings to be less of a risk than removal to a hospital for better medical treatment.

For competent elderly research subjects, these problems are not insuperable. With extra effort by the investigators to explain the nature of the research project, and to make sure that the participants understand what they have been told and do not feel coerced to take part, the requirements for informed consent can be met. There is need, however, for research into how best to facilitate and increase participation of elderly persons in research projects (Canadian Coalition, 1991, 39-41).

The participation of incompetent elderly patients in research studies is a much more difficult problem. A case in point is Alzheimer's-type dementia. Unlike most other diseases, this one affects only human beings, and so research on animals is of little or no help in understanding its causes or testing new treatments. Moreover, at the present time, most Alzheimer's research is unlikely to benefit those who are now affected by this disease, but only future sufferers. The dilemma that researchers (and society in general) face is, therefore: is it ethical to do research on incompetent patients that is not for their own benefit, or is it ethical to forego such research when there is no other way to obtain information that can lead to an understanding of how the disease can be prevented or cured?

The current Medical Research Council of Canada *Guidelines on Research Involving Human Subjects*, which will be discussed in the next chapter, are generally interpreted as forbidding all research on incompetent patients that does not benefit them directly. It has been strongly argued that this restriction is inappropriate for Alzheimer's disease, and that guidelines can be developed that will both promote research on this disease and protect research subjects from harm (Berg, 1991).

DUTIES AND RESPONSIBILITIES

In the light of these facts about Canada's aging population and its health care needs, many questions are being asked about how these needs can be met, and who should meet them. Do children have an obligation to care for their parents in old age? If so, to what extent: providing accommodation, meeting their physical requirements, or, if this is not possible, paying for these services? What obligations does society have towards the elderly? Can the government afford to provide all needed health and social services for them? These are ethical issues, since they involve the balancing of the rights and responsibilities of different individuals and groups in society.

The principle of respect for persons is a useful criterion for dealing with the medical problems of the elderly. However, it is not very helpful for the resolution of the question of who is responsible for the care of the elderly. In view of the changing family patterns in our society, it can no longer be assumed that there will be children around to look after their parents in their old age. For much of the twentieth century, governments have provided pensions and other services, so that senior citizens can enjoy an adequate standard of living and health care until they die. These programmes have been funded, for the most part, from general tax revenue. However, as the percentage of taxpayers declines in relation to the number of seniors to be supported, it is uncertain whether society will be able or willing to continue these support programmes.

There are no easy answers to this dilemma. Governments are encouraging people to save for their retirement through registered retirement savings plans and other such programmes. However, only those with disposable income can afford to do this. All others face an uncertain old age, in which the medical care that we take for granted now may no longer be available, just when it is most needed.

Even when finances are not at issue, the care of the elderly often involves major hardships on the part of caregivers. Family members may feel trapped by the need for round-the-clock attention to an elderly patient. For both family and professional caregivers, the physical and emotional requirements of their work can be extremely burdensome. Severely demented patients must be fed, clothed, and toileted, and can provide little if any positive feedback to those who look after them. Caregivers in these situations are subject to considerable stress, which can lead either to burnout or to withdrawal from, and neglect of, their patients. To prevent this from happening, there is a great need for respite programmes for caregivers, whereby they can be relieved of their duties before problems develop. Also helpful are mutual support groups, such as those organized by the Alzheimer's Society.

More than most other bioethical issues, the care of the elderly calls for a greater realization that individuals are interdependent and in need of each other. The ideal of "seniors independence" (the name of a federal government grants programme) is laudable to a certain extent, but it should not be treated as an absolute. It is perfectly normal to become more dependent as one enters old age, and this should not be regarded as a failure. Instead, the elderly should be encouraged to seek help from family members, community groups, health care institutions, and government when they need it. And society, in its turn, should encourage and facilitate efforts to anticipate these needs and develop programmes to meet them.

CONCLUSION

The ethical problems of the elderly affect all Canadians. Most of us will live into our 70s, and many of us into our 80s and beyond. We may have elderly parents and other relatives to care for, even after we reach retirement age. If we enter any of the health care professions, we will be faced with a steadily growing elderly clientele for most of our careers. As citizens and taxpayers, we will need to make decisions about the allocation of public resources to the rapidly expanding health care needs of the elderly, vis-à-vis the educational needs of youth, the social needs of the poor and other disadvantaged groups, and many other worthy causes.

The broad range of ethical issues in the care of the elderly requires the full complement of resources of bioethics as public, clinical, and research ethics

(Thornton, 1988). Within each of these fields, the first principle in dealing with the elderly is respect for them as persons. Just as we want to be seen as more than a "crabbit old woman" or man when we turn 65, so do we owe the elderly respect and care, in each of our roles as health care professionals, researchers, family members, and citizens.

REFERENCES

Battin M.P. "Choosing the Time to Die: The Ethics and Economics of Suicide in Old Age." In: S. Spicker et al., eds. *Ethical Dimensions of Geriatric Care: Value Conflicts for the 21st Century.* Dordrecht/Boston: D. Reidel, 1987, 161-189.

Berg J., **Karlinsky H.** and **Lowy F.**, eds. *Alzheimer's Disease Research: Ethical and Legal Issues.* Toronto: Carswell, 1991, 333-354.

Brillon Y. *Victimization and Fear of Crime Among the Elderly.* Toronto and Vancouver: Butterworths, 1987.

Butler R.N. *Why Survive? Being Old in America.* New York: Harper & Row, 1975.

Callahan D. *Setting Limits: Medical Goals in an Aging Society.* New York: Simon & Schuster, 1987.

Canadian Coalition on Medication Use and the Elderly *Drug Utilization Related Problems in Elderly Canadians: Proceedings of an Invitational Consensus Conference on Research Priorities.* Ottawa: Canadian Public Health Association, 1991.

Canadian Medical Association *Challenges and Changes in the Care of the Elderly.* Ottawa: CMA, 1991.

Canadian Medical Association *Health Care for the Elderly: Today's Challenges, Tomorrow's Options.* Ottawa: CMA, 1987.

Daniels N. *Am I My Parents' Keeper? An Essay on Justice Between the Young and the Old.* New York: Oxford University Press, 1988.

Fry S.T. "New ANA Guidelines on Withdrawing or Withholding Food and Fluid from Patients." *Nursing Outlook* 1988;36/3:122-123, 148-150.

Gee E.M. and **Kimball M.M.** *Women and Aging.* Toronto and Vancouver: Butterworths, 1987.

Horne J.M. "Beyond 'De-Institutionalizing' the Elderly: Financial Savings from a More Radical Approach to Alternative Health Care Delivery Methods by the Year 2021." In: Economic Council of Canada *Aging with Limited Health Resources.* Ottawa: Minister of Supply and Services, 1987.

Kapp M. "Rationing Health Care: Legal Issues and Alternatives to Age-Based Rationing." In: R.L. Barry and G.V. Bradley, eds. *Set No Limits: A Rebuttal to Daniel Callahan's Proposal to Limit Health Care for the Elderly.* Urbana and Chicago: University of Illinois Press, 1991, 71-91.

McDaniel S.A. *Canada's Aging Population.* Toronto and Vancouver: Butterworths, 1986.

Moss R.J. and **La Puma J.** "The Ethics of Mechanical Restraints." *Hastings Center Report* 1991;21/1:22-25.

Royal College of Physicians and Surgeons of Canada "Informed Consent: Ethical Considerations for Physicians and Surgeons." *Annals of The Royal College of Physicians and Surgeons of Canada* 1988;21/2 (insert).

Schiedermayer D.L. "The Decision to Forgo CPR in the Elderly Patient." *Journal of the American Medical Association* 1988;260/14:2096-2097.

Taub H.A. "Comprehension of Informed Consent for Research: Issues and Directions for Future Study." *IRB: A Review of Human Subjects Research* 1986;8/6:7-10.

Thomasma D.C. "Freedom, Dependency, and the Care of the Very Old." *Journal of the American Geriatrics Society* 1984;32/12:906-914.

Thornton J.E. and **Winkler E.R.**, eds. *Ethics & Aging: The Right to Live, The Right to Die.* Vancouver: University of British Columbia Press, 1988.

13

WHEN TREATMENTS ARE UNCERTAIN: THE ETHICS OF RESEARCH WITH HUMAN BEINGS

The title indicates this chapter's focus and its limits. The focus is on the conditions for ethically acceptable biomedical research with human beings. Human beings participate as subjects in many different kinds of biomedical research, as well as in behavioural and social research. However, in this chapter we focus on research undertaken to test and perfect treatments for human disease. For this reason, controlled clinical trials, the current leading strategy for the study of medical and surgical treatments, will be the central point of reference for our discussion of research ethics.

Although the ethical issues specific to behavioural and social research are an important subspecialization of the field of research ethics in bioethics, they will not be discussed in this chapter or in this book, for reasons we have already given in the introduction. A similar limitation applies to the ethics of research with animals. We do not have the space available that would be required to describe and discuss the various positions that have been taken for and against the use of animals in pharmaceutical, surgical, behavioural, and consumer-product research. Yet we cannot bypass this topic completely, since prior experimentation with animals is one of the conditions, as we shall see, for the ethical acceptability of drug and surgical research with human beings.

This chapter has a central guiding assumption. If the practice of medicine is both morally mandatory and inherently experimental, then research with human beings, undertaken to obtain reliable knowledge about the safety and effectiveness of diagnostic, preventive, and remedial procedures, cannot be inherently unethical. Such research will be unethical to the extent that it fails to honour a set of necessary and sufficient conditions. The primary purpose of this chapter is to set out and explain what these conditions are.

UNCERTAINTY, EXPERIMENTATION, AND KNOWLEDGE IN MEDICINE

The first words of the chapter title, "When Treatments Are Uncertain," draw attention to one of the components in the chapter's guiding assumption, namely, that the practice of medicine, and the knowledge in terms of which the standards of medical practice are defined, are inherently experimental. Medical knowledge about the causes and treatments of disease, and the specific knowledge about how best to treat this or that particular patient, *ultimately* come from experimentation. The word *ultimately* is emphasized, because experiments have to be carefully prepared and conducted, and they have to be guided by clear hypotheses, if they are to result in reliable knowledge. Precise observation and description of the frequency, distribution, characteristic symptoms, and course of a disease, and the drawing of inferences from these observations, are the preliminary steps leading to the formulation of hypotheses to be tested by experiments.

The hypothesis may centre on the cause of a disease. Scientists, for example, are still uncertain about whether the human immunodeficiency virus (HIV) is a necessary and sufficient cause of the collapse of the body's defence system, as manifested in the acquired immunodeficiency syndrome (AIDS). The hypothesis may also relate to the mechanism of a disease. For example, what is the mechanism of cancer metastasis? How does a cancer spread from one spot to other, distant sites in the body? Other hypotheses are concerned with the question about how best to prevent a disease. For example, the drug tamoxifen has been used for about twenty years to treat women with breast cancer. This drug has many effects, some beneficial, others harmful, and the results of using this drug depend, in part, on the variable characteristics of individual women's bodies. But the drug will now be given to healthy women in the context of a research project, to test the hypothesis that it can prevent breast cancer. The question of how best to treat diseases generates the hypotheses involved in the thousands of medical research projects conducted yearly throughout the world. For example, a preliminary study has been conducted to test the hypothesis that the drug thalidomide is a safe and effective way to treat graft-versus-host disease (the transplantation tissue leads to infections in the recipient) in people who have received donor bone-marrow transplantation for blood cancer or certain forms of anemia. Thalidomide, by the way, was the drug that, inadequately tested at the time, caused severe arm and leg defects in babies whose mothers had taken the drug as a sedative during pregnancy, in the 1950s and 1960s.

The kinds of hypotheses mentioned are provisional, possibly true or partially true, answers to important questions about health and disease. Hypotheses are born out of uncertainty, and experimentation is the only way to find out how probably the proposed answers framed in the hypotheses approach the truth. Rarely, however, are the results of experimentation in medicine so black and white as to totally clear up the uncertainty that gave rise to the hypothesis. For example, in the thalidomide study mentioned above, of the 44 patients with graft-versus-host disease who were treated with the drug, 14 had a complete response, 12 patients showed a partial response, and 18 patients showed no response at all. Response, here, means that the drug had an effect on control of the infections. So, is thalidomide a safe and effective way to treat the particular disease in question? Possibly for some patients, and not for others. Is it safer and more effective than treatments currently used? Only further experimentation will tell. Sometimes many experiments, involving thousands of patients, are needed to produce reliable knowledge. Even then, the treatment that has been shown to be beneficial may well be beneficial only for a certain percent of the patients affected by a given disease.

There are many sources and kinds of uncertainty in medicine (Beresford, 1991). In this chapter, we are concerned mostly with two: first, the uncertainty of medical knowledge that is due to the sheer complexity of the human body and its diseases; second, the uncertainty that results from the utter individuality and variability, genetic, physiological, and biographical, of each body and patient, regarding susceptibility to disease and response to treatment, whether it be preventive or remedial in intent.

Uncertainty in medicine, coming from these two sources, involves matters of fact, and such uncertainty cannot be reduced or cleared away by discourse, debate, and argument. Neither can it be cleared away by observation alone, however careful, methodical, and sustained that observation may be. Nature — in medicine, the human body — is the one and only source of medical knowledge, and experimentation is the mode of questioning that will prod nature to reveal how it works and, when there is a breakdown, how these workings can be repaired and restored.

The experimental character of medical knowledge was not always recognized. A system of medical thought based on the authority of Galen (138-201 B.C.E.) influenced, if not dominated, medical practice for centuries. Even as late as the 1500s, some university physicians, who were convinced Galenists, preferred authority to evidence, and rejected Andreas Versalius's findings. Based on his dissections of the human heart, Versalius found that, contrary to Galen's teaching, there were no pores perforating the wall separating the chambers of the heart. Nearly a century later, Galenist physicians opposed William Harvey's 1628 discovery of the circulation of the blood, because that discovery did not agree with Galen's theory about blood flow (Silverman, 1985, 2).

There is little or no progress in medicine when new generations of doctors, as Professor G.W. Pickering has emphasized, simply subscribe and assent to the views held by an earlier generation, who had been themselves subjected to the same process of screening (Pickering, 1949, 2). Reliable medical knowledge has no foundation in dogmatism. Yet, recognition of the experimental character of medical knowledge requires also that doctors do more than tinker from patient to patient, make observations, and collect anecdotal evidence. Empirical physicians, as Claude Bernard, the recognized father of experimental medicine, said in 1865, should strive towards science. Science here means the kind of methodically organized experimentation that will allow doctors to prove that their interventions, and not nature on its own or some other factors, have brought about the prevention and cure they claim to have achieved (Bernard, 1949, 204).

Because medical knowledge is experimental in nature, progress is inevitably incremental. Discoveries and new knowledge are achieved step-by-step, experiment-by-experiment, with some research confirming, other research modifying, and still other research disproving the results of earlier studies (McIntyre, 1983).

Some who recognize the inherently experimental character of medical knowledge, and who also recognize that doctors should *know* what they are doing when they intervene into the bodies and lives of sick people, still shy away from wholeheartedly accepting that research with human beings is essential, if we are to increasingly reduce the number of people who suffer needlessly and die prematurely. Part of the task of this chapter is to examine why research with human beings has acquired the reputation of being hardly better than a tolerable evil. If we then move on to argue, as we shall, that research with human beings is ethically imperative, we will also have to show how such research can be conducted in an ethically justifiable manner. These are the core tasks of the chapter. We prepare their discussion now, by considering how medical research is conducted today.

HOW MEDICAL RESEARCH IS CONDUCTED TODAY

Research, in whatever field, is a methodological and systematically planned investigation, undertaken with specific safeguards to reduce bias, so that the results of the research have a high probability of being valid and reliable. Only such results merit to be called new *knowledge*. Research, then, is undertaken to produce new knowledge, to reduce uncertainty, and to resolve controversies over matters of fact by producing accumulations of reliable data that offer decisive evidence. The overall goal of research, to take up a theme reaching back to ancient philosophy, is to distinguish reality from mere appearances. Research undertaken to evaluate the safety and efficacy of treatments to prevent or remedy disease is the focus for this chapter's discussion of the ethics of research with human beings.

Descriptive and Comparative Research

The classification of the many kinds of research undertaken in medicine, and the analysis of their various methods, structures, and functions is itself a specialty within medical science. This specialty has come, in recent years, to be called clinical epidemiology (Feinstein, 1985; Sackett, 1985). When medical research, following this recent work, is classified according to its purposes, the research may be either descriptive or comparative.

Descriptive research may be undertaken, for example, to produce knowledge about the way a disease is distributed in a population. Reference was made in Chapter 10, on HIV disease and AIDS, about studies to measure the prevalence and clustering of HIV infection in various communities, and we briefly discussed the need for such research, and some of the ethical issues raised by such studies.

Our focus in this chapter is, rather, on comparative research, more specifically on cause-effect research. Some cause-effect research, for example, research on the causes and the co-factors responsible for disease, is observational. Groups of people, some who are subjected to a factor suspected to be causative of disease and others who are not, are systematically observed over a period of time. Depending on the eventual incidence of disease in one or another of these groups, reliable conclusions can or cannot be drawn about whether the factor under study is really a cause of the disease in question.

Another kind of comparative cause-effect research is experimental, and employs the induction of controlled changes in the bodies of healthy or sick volunteers to obtain a desired research result. The knowledge sought may be *explicatory*, for example, regarding a drug's mechanism of action on the body; or regarding the physiological, cellular, or genetic mechanisms involved in a disease. The knowledge sought may also be *evaluative*, for example, regarding the comparative safety and efficacy of two or more treatments for a disease. Research undertaken to distinguish superior from inferior treatments is sometimes called *managerial*, in contrast with *explicatory* research. The immediate goal of managerial research is the best possible care of individual patients.

The Phases of Research on Drug Therapies

Explicatory and managerial research, when conducted in an experimental manner, both involve the induction of controlled changes into the bodies of human beings. However, the intent of the experiments is quite different in each of these forms of research (Feinstein, 1974).

In explicatory research, there is not intent to treat a patient's underlying disease. In fact, healthy volunteers are often, though not always, the human subjects used for such research. The changes introduced into the bodies of these subjects, for example, by the administration of a drug, are intended to be transient. The changes are induced, not for the sake of the volunteer subject, but to obtain information about the human body's reaction to a drug that may, based on previous animal studies, offer some promise as an eventual treatment for a human disease. These are the kinds of experiments conducted in human beings in Phase I studies of a drug. The studies are conducted to learn about the dosages required to produce a response in the human body; about how the human body processes the drug; and to learn whether the drug produces toxic or harmful effects, and at what dosages.

In Phase II studies, a drug under consideration as a possible treatment for a disease is tested on a group of patients who have that disease. The drug at this phase is not a treatment, and is not being given to patients as a therapy, but rather as an object of study. Though both physicians and patients participating in Phase II studies hope that the drug will exert beneficial effects on the disease, the goal of these studies, nevertheless, is primarily explicatory. There is great uncertainty at this stage, and the studies are undertaken to acquire knowledge about whether the drug has any beneficial effect at all on the disease and, if so, at what dosages that do not cause harmful side effects. If there is no evidence of effect or benefit, or if there is evidence of harm disproportionate to any benefit achieved, study of the drug halts there. If the drug appears to be effective and relatively safe, the stage is set for Phase III of the research.

The experiments undertaken with drugs in Phase III studies differ in intent from those carried out in explicatory research. The intent of the drug experiment in Phase III research is to introduce a lasting beneficial change in the patients participating in the study. The intent is to prevent, or to reverse, the progression of a disease. However, it is still uncertain at this Phase III stage that the drug will prove to be either a truly effective and safe treatment (a real therapy), or a treatment superior to others already in use for a given disease. So the treatment experiments undertaken with patient participants in Phase III research are organized according to a research strategy, to produce reliable and generalizable knowledge about the worth of the drug as a treatment for a whole population of patients affected by a given disease. We shall examine, in a later section, how the treatment experiments of Phase III clinical research differ from the treatment experiments doctors carry out in everyday clinical practice, and why this difference is important for the ethics of research. Prior to that, we consider the controlled clinical trial, the strategy used for Phase III research on drug treatments, and also for clinical research in surgery.

The Controlled Clinical Trial

Clinical research on drug or surgical treatments is undertaken to provide reliable answers to questions such as:

- Will this treatment prevent or remedy a particular disease?
- Will this treatment do more good than harm to patients with this particular disease?
- Will this treatment do more good than available alternative treatments?

These questions may seem to be direct and simple, but the research procedures required to obtain reliable evidence and convincing answers to these questions are complex, difficult, time-consuming, expensive, and, for their implementation, depend upon the collaboration of many hospitals, universities, drug companies, scientists, physicians, surgeons, nurses, and patients. Careful strategies are needed for research, set up to produce the knowledge for reliable recommendations about how best to treat hundreds and thousands of patients afflicted with, perhaps, seriously incapacitating or fatal diseases.

The strategies have been contrived to counter bias. *Bias* is used in a technical sense here, and may be defined as any of the many processes that can inadvertently skew research towards results or conclusions that differ systematically from the truth (Murphy, 1976). Strategies are required, because bias is pervasive in research, in the sense that there are many sources of accidental bias, and they can distort the scientific process at any stage of clinical research, from design of the research protocol, through selection of patients and conduct of the clinical study, up to analysis, interpretation, and reporting of research results. Dr. David Sackett and colleagues at McMaster University have identified at least sixty-five sources of bias that can distort the research process (Sackett, 1979). Bias, if unsuccessfully countered, can vitiate a study of therapies to a point that the research results are worthless, and the whole research exercise ends up offering no reliable guidance at all about how sick people should be treated. At worst, undetected bias can create a false belief that ineffective or harmful treatments are therapeutic.

The strategy most widely used today, to protect clinical research against the potential ravages of bias, is the *controlled clinical trial*. The word *trial* is used when a comparison is set up between two available treatments for a disease, and the goal of the research is to determine whether one is superior (safer and more effective) to another. When only one treatment is available, for example, for a newly discovered disease, the comparison may be set up between that treatment and no treatment at all; or between that treatment and an inactive substance called a placebo (or, in popular terms, a sugar pill). This kind of a trial is called *clinical* (from the Greek word for bed), because it seeks to discover the best way of treating patients, the best way of managing care "at the bedside." The trial is said to be *controlled*, when the results of one treatment are being monitored by comparison with the results of another treatment (or of no treatment or of a placebo) on similar groups of patients affected by the same disease or disorder.

The *strategy* of the controlled clinical trial uses certain *tactics* to eliminate, or at least minimize, the distortion of bias on the results of research to evaluate the safety and efficacy, or the relative worth, of treatments.

Randomization is one such tactic, and it is used to block *selection bias*, the bias that can distort a research project on treatment, if the patients participating in the project are not similar. Consider, for a moment, a research project in which surgery will be compared to a medication, as treatments for a disease condition; for example, a heart problem linked to blocked arteries. The results of such a clinical trial would be highly untrustworthy and invalid if doctors regularly assigned their sickest patients to medication, and their least sick patients to surgery, or vice-versa. The results of such a trial would be biased for or against one of the treatments, depending upon how patients were selected for one or another of the treatments by their physicians. To avoid this bias, patients in a controlled trial are randomly assigned, by some lottery system, to receive one or another of the treatments under study.

Double-blinding is another tactic used, whenever possible, in controlled clinical trials. This means that the patient and the treating physician participating in such a trial are "blinded," that is, kept in ignorance of which of two treatments (and one "treatment" may be a placebo) the patient is receiving during the course of the trial. The tactic of double-blinding is particularly useful when the treatment outcomes that will be used to judge the efficacy or relative worth of treatments are not of the either-or kind, such as death, or objectively measurable, such as the growth of a tumor or the spread of an infection. Subjective measures are such matters as how patients say they feel, and how well observers find them to be functioning.

Randomization and double-blinding are two of the very important tactics employed in controlled clinical trials, to minimize bias and increase the probability of producing reliable results. Because uncertainty is inherent in medical science, and because the reliability of research results is measured in terms of probabilities, and rarely in terms of absolute certitude, there are also crucially important statistical conditions that have to be respected if a clinical trial is to produce both valid and credible results. Sample size, or the numbers of patients to be enrolled in the trial, is an example, since a clinical trial conducted on too few patients can prove nothing (Sackett, 1979, 61).

Clinical Research and Clinical Practice

Some people may think that there is little ethical difference between clinical practice and clinical research, because doctors conduct experiments on patients both in practice and in research. But the experiments of everyday clinical practice differ considerably from those conducted in a controlled clinical trial, and the differences are ethically significant.

Physicians conduct experiments daily, in routine clinical practice. One such kind of experiment we might call "tailoring the treatment to the patient." Even when drug treatments are available that have proven to be effective in specific dosages for a given disease, the effectiveness often has to be qualified as "effective by and large," because individual patients vary widely in their responses to drugs. So a doctor may have to vary dosages of a drug and the frequency of its administration, or combine one drug with others until a beneficial effect is achieved for a given patient.

"Tailoring the treatment to the patient" is precisely what doctors are not supposed to do, when they are treating their patients within a controlled clinical trial. A trial, set up to provide reliable conclusions about the potential superiority of one drug over another, requires that observations and measurements of patient responses to the study drugs can be made under controlled conditions. And the conditions that have to be controlled include dosage, frequency and route of administration, and combination of the drugs under study with other drugs. If doctors tailored drug treatments to best fit the day-to-day responses of their patients who are participating in a controlled clinical trial, there would be no way to determine if the harms and benefits observed during the trial were due to the drugs under study, or to all the variations, including combination with other drugs, that doctors would have introduced during their treatment-tailoring experiments.

Achieving a rapid beneficial response from each patient treated is the immediate goal of the physician's daily "tailoring of the treatment to the patient" experiments. In controlled clinical trials, the purpose of each drug treatment experiment is to better each patient, but these experiments serve the more comprehensive and governing goal of producing reliable knowledge about the long-term superiority of one or another of the treatments under study, for a population of patients affected by a given disease. Though both the routine clinical experiments and those conducted in a clinical trial deliver treatment, in the controlled clinical trial, tailored treatment for immediate, optimal, individual care is sacrificed, in favour of controlled treatment for optimal scientific results about the relative efficacy and safety of two treatments for a population of patients.

Patients have every right to know about this difference, when they are asked to participate in controlled clinical trials. They, at times, do not, as we shall point out later in the chapter, when we discuss the "therapeutic misconception" some patients have about controlled clinical trials.

The fact that experiments are conducted both in everyday clinical practice and in formally organized clinical research is, then, not a justification for slipping to the conclusion that there is no ethical difference between clinical practice and clinical research. The preceding discussion has highlighted one difference. There are others.

It would be incorrect, for example, to infer from the preceding discussion that patients always fare better in the "tailoring" experiments of everyday practice than they do in the "controlled" experiments of clinical research. Often, quite the contrary is true. Some patients even make considerable effort to enroll in clinical research projects, because they expect, at times rightly so, that the close supervision and overall care they will receive in the trial will be superior to the care they would generally receive in everyday clinical practice.

There is another important dimension to this discussion. Some of the treatments used in everyday clinical practice, and that have acquired the reputation of being standard and established therapies, have never been subjected to the methodological evaluation given to treatments in a controlled clinical trial. The reputation of being a standard or established therapy is often based on little more than clinical rumour, anecdotal evidence, or fashion (McKinlay, 1981; Burnum, 1987). In the past, a number of such "standard" treatments, as we shall note again later in the chapter, had to be abandoned because they were eventually shown, under careful study, to have been either useless or definitely harmful.

New treatments are not necessarily, and often are not, "the best," or even better than available treatments; and treatments long in use are not necessarily either safe or effective. The purpose of controlled clinical trials is to validate such treatments, which, without scientific scrutiny, could be used for years, all the while achieving no good, and even causing harm, without anyone being the wiser.

Research on Therapy, not "Therapeutic Research"

The distinction between "therapeutic" and "non-therapeutic" research, used quite extensively in the literature on the ethics of research, has now been largely abandoned. These adjectives cause confusion, and serve no useful purpose.

Labelling research on therapies as "therapeutic" suggested that such research was generally of direct benefit to the health of patients; was much more benign than other kinds of research; and was, therefore, much less in need of rigorous ethical evaluation and monitoring than explicatory research. That suggestion does not square with the realities of medical research (Levine, 1979; Rolleston, 1981).

Controlled clinical trials are set up to measure the safety and efficacy of new treatments, or to evaluate the worth of treatments already in use, because there is uncertainty, or controversy, or simply little reliable information at all about the power of these procedures (whether they be drug treatments or surgical operations) to remedy disease. Patients enrolled in these trials may receive benefit, or they may receive no benefit whatsoever regarding reversal or halting of the progression of their disease. If one of two treatments under study eventually proves to be decidedly inferior to the other, patients may even have been harmed during the course of the study. The harm can range from moderate and transient to severe and irreversible, and may even consist in death, depending on the disease for which the treatments under study are being proposed.

The adjective *therapeutic*, when applied to research on therapies, tends to mask these realities. The adjective also tends to mask the fact, already mentioned in the discussion above of "tailoring the treatment to the patient" experiments of everyday clinical practice, that doctors participating in controlled clinical trials have to follow research rules, such as being blinded to the treatments their patients are receiving, that limit the ordinary clinical manoeuvrability they have in clinical practice. Moreover, use of this adjective, *therapeutic*, can lead to the impression that painstaking education of patients about the realities of the research, and about the treatment under study and existing alternative treatments, is really not altogether that necessary, because, after all, the research is "therapeutic."

These considerations are not a critique of research and of the controlled clinical trials undertaken to validate new and existing therapies. Quite the contrary! They are intended, rather, as a critique of terms, such as "therapeutic research," likely to imply, however subtly, that there is no uncertainty or controversy about treatments for a disease, or that a process to validate these treatments is not underway. One of the central requirements of research ethics, as we shall discuss in a later section of this chapter, on informed and voluntary consent, is that patients be told the truth, and that they be brought to face existing clinical uncertainty or controversy about the value of treatments. The ethics of research, however, has a long history, and we will now consider the major turning points in that history, before focusing attention on why controlled clinical trials are ethically imperative, and on the conditions for conducting such trials in an ethically justifiable manner.

CONTROLLED CLINICAL TRIALS ARE ETHICALLY IMPERATIVE

It is not obvious to many people that controlled clinical trials are as necessary ethically as they are scientifically. These trials have been criticized, in terms that pit against each other realities that belong together, but can only exist together in tension. For example, controlled clinical trials have been criticized on ethical grounds, because they presumably sacrifice the good of individual patients to the good of society or the good of future patients. Or these trials have been criticized because physicians who participate in them as clinical investigators are forced, it is assumed, to subjugate their loyalty to individual patients, which should be prime, to the scientific exigencies of conducting valid research.

There *are* judicious criticisms directed against the way certain tactics, such as randomization, use of placebos, and the monitoring of clinical trials, are implemented, and we shall consider some of these criticisms carefully, in a later section of this chapter on controversies in research ethics. However, simplified polarizing critiques, such as those mentioned above, gloss over or outrightly ignore some of the inescapable ethical tensions and scientific realities of contemporary medicine.

A doctor has a therapeutic obligation never to recommend a therapy that would be known to be inferior to an available alternative treatment, or that would be inferior (more harmful or less beneficial) to no treatment at all. But a doctor cannot fulfil that obligation, when it is precisely the relative superiority or inferiority of available treatments that is uncertain and unknown. This is the situation in which controlled clinical trials are both ethically justifiable and ethically imperative.

A physician's professional and ethical obligation to offer each patient the best available treatment cannot be separated from the twin clinical and ethical imperative of basing the choice of treatment on the most reliable available or obtainable evidence. The tension between the interdependent responsibilities of giving patients personalized, compassionate care, as well as scientifically sound and validated treatment, is a tension inherent to the practice of medicine today.

Some confuse this tension between a physician's co-equal responsibilities with a conflict of interest. A conflict of interest occurs when activities for one's own gain or good, or the good of one individual or group, imperil the fulfilment of one's responsibility to act for the good of others. However, the tension between a physician's correlative responsibilities of giving personal, compassionate care and scientifically sound and validated treatment exists independently of any potential conflict, which can occur in medicine as well as in any other profession, between a physician's personal agenda and his or her professional responsibilities.

Moreover, this tension is localized at the bedside of individual patients, and not out in some space where the good of an individual patient conflicts with the good of society. It is a clinical tension between two goods, individually tailored *and* scientifically validated care, that a physician owes each patient.

When there is uncertainty or definite doubt, or controversy about either the safety or efficacy (or both) of new or established treatments, there is an ethical obligation to test these treatments critically, rather than to prescribe them, day after day, on the basis of custom, fashion, unreliable anecdotal evidence, or clinical rumour. When large numbers of innovative treatments are continuously introduced into clinical practice, as is the case today, rigorous testing of these is ethically mandatory, both for the protection of individual patients and for the just use of scarce resources. This holds true with even greater force in the light of evidence that many innovations show no advantage over existing treatments, when submitted to properly controlled study (Gilbert, 1977). They may be even less effective, or harmful. Neither is the fact that a treatment has been prescribed by many doctors, over a considerable period of time, any guarantee of its real therapeutic worth. Several years ago, Dr. Howard Hiatt compiled a list of treatments (for ulcer, epilepsy, pelvic hemorrhage, kidney failure, asthma, coronary artery disease, and hypertension) that later had to be abandoned, because they were found to be either harmful or useless (Hiatt, 1975).

Controlled clinical trials — randomized and properly blinded, when these tactics to minimize bias are feasible, scientifically appropriate, and ethically achievable — are an integral part of the ethical imperative that physicians should *know* what they are doing, when they intervene into the bodies, minds, and lives of sick people. However, controlled clinical trials can be an *ethical* imperative, only if it is possible to conduct them in an ethically justifiable manner. It has, though, taken many years, often years of intolerable abuse of human beings in research, to arrive at a clear grasp of what these conditions for ethically justifiable research with human beings really are.

RESEARCH ETHICS: HISTORICAL BACKGROUND

The trials held at Nuremberg, Germany, shortly after the end of World War II, to prosecute war criminals, included the trial of twenty doctors who had carried out deadly medical experiments on human beings between 1939 and 1945. These experiments violated the laws of humanity and the ethics of the medical profession. The judgment on these doctors, while admitting that medical research with human beings can conform to medical ethics, specified that ethically and legally justifiable research must honour at least ten principles. These ten principles, outlined in the judgment of the Nuremberg trials, are now known as the *Nuremberg Code*.

The *Nuremberg Code* marks a major turning point in the history of the ethics of research with human subjects. The Code emphasized respect for human beings and the protection of their health, lives, dignity, rights, needs, and interests in any conduct of medical research and experimentation. The Code also crystallized the essential characteristics of *consent* required to protect the autonomy of human beings in research. Consent of patients and volunteers involved in medical research has to be *competent, voluntary, informed*, and *comprehending*.

Before Nuremberg

The demands of the *Nuremberg Code* are basic. They arose out of the crushing evidence of experiments in which human beings were treated as objects or things, or treated with less solicitude than one would treat animals, in medical research conducted during the Nazi period.

However, the inhuman or unethical treatment of human beings in research both preceded and followed the practices of medical researchers under the Nazi regime.

When a Russian doctor, Vikenty Veressayev, wrote his *Memoirs of a Physician* — the English translation was subsequently published in 1916 — venereal or sexually transmitted diseases, such as gonorrhea and syphilis, had been the focus of medical-research interest for some years. Veressayev's *Memoirs* document numerous utterly unethical experiments that were conducted on human beings, by eminent and respected physicians, in the late 1800s in Germany, France, Russia, Ireland and the United States. This research was not carried out clandestinely, but published in some of the world's leading medical journals. In a number of these experiments, active gonorrheic or syphilitic microorganisms were injected into patients, often very sick and dying patients or severely ill infants, without their knowledge and consent, or the consent of their parents. Painful inflammation and death were the price many patients paid for the experiments doctors conducted to test theories about venereal diseases.

Dr. Veressayev was astonished that publication of these terrible experiments did not result in the immediate banishment of the researchers from the medical community: "But, unfortunately, this is not so. With heads proudly erect, these bizarre disciples of science proceed upon their way without encountering any effective opposition, either from their colleagues or the medical press..." The *Memoirs* direct a plea to society, a plea not to wait for the conscience of medical scientists to awaken, but rather "to take its own measures of self-protection against those zealots of science who have ceased to distinguish between their brothers and guinea pigs..." (Veressayev, 1916).

After Nuremberg

In 1966, just about twenty years after Nuremberg, Dr. Henry K. Beecher, Dorr Professor of Research in Anesthesia at Harvard University Medical School, published a critical survey of twenty-two medical research projects done in the United States after World War II. Many of the patients used in these research projects never had the risks satisfactorily explained to them; many never realized they were involved in research; and many never were asked to consent to their involvement. Some of the patients suffered grave consequences, or death, as a result of the experiments. Dr. Beecher cited the belief, then prevalent in some sophisticated circles, that attention paid to adequately informing human subjects, and attention and time given over to preparing subjects for comprehending and voluntary consent, would "block progress." Dr. Beecher countered this belief with a quotation from Pope Pius XII, to the effect that "... science is not the highest value to which all other orders of value ... should be subordinated." (Beecher, 1966, 1354)

Dr. Beecher emphasized two most important components in the ethical approach to research with human subjects. The *first* was informed consent. But it is often difficult, in Beecher's view, to achieve adequately informed consent. So Beecher emphasized a *second* component, one he believed offered patients a more reliable safeguard, namely: "the presence of an intelligent, informed, conscientious, compassionate, responsible investigator." (Beecher, 1966, 1360)

Dr. Beecher's article in *The New England Journal of Medicine* was another major turning point in the evolution of the ethics of research with human subjects. But it was not the last. A key question arose: does or can science produce the ideal medical researchers Dr. Beecher put forth as the real safeguard of patient's health, life, and interests in research? (Katz, 1972, 307)

The Need for Ethical Review of Research

People have reached a widespread consensus in North America and Europe, over the past twenty years, that sole reliance on Dr. Beecher's ideal medical researchers is insufficient to protect adequately the health, life, and dignity of persons involved as subjects in medical research. An independent ethical review of research projects using human subjects is now considered essential.

The World Medical Association in its *Declaration of Helsinki* specified that experimental procedures involving human subjects should be clearly formulated in a research protocol, and should be transmitted to a specially appointed independent committee for consideration, comment, and guidance (World Medical Association, 1975).

In the mid-1970s, the United States established the National Commission for the Protection of Human Subjects of Biomedical and Behavioral Research. That Commission's *Report and Recommendations on Institutional Review Boards* (IRBs, the American expression for research ethics committees, also called research ethics boards, or REBs, in Canada) emphasized that the ethical conduct of research involving human subjects requires a balancing of society's interests in developing beneficial medical knowledge, and in protecting human beings in research. The key point is that investigators and researchers cannot achieve that balance all by themselves. People not involved in the conduct of research should be involved in the ethical review of proposed research, so that potential conflicts of interest can be detected and controlled.

Research ethics committees (IRBs or REBs) wield considerable power. They have the authority to approve, reject, or demand modifications of protocols for research with human subjects. These committees typically examine research protocols to assure that they demonstrate: sound scientific method and design; acceptable balance between risk of harm and probability of benefit; importance of scientific objective; adequate procedures to assure that consent is informed and voluntary; equitable selection of subjects; adequate protection of subjects who are particularly vulnerable; avoidance of discrimination; and protection of confidentiality.

The question of consent offers an example of an emerging controversy, regarding the degree of power research ethics committees should exert on the research process. Research ethics committees generally confine their attention to the information sheets and consent forms included in protocols, and prepared by clinical investigators to help participants understand the objectives, procedures, as well as the potential risks and benefits, of the project. The focus of research ethics committee review is usually on the clarity and comprehensibility of the consent form and information sheets.

Even if the *Nuremberg Code* is not explicitly cited, the emerging controversy centres on the Code's statement that responsibility for ascertaining the quality of research subjects' consent rests with each individual who initiates, directs, or engages in the experiment. Some scientists still look upon "obtaining informed consent" as a legally imposed and obstructive ritual. They have to "get" the patient's or subject's consent, as something *they* need for *their* research. An ethically adequate research protocol and a comprehensible consent form offer no guarantee or evidence that careful communication, designed to maximize the research subject's understanding, will take place. Dr. Beecher rightly emphasized, over twenty years ago, that researchers' statements about having obtained patients' consent are meaningless, unless something is known about what actually transpired between investigator and subject.

How can one know about what transpires between physician-investigators and patient-subjects? Should the responsibilities of research ethics committees extend beyond the review of research protocols, to include the monitoring of consent conversations and the actual conduct of research with human subjects? (Robertson, 1982; Christakis, 1988) Even the *Medical Research Council of Canada 1987 Guidelines*, which advocate such monitoring, at least for certain research projects, recognize that such a monitoring process could present significant problems. The Guidelines identify some of the potential problems, but offer little concrete advice about how these problems could be prevented or solved if they occur (Medical Research Council of Canada, 1987).

Others in this controversy wonder if the moment has not arrived to brake the evolution of research ethics in the direction of ever more elaborate mechanisms of external supervision of clinical investigators, and to accelerate the development of awareness among clinical investigators that ethics is an integral function of scientific intelligence and judgement.

THE CONDITIONS FOR ETHICALLY JUSTIFIABLE MEDICAL RESEARCH WITH HUMAN SUBJECTS

If medical research with human subjects, and controlled clinical trials were inherently unethical, research ethics would be quite simple and absolute. However, as implied in the guiding assumption at the beginning of this chapter, research ethics is conditional ethics. Research with human subjects will be unethical, to the extent that it fails to fulfil a set of necessary and interrelated conditions. *Ethical justifiability* means consistency with the beliefs and values, with the ethos and morality of a community. Of course, communities vary from one culture and society to another, not only in their customs and art, but also in their governing perceptions and values regarding the body, health, disease, suffering, death, and a host of other realities affecting the practice of medicine.

The conditions, which we are now about to discuss, for ethically justifiable research with human subjects, reflect a consensus widely shared in North America and Europe. In a later section of the chapter, we open a discussion of how some of these conditions are interpreted differently in various cultures than they are in Western societies.

Scientific Adequacy

The *Nuremberg Code* and the *Declaration of Helsinki* have stated that research with human subjects must, as a general condition of ethical justifiability, conform to the canons of scientific methodology. Both insist on respect for accepted scientific principles, knowledge of the natural history of the disease or problem under study, adequate preliminary laboratory and animal experimentation, and the proper scientific and medical qualifications of investigators.

This emphasis, though covering the basic preconditions for valid, credible research, ethically justifiable research, may seem to be an overemphasis of the obvious.

However, the attempt, in the early 1980s, to treat two betathalassemic patients (betathalassemia being a disease, due to a genetic defect, that affects the blood and causes anemia) with human beta-globin gene implants was widely criticized as premature and unethical, chiefly on two grounds. The treatment was tried without adequate preliminary experimentation with animal models of betathalassemia, and without the solid foundation of adequate scientific knowledge about the regulation of beta-globin gene expression.

David R. Rutstein's maxim, "a poorly or improperly designed study involving human subjects ... is by definition unethical" (Rutstein, 1970, 384), directs attention to the general rule of proportionality ethics. Inviting human beings to submit themselves to possibly heightened risk of discomfort, inconvenience, harm, or death, consuming scarce precious resources, and raising hopes, particularly in situations when hope is about all that patients have left, demands the balancing weight of a clinical trial that exhibits a high probability of achieving three objectives identified by David L. Sackett as: "validity (the results are true), generalizability (the results are widely applicable), and efficiency (the trial is affordable and resources are left over for patient care and for other health research)." (Sackett, 1980, 1059)

Protection of Subjects

Henry K. Beecher's statement, "Ordinary patients will not knowingly risk their health or their life for the sake of science," is as true today as it was in 1966 (Beecher, 1966, 1360). Sick people come to doctors for care, relief, and cure. The expectation that doctors will help, and not harm, is the basis of the patient-doctor relationship, the primary content of the medical profession's societal mandate, and the guiding norm of one of medicine's most ancient ethical maxims. Fidelity to this expectation is an essential condition for ethically acceptable clinical research.

Claude Bernard gave precision to the meaning of this fidelity in his statement of a principle of medical and surgical morality:

> It is our duty and our right to perform an experiment on man whenever it can save his life, cure him, or gain him some personal benefit. The principle of medical and surgical morality, therefore, consists in never performing an experiment which might be harmful to him to any extent, even though the result might be highly advantageous to science, that is to the health of others. (Bernard, 1949, 101)

This principle, establishing a basic right of patients, and a corresponding fundamental duty of doctors, takes precedence over any utilitarian calculus that would tolerate a sacrifice of the health or lives of individuals today for the putatively greater good of society, or the patients of tomorrow.

This "Bernard" principle, though clearly essential for the ethical justifiability of clinical research with human subjects, is, as worded, too pure and absolute to be realistic. Medicine is inherently experimental. It is clearly impossible, either in everyday clinical practice or in controlled clinical trials, to abstain totally from interventions that might be harmful "to any extent." The factors of uncertainty and risk of harm, attendant upon any clinical intervention into the body, have to be recognized in this principle of the primacy of the therapeutic obligation.

Distinctions also have to be made, to grasp properly what are the risks of physical harm to subjects and patients in the various kinds and phases of medical research.

First, it would be a serious mistake to imagine or claim that the terrible and humanly insensitive experiments, dangerous to the health and life of human beings, that were carried out during the last century, earlier in this century, and during the Second World War, are still being done on human beings today. The undeniable progress of the past forty years, in clarifying and achieving the theoretical, practical, and institutional requirements for ethically justifiable research with human subjects, serves as a generally effective bulwark against the destructive and inhuman *use* of human beings in research.

Second, the occurrence of physical or psychological injury to human beings in explicatory research generally, and in the early phases of research in therapies (Phases I and II of drug studies) in particular, is very rare. Dr. Robert Levine has reviewed studies done on the incidence of injury to human beings in research carried out over a twenty-year period, and concludes that all available evidence indicates that playing the role of research subject is not a highly perilous business (Levine, 1986, 40).

Third, one has to be quite clear on the fact that some patients afflicted with high-mortality and high-morbidity diseases are inevitably going to die, or suffer progression of their disease, during the course of clinical trials set up either to discover a first effective treatment for such a disease, or to discover which of several available treatments is the safest and most effective. Patients who die, or suffer harm from the progression of their disease, because they have, in clinical trials, received treatments that eventually prove to be inferior, would also have died or have suffered harm under the same treatments had they been administered in the context of clinical practice. Suffering death or harm, in the context of clinical trials conducted to discover or validate therapies for high-mortality diseases, is due not to the research, but to the fact that research has not advanced far enough to have discovered either a cure or an effective way of halting progression of the disease. When there are no validated treatments for high-mortality diseases, controlled clinical trials are no more dangerous than uncontrolled use of these unvalidated treatments in clinical practice.

There are, however, two procedures established to maximize protection of patients who have enrolled in clinical trials, particularly in randomized, double-blinded clinical trials. The first consists in withdrawal from the trial of any patient who is deteriorating under the treatment he or she has received under the randomization code. The code is broken for such a patient, the patient's physician is unblinded, and treatment is then tailored to meet the patient's need in the best possible way.

The second procedure utilizes a *safety and data monitoring board*, sometimes also called a safety and efficacy review committee. This committee, the membership of which usually includes physicians, biostatisticians, ethicists, and representatives of patients with the disease under study in the trial, has the responsibility of periodically examining accumulating data as the clinical trial progresses, and of recommending cessation or modification of the trial as soon as there is solid evidence of the superiority of one treatment over another.

The harms patients may suffer and the benefits they may receive in controlled clinical trials are not always precisely measurable and quantifiable. It is really quite impossible to determine that a proportion between possible harms and benefits holds for particular patients, without giving due attention and weight to their personal interpretations of the total impact of a clinical intervention on their lives. Judging the efficacy of a treatment, in terms of its power to avert death, is obviously important. It is also important to judge the worth of treatments in terms of their impact on patients' quality of life. A treatment that prolongs life, for example by shrinking tumors, may rank low in patients' estimation, if the life prolonged is a life of misery. For this reason, adequate evaluation of a treatment's worth must not be made on the basis of a dehumanized array of data. That evaluation must include data on patients' symptoms, severity of illness, disability, and all the distinctively human experiences that, as Feinstein has emphasized, differentiate people from animals or molecules (Feinstein, 1987).

Informed, Comprehending, and Voluntary Consent

The *Nuremberg Code* crystallized the essential characteristics of consent required, to respect the autonomy and liberty of human beings participating as subjects in medical research. Their consent has to be competent, voluntary, informed, and comprehending. These are basic demands.

The Code emphasized that persons asked to participate in research should have sufficient knowledge and comprehension of the research as to be able to make an enlightened decision. The Code then specifies that research subjects need to know the nature, duration, and purpose of the experiment; the method and means by which it is to be conducted; all inconveniences and hazards reasonably to be expected; and the effects upon health or person that may come from participation in the research.

The *Medical Research Council of Canada Guidelines* are even more specific about the scope of consent, and provide a checklist of items about which patients must be informed. These guidelines wisely emphasize two items that are particularly important in controlled clinical trials of therapies. Patients, whose enlistment in such trials is sought, need to know about their prognosis, if no treatment of their disease is undertaken; about the availability of treatments, other than those to be studied in the clinical trial; and about treatments that will not be available to them, if they decide to participate in the trial.

The obvious often needs emphasis, and so we here emphasize that the very first thing patients must be told is that they are being asked to participate in research. One of the most egregious offences against the ethics of research is to treat patients according to the procedures of a controlled clinical trial, without even informing them that a trial is being conducted. That offence has been committed several times in the quite recent past (Nicholson, 1986; Gerber, 1989).

It is very important that physicians and clinical investigators take pains to assure that patients really do understand what randomized, double-blinded clinical trials involve. Patients affected by what has been called the "therapeutic misconception" do not have such understanding. That misconception resides in the tendency of research subjects who are patients to misinterpret the harm-benefits ratio of participating in research. The misinterpretation derives from an overly optimistic expectation patients have, even after being told about randomization and double-blinding, that in their own case physicians involved in the trial will make treatment decisions in terms of a precise consideration of their own needs and best interest. Some patients need special help to understand that, in a controlled clinical trial, their physicians will not be tailoring treatment to their precise personal needs, as physicians normally do in everyday clinical practice (Appelbaum, 1987).

Doctors who are clinical investigators involved in controlled clinical trials are as much in need of knowing every essential of the life plans, concerns, and bodily condition of patients and subjects as the latter are in need of knowing every essential of the research procedures to be used, and of the treatments to be studied, in the controlled clinical trial.

Physicians and clinical investigators bear primary responsibility for organizing consent conversations, and making certain that this mutually informing process really takes place. Insecure and vulnerable patients and subjects may easily be cowed into silence, or even acquiescence, by the awesome environment of the hospital and the authority-laden image of the doctor. The hospital is the doctor's daily domain and home territory, which the patient enters as a frightened and dependent stranger. In these circumstances, voluntary consent does not come naturally. It requires sensitive perception and dedicated commitment on the part of physicians and clinical investigators, if they are to serve the needs and goals of those who come to them for care and cure.

When Consent Negotiations Are Defective: Two Canadian Cases

In August 1961, Walter Halushka, a student at the University of Saskatchewan, agreed to be a volunteer subject in a medical research project set up to test a new anaesthetic drug. Mr. Halushka suffered a cardiac arrest during the experiment and, though successfully resuscitated, he was left with some brain damage and a diminution of mental ability. He could no longer continue his university studies. The Court of Appeal found that one of the physician-researchers had told the student that the test was safe and there was nothing to worry about. The physician-researchers had failed to inform Mr. Halushka that the test was of a new drug, that they had little previous knowledge about this drug, that the drug was an anaesthetic, and that there was, accordingly, risk involved in its use. The physician-investigators also failed to tell this student that the test would also involve passage of a catheter up a vein in his arm into his heart.

In finding the doctor-researchers guilty of failing to inform Mr. Halushka adequately about the risk of harm involved in this research, the Court of Appeal clarified the requirements for consent in the research setting:

> There can be no exceptions to the ordinary requirements of disclosure in the case of research as there may well be in ordinary medical practice. The researcher does not have to balance the probable effect of lack of treatment against the risk involved in the treatment itself. The example of risks being properly hidden from a patient when it is important that he should not worry can have no application in the field of research. The subject of medical experimentation is entitled to a full and frank disclosure of all the facts, probabilities and opinions which a reasonable man might be expected to consider before giving his consent. (*Halushka*, 1965)

Some investigators speak and behave as though *obtaining* consent is the ethical be-all and end-all of research with human subjects. The attitude frequently seems to be: if only I can get that consent, I can get on with what is really important, my research. This attitude ignores the ethically important fact that the real consent of subjects is an element in a process of shared decision-making, not just a ritual password required by law before research can proceed. Clinical investigators demonstrating this attitude fail to grasp that adequate information is primarily the need of the patient, and that adequately informing patients about research is a moral requirement of integrity in the human relationship between physician-investigator and patient-subject.

Though patients are rarely harmed seriously in explicatory research, as already mentioned earlier in the chapter, such harm, even death, can occur. It is particularly tragic when a research-related death occurs that could have been avoided, if consent negotiations had been adequate.

On October 13, 1981, Mr. Julius Weiss, 62 years old, died in a Montréal hospital, while participating in a research project conducted to test the efficacy of a drug (indomethacin, administered by eye drops) to reduce swelling in the eye after cataract surgery. This project also required that Mr. Weiss undergo fluorescein angiograms, to gauge the effects of the indomethacin eye drops. Angiograms involve injection of a fluorescent dye (fluorescein) into a vein.

Mr. Weiss had a history of heart problems, and went into convulsions following a drop in blood pressure after the first injection of dye. Mr. Weiss's heart stopped, resuscitation attempts failed, and he died.

Mr. Weiss's wife and children sued the two physicians involved in the clinical study, and the hospital where the study was conducted. In his judgment on this case, rendered on February 23, 1989, Judge De Blois of Québec Superior Court found that Mr. Weiss would not have agreed to be in this project, had he known it carried even a small risk of cardiac arrest and death. It also seems that the key physician-investigator in the project was not aware of Mr. Weiss's weak-heart condition. It is likely, or at least possible, that the physician-investigator, had he known of Mr. Weiss's condition, would have discussed risk with Mr. Weiss in greater detail and with greater precision. The physician-investigator might not even have considered Mr. Weiss as a participant for this project.

This tragic case raises many legal issues, too complex to discuss in this chapter (Freedman, 1990). It also emphasizes that informed consent is a two-way transaction (Dickens, 1982). Physicians-investigators need information about patients, as much as patients need information about the trial.

Telling Patients about Randomization

One of the conditions for the ethical acceptability of using randomization, as the way of determining which of two or several treatments patients will receive in a clinical trial, is that physicians really do not know whether one treatment is superior to another. This is called the condition of clinical equipoise, when one group of physicians may favour one treatment and other physicians favour another treatment, but both groups of physicians recognize that there is real uncertainty and reasonable controversy about the relative merits of the treatments under study (Freedman, 1987).

However, the ethical justifiability of randomization does not hinge only on the ability of physicians "to live with" randomization. The existence of clinical equipoise regarding two treatments does not justify the inference that patients will be, or should be, indifferent about the treatments that will be allotted them under the randomization procedure. Treatments have many effects, and possible prolonged survival is only one such effect. Even when there is clinical equipoise or equivalence at the beginning of a trial regarding the effect of two treatments on survival, these treatments may not be in "patient equipoise" regarding their effects on quality of life.

In earlier clinical trials of treatments for breast cancer, some women preferred not to have the total surgical removal of the breast (mastectomy) but, rather, the treatment that excised only the tumor from the breast (lumpectomy). Clinical equipoise of these two treatments at the beginning of the trial, with respect to the prolongation of survival time, did not imply that women were capricious in preferring one treatment over the other, for reasons and purposes clear to them.

Failure to tell patients about randomization, and the associated additional concealments of information this would often entail, can bar patients from what they need to know to make the choices they consider most important for their lives. This is ethically unjustifiable in a trial that would otherwise be ethically acceptable. As a rule, patients should be informed about randomization. Exceptions will have to be justified.

THE ETHICAL USE OF ANIMALS IN RESEARCH

It is generally, and correctly, assumed that the ethical justifiability of research with human subjects depends on adequate prior experimentation with animals. Both the *Nuremberg Code* and The World Medical Association *Declaration of Helsinki*, for example, mention that animal experimentation should precede research with human subjects, in the testing of new drugs and surgical operations. This does not mean that the use of animals in research requires no further justification. However, a comprehensive response to the question about whether we are morally justified in imposing suffering on, or taking the lives of, other species solely for our own benefit would require an analysis of the expanding and unfinished debate on these issues. Since such an analysis would exceed the boundaries of this chapter and book, two major points have been selected for discussion.

First, differences between species do have moral significance. Ethical constraints on what we may impose on other animals, to satisfy our own good and our own needs, increase as the capacities and needs of the animals approach those of human beings. Second, the critical question is not whether, but under what conditions, may we use animals in research.

Effective measures to assure the humane treatment of animals in research, and to protect animals against wanton disregard of their needs and welfare are essential requirements of civilized scientific behaviour. Fulfilling these requirements does not necessitate acceptance of any of the following positions:

- humans have no right to treat animals any differently than they would treat any member of their own species;
- animals should be used in research projects only when the results will directly benefit the animals themselves;
- there should be an immediate replacement of all animals used in experiments by alternative systems (McIntosh, 1985; Rowan, 1983).

Sensitivity to the needs of animals, and to their differential capacities for suffering from pain, constriction, and deprivation, does necessitate careful attention to Lane-Petter's five basic questions:

- Is the animal the best experimental system for the problem?
- Must the animal be conscious at any time during the experiment?
- Can the pain and discomfort associated with the experiment be lessened or eliminated?
- Could the number of animals involved be reduced?
- Is the problem under study worth solving? (Lane-Petter, 1972)

Necessity of experiment, humaneness of design, and a standard of pre- and post-operative care that is at least as good as that required for acceptable clinical veterinary practice summarize the conditions for the ethical justifiability of using animals in research. A more complete discussion of these conditions can be found in both Canadian and international guidelines (Canadian Council on Animal Care, 1980, 1984; CIOMS, 1985).

ETHICS OF RESEARCH AND CULTURAL DIVERSITY

Though science is largely transcultural, the human community has not yet developed a completely corresponding transcultural ethics. Differing views about what is normative in person-person, doctor-patient, and investigator-subject relationships may create the need for ethical compromise or accommodation in some multicentre trials, particularly when the collaborating centres are situated in different nations.

A Japanese physician-investigator may find it difficult to honour North American insistence on detailed disclosure to patients, about the randomization process used to select treatment in a clinical trial for breast cancer or cancer of the prostate. Both physicians and patients, in a culture that places great emphasis on trust in the physician as an integral part of the healing process, may find an open admission of physician ignorance or uncertainty to be therapeutically damaging, or even absurd.

North American culture emphasizes the value of individual autonomy. Chinese culture emphasizes the value of the family and the community. The approach to informed, comprehending, and voluntary consent may be quite different in each of these cultures. Sensitivity to the dominant values of other cultures should be an ethical requisite of international collaboration in multicentre trials. Accommodating cultural differences, even in ethnic groups within the pluralistic society of Western nations, will usually require a flexibility in procedures, rather than the compromise of fundamental principles.

This position may be put to an acid test in the context of research carried out in developing countries, on the prevention and treatment of HIV infection and disease. We have already discussed the tension, inherent in the contemporary practice of medicine, between the correlative responsibilities of giving personal, compassionate care *and* scientifically sound and validated treatment. The tension between maintaining the principles of research ethics *and* making respectful accommodations to cultures that do not emphasize individuality, as does Western culture, sets up the dilemma of choosing between ethical imperialism and ethical relativism. How do we respect the ethics of a culture very different from our own, without abusing people, when we carry out a research project in a country with a research ethics that is much less demanding than our own?

CONCLUSION

There is a time and a place for everything, but times change. The ethics of research with human beings has a history, and that history demonstrates the development, throughout this century, of a consciousness of the need to protect human beings from abuse, indeed, from simply being *used*, in medical research. The time for vigilance will never pass away. But we should also now move beyond the ethics of vigilance and protection. People will, in fact, be better able to protect themselves against abuse in medical research, the more they are able to understand the purposes and methods of this research. The goal should be the promotion of intelligent and active collaboration of patients and doctors with scientists, in developing safe and effective treatments for incapacitating and deadly diseases. Young children, of course, cannot collaborate in this way in research on treatments for childhood diseases. So research involving children presents special ethical difficulties and requirements, the discussion of which goes beyond the purposes and space of this chapter (National Council, 1992).

We would not have effective treatments for many diseases today, if earlier generations had not participated as subjects in medical research. Some, as we have seen, did not *participate*. They were simply used, without their knowledge and consent. Patients and volunteers have every right, one may even argue that they have a duty, to refuse to participate in unethically designed research.

This coin also has another side. Developing treatments for diseases that cause great suffering and death depends on maintaining and increasing excellent and ethical medical research. Much of this research will have to be done with human subjects, since animal models are frequently lacking or inadequate. Does this mean that a new duty is emerging in the moral consciousness of people at the end of this century, a moral duty to participate in medical research? (Caplan, 1984) Some would say the term *moral duty* is too strong. Perhaps, but is participation in medical research an intrinsic component of the responsibility we bear towards future generations, the generations of our children?

REFERENCES

Appelbaum P.S. et al. "False Hopes and Best Data: Consent to Research and the Therapeutic Misconception." *Hastings Center Report* 1987;17/2:20-24.

Beecher H.K. "Ethics and Clinical Research." *The New England Journal of Medicine* 1966;274:1354-1360.

Beresford E.B. "Uncertainty and the Shaping of Medical Decisions." *Hastings Center Report* 1991;21:6-11.

Bernard C. *An Introduction to the Study of Experimental Medicine.* Originally published in French in 1865, and translated by H.C. Greene. New York: Henry Schuman, 1949.

Burnum J.F. "Medical Practice à la Mode: How Medical Fashions Determine Medical Care." *The New England Journal of Medicine* 1987;317:1220-1222.

Canadian Council on Animal Care *Guide to the Care and Use of Experimental Animals.* Ottawa: The Council. Vol. I, 1980; Vol. II, 1984.

Caplan A.L. "Is There a Duty to Serve as a Subject in Biomedical Research?" *IRB: A Review of Human Subjects Research* 1984;6:1-5.

Christakis N.A. "Should IRB's Monitor Research More Strictly?" *IRB: A Review of Human Subjects Research* 1988;10/2:8-10.

CIOMS *International Guiding Principles for Biomedical Research Involving Animals.* Geneva: Council for International Organizations of Medical Sciences, 1985.

Dickens B.M. "The Modern Law on Informed Consent." *Modern Medicine of Canada* 1982;37:706-710.

Feinstein A.R. "The Intellectual Crisis in Clinical Science: Medaled Models and Muddled Mettle." *Perspectives in Biology and Medicine* 1987;30:223.

Feinstein A.R. "Clinical Biostatistics: XXVI. Medical Ethics and the Architecture of Clinical Research." *Clinical Pharmacology and Therapeutics* 1974;15:316-334.

Feinstein A.R. *Clinical Epidemiology. The Architecture of Clinical Research.* Toronto: W.B. Saunders Company, 1985.

Freedman B. and **Glass K.C.** "Weiss v. Solomon: A Study in Institutional Responsibility for Clinical Research." *Law, Medicine & Health Care* 1990;18:395-403.

Freedman B. "Equipoise and the Ethics of Clinical Research." *The New England Journal of Medicine* 1987;317:141-145.

Gerber P. and **Coppelson M.** "Clinical Research after Auckland." *The Medical Journal of Australia* 1989;150:230-233.

Gilbert J.P., McPeek B. and **Mollester F.** "Statistics and Ethics in Surgery and Anesthesia." *Science* 1977;198:684-689.

Halushka v. The University of Saskatchewan et al. (1965), 53 Dominion Law Reports (2d) 444.

Hiatt H.H. "Protecting the Medical Commons: Who is Responsible?" *The New England Journal of Medicine* 1975;293:236-237.

Katz J., ed. *Experimentation with Human Beings.* New York: Russell Sage Foundation, 1972.

Lane-Petter W. "The Place and Importance of the Experimental Animal in Research." *Proceedings of the Royal Society of Medicine* 1972;65:343-344.

Levine R.J. "Clarifying the Concepts of Research Ethics." *Hastings Center Report* 1979;9:21-26.

Levine R.J. *Ethics and Regulation of Clinical Research.* Baltimore-Munich: Urban & Schwarzenberg, 1986.

McIntosh A. "Animal Rights and Medical Research." *Future Health* Winter 1985:10-11.

McIntyre N. and **Popper K.** "The Critical Attitude in Medicine: The Need for a New Ethics." *British Medical Journal* 1983;287:1919-1923.

McKinlay J.B. "From 'Promising Report' to 'Standard Procedure': Seven Stages in the Career of a Medical Innovation." *Milbank Memorial Fund Quarterly* 1981; 59:374-411.

Medical Research Council of Canada *Guidelines on Research Involving Human Subjects.* Ottawa: Medical Research Council, 1987.

Murphy E.A. *The Logic in Medicine.* Baltimore, London: The Johns Hopkins University Press, 1976, 239-262.

National Council on Bioethics in Human Research Consent Panel Task Force *Report on Research Involving Children.* Ottawa: NCBHR Consent Panel Task Force, 1992.

Nicholson R.H. "Medical Research Council Multi-Centre Trial of Orchiectomy in Carcinoma of the Prostate." *IRB: A Review of Human Subjects Research* 1986;815:1-5.

Pickering G.W. "The Place of the Experimental Method in Medicine." *Proceedings of the Royal Society of Medicine* 1949;42:229-234.

Robertson J.A. "Taking Consent Seriously: IRB Intervention in the Consent Process." *IRB: A Review of Human Subjects Research* 1982;4:1-5.

Rolleston F. and **Miller J.R.** "Therapy or Research: A Need for Precision." *IRB: A Review of Human Subjects Research* 1981;3/7:1-3.

Rowan A.N. and **Rollin B.E.** "Animal Research - For and Against: A Philosophical, Social and Historical Perspective." *Perspectives in Biology and Medicine* 1983;27:1-17.

Rutstein D. "The Ethical Design of Human Experiments." In: P.A. Freund, ed. *Experimentation with Human Subjects.* New York: George Braziller, 1970, 383-401.

Sackett D.L. "Bias in Analytic Research." *Journal of Chronic Diseases* 1979;32:51-63.

Sackett D.L. "The Competing Objectives of Randomized Trials." *The New England Journal of Medicine* 1980;303:1059-1060.

Sackett D.L., **Haynes R.B.** and **Tugwell P.** *Clinical Epidemiology: A Basic Science for Clinical Medicine.* Boston: Little Brown, 1985.

Silverman W.A. *Human Experimentation: A Guided Step into the Unknown.* Oxford, New York, Tokyo: Oxford University Press, 1985.

Veressayev V. *The Memoirs of a Physician.* Translated from the Russian by S. Linden. New York: Knopf, 1916, 332-366. Quoted from J. Katz, ed. *Experimentation with Human Beings.* New York: Russell Sage Foundation, 1972, 291.

World Medical Association *Declaration of Helsinki. Recommendations Guiding Medical Doctors in Biomedical Research Involving Human Subjects.* Adopted by the 18th World Medical Assembly, Helsinki, Finland, 1964, and revised by the 29th World Medical Assembly, Tokyo, Japan, 1975.

14

WHEN RESOURCES ARE LIMITED: THE ETHICS OF ALLOCATION

In Chapter 4, we described the future of the Canadian health care system as uncertain, if not perilous. The main reason for this uncertainty is financial in nature — the already large and rapidly growing gap between society's demand for health services and its ability or willingness to pay for them. In this chapter, we will explain in some detail the extent of this problem, the ethical issues that it raises, and the alternative solutions from which Canadians will have to choose, in dealing with these issues.

Our discussion of this topic will reflect, in a very direct manner, the Canadian context of health care. For example, in the United States a major topic in the bioethical literature dealing with the allocation of health care resources is the "right" to health care — whether there is such a right, how extensive is it, and who should satisfy it. In Canada, this is not an issue; we may not call it a right, but we all know that health care is available to all who require it. We can, therefore, skip over this matter, and go on to discuss how scarce resources should be distributed to those in need.

Although the allocation of health care resources is a concern of bioethics in each of its three fields — clinical, research and public ethics — it is within public ethics that the major discussion of this topic occurs. In this chapter, we will refer only in passing to research and clinical ethics. Our principal focus will be the allocation issues facing the various decision-makers in the health care system: government, institutions, health care professionals and patients.

THE PROBLEM

The health care system that Canadians have possessed since the 1960s is regarded by many as the best in the world. Access to the system is guaranteed, through a national health insurance programme that is supposed to provide all needed services to every citizen, regardless of their financial circumstances. The system has been very satisfactory in most respects but, in recent years, Canadians have begun to experience serious difficulties in obtaining medical services. Consider the following examples:

- Ambulance drivers often have to try several hospitals, before they find one that can provide emergency care to their patients.
- Delays of up to one year are not uncommon for certain heart operations; some patients die before their turn comes.
- In some communities, it takes many months before one can have an appointment with a local medical specialist.
- Doctors, nurses, and other health care professionals have seen their incomes frozen in recent provincial budgets; this has caused much anger and loss of morale.

These are only a few examples of the large and increasing gap between the demand for, and the supply of, health care resources in Canada. This gap, which will be described in greater detail below, has led many people to speak of the need to *ration* the resources that are currently available, since there is simply not enough to satisfy everybody's requirements or desires. *Rationing*, however, is originally a war-time concept. It referred to the daily portion of supplies issued to each soldier; later, to the basic allowance of commodities citizens could obtain, by use of ration books of coupons. Use of the concept *rationing* has been quite convincingly criticized as incorrect for the process of distributing limited health care resources, the focus of this chapter (Office of Health Economics, 1979). So, we use the term *allocation* rather than *rationing*, and point out straightway that allocation of scarce health care resources raises important ethical issues, especially the role of justice or equity in determining who should benefit from the resources, when not everybody can. These decisions are often *tragic*, in that they result in pain and suffering, and even death, for some patients. Allocation issues pose challenges to everyone involved in the health care system — doctors, nurses, hospital administrators, politicians and other public health officials, and ordinary citizens. In this chapter, we will examine how each of these groups is required to cope with the inevitable shortage of resources in health care.

These resource shortages are bound to get worse in the years to come. The reasons for this are many:

- People are living longer than ever before. At first glance, this would seem to be a result of better health, which should reduce the demand for health services. However, as we saw in Chapter 12, elderly persons consume far more medical care than do others. As the numbers of senior citizens continue to increase, so, too, will the overall costs of their health care.

- Medical science and technology is continually producing new diagnostic tests, vaccines, and treatments for diseases. The equipment and materials for these services are almost always more expensive than those that are being replaced (McGregor, 1989).

- Just when some diseases, such as smallpox, have been eradicated, others come along to take their place. AIDS, for example, is proving to be an enormous drain on the health care budgets of research-funding agencies, public health services, and many hospitals. The rates of certain cancers, especially skin cancer, have risen dramatically in recent years, as a result of environmental and lifestyle changes.

- Another important factor in the rise of health costs, up to now, and one that may well continue in the future, is the fear of malpractice suits by physicians, and the resultant use of all available tests, no matter what the cost, to ensure that their diagnoses are as accurate as possible.

Throughout the 1960s and 1970s, large increases in Canada's national and provincial health budgets were absorbed without much difficulty, thanks to generally good economic conditions. From the 1980s on, however, governments have introduced harsh restraint measures, in order to limit budget deficits. Since health care is one of the largest budget categories, it has been a particular target of cost-cutting initiatives. Even with these cutbacks, though, health costs have continued to rise at a rate greater than inflation. As we saw in Chapter 4, the percentage of the Canadian gross domestic product spent on health care rose from 7.4% to 8.7% between 1980 and 1989. The increase would have been much greater, if all the needs of patients and health care providers had been satisfied.

ECONOMICS AND BIOETHICS

Throughout this book we have seen how bioethics must be interdisciplinary, if it is to answer the questions: what must we do, what should we permit, what can we tolerate, and what must we prohibit, among all the new things that biomedical science and technology now enable us to do with human beings, and other forms of life on this planet. One of the key disciplines with which bioethics as public ethics interacts, when dealing with the allocation of health care resources, is economics. The terms of this relationship are a matter of dispute. Ethics and economics are often considered to be opposing forces, rather than complementary. Which view is correct?

To answer this question, we have to know that economics is viewed, by some of its practitioners, as strictly an *instrumental* discipline, i.e., a means for achieving a predetermined end, and by others as both an instrumental and a *normative* discipline, one that determines the ends. As an instrument of a public policy, such as the Canadian health care system, economics can help government officials determine how the principles of this system can be achieved within a fixed budget. As a normative discipline, however, economics evaluates the policy itself, as well as suggesting ways to implement it. A very powerful school of current economic thought holds that the free-market system of allocating resources is the only rational and efficient system there is. According to this school, national health insurance should be abolished, in favour of a free market in health services.

Ethics and economics interrelate at both the normative and instrumental levels. At each level, there is potential for conflict as well as for complementarity, not between the disciplines as such, but between different schools within each discipline. For example, at the normative level, the free-market economists have much in common with certain ethicists who give priority to individual autonomy. An example of their agreement on a particular bioethical issue will be found in the following chapter, in the section on the sale of organs for transplantation. Conversely, this school of economics is strongly opposed by other ethicists, some of whom feel that economics is not a normative discipline at all, and that free-market economists are simply pseudo-ethicists in disguise.

At the instrumental level, there is potential for conflict between ethics and economics, because each invokes different criteria for allocating health resources. The criteria of ethics, namely justice, equality, and equity, will be discussed in the next section of this chapter. Economic criteria include efficiency, cost-effectiveness, and cost-containment. Although these two sets of criteria are not necessarily opposed in principle, in practice there is often need to choose between them. We will deal with this potential conflict in the sections of this chapter on allocation by governments, institutions, and health care professionals.

JUSTICE, EQUALITY, EQUITY

Health care resources can be distributed (allocated) in any number of ways. In this chapter, we want to know how they are actually distributed in Canada at the present time and, more importantly, how they *should* be distributed. The latter question is likely to receive different answers, depending on the background of the respondent. A legal expert will say that, at the very least, distribution must be in accordance with the law (for example, the anti-discrimination sections of the *Canadian Charter of Rights and Freedoms* and of provincial human rights codes). Economists, as we have just seen, will invoke such criteria as efficiency and cost-effectiveness, for determining how resources should be allocated. The political scientist will tell us that the relative strength of political pressure groups, such as business and consumer associations, doctors, nurses, other health care workers and patient organizations, is the principal factor in the distribution of health care resources. Finally, ethicists invoke the concepts of justice, equality, and equity as criteria that should be used in allocation decisions.

Although these three concepts are related, they are not identical. Justice, like law, is an extremely rich term; at its most basic level, it is equivalent to fairness, but it also signifies the entire system of defining and enforcing fairness in a society ("the justice system"). One frequently cited maxim of justice is "equal cases should be treated equally." In modern, democratic societies, the equality of all citizens is a fundamental principle. However, when putting this principle into practice, major problems arise. In the health care setting, it is obvious that all patients are not equal; indeed, every case is different. If health care resources were to be distributed equally among all citizens, some would receive far more than they need, and others far less. For this reason, the concept of *equity* is considered to be more appropriate than equality, in the application of justice to health care. An equitable distribution of resources is geared to the differing needs of individuals and groups within society. In what follows, we will focus on the concept of justice, while realizing that equity is a key factor in the just distribution of health care resources (Daniels 1985).

In recent years, there has been an explosion of interest in justice. In the academic world, theologians, philosophers, social scientists, and jurists have produced an already large, and rapidly growing, body of literature on this topic. At the same time, numerous human rights organizations, both governmental and independent, have been formed to seek greater justice for disadvantaged individuals and groups — racial minorities, women, elderly persons, prisoners, refugees, the unborn, animals, the environment, and so on.

Although justice is almost universally recognized as a basic social value, there is widespread disagreement about its meaning. Even if we restrict our analysis to *distributive* justice, which is concerned with the fair distribution of rights and privileges (including access to health care resources), we encounter a bewildering variety of theories of justice, each of which comes to very different conclusions about how resources should be distributed (Sterba, 1986).

Some of the most important philosophical theories of distributive justice are the following:

- *utilitarianism*: distribute resources according to the principle of maximum benefit (utility) for all citizens. This is the approach used most often by governments in a pluralistic society, as will be shown below.

- *libertarianism*: distribute according to what individuals freely choose to do with their property (i.e., resources should be bought and sold on the free market). This approach is favoured by proponents of extreme free-enterprise capitalism, who want to reduce to a minimum the role of government in the affairs of individual citizens, including health care.

- *socialism*: distribute to each according to their need; receive from each according to their ability to contribute. Attractive in theory, this approach has been difficult to apply in practice.

- *merit standard:* distribute to each according to what they deserve. This approach is used fairly widely in our society (e.g., in education and business), but is difficult to apply in the field of health care.

Although there are proponents of all these theories of justice in Canada, utilitarianism has, until recently, been dominant. The extreme libertarian view, which considers that any government restraint of individual freedoms is suspect, has never been very popular here. Unlike the United States, where universal medical insurance and equal access to medical services are widely regarded as unfair constraints on the freedom of patients to buy whatever services they can afford, and of doctors to charge whatever patients are willing to pay, Canadians are quite willing to accept restrictions on these freedoms, in return for equity of access. In the words of Robert Evans, a leading Canadian health economist:

> ... the Canadian health care system reflects a strong commitment to egalitarianism combined with a strong respect for, and substantial confidence in, duly constituted authority. This authority includes both the politically legitimate authority of the state and the professionally legitimate authority of the providers of care. These attitudes stand in sharp contrast to those lying behind the American approach, where the health care funding system, like many other institutions, responds to a combination of individualism and suspicion of authority. (Evans, 1988, 171f.)

Many commentaries on the Canadian character have endorsed this view, especially its contrast between American individualism and Canadian communitarianism (Kilbourn, 1988, 22). This combination of egalitarianism and communitarianism is manifest in Canadians' acceptance of less-than-optimal medical services, particularly the latest technological developments, in order that a basic level of care can be provided to all in need.

Despite the incompatibility of the libertarian view of justice with the Canadian ethos, and especially with our system of national health insurance, there are strong forces at work to introduce it here, led by certain business groups and conservative political forces. Proponents of this approach consider health care to be a commodity like food or housing, and they see nothing wrong with making its provision more businesslike, both for providers (including greater recourse to the profit motive) and for consumers (allowing them to purchase whatever services they want and can afford). For many, if not most, Canadians, the commercialization of health care is wrong, because it will inevitably result in inferior medical treatment for the poor.

Utilitarianism seeks to maximize the welfare of the majority, without unduly restricting the rights of minorities. It appeals to politicians, civil servants, and administrators, because it saves them the trouble of deciding which moral principles should prevail when two or more are in conflict. The abortion issue, for example, is solved, not by evaluating the rights of fetuses and of pregnant women, but by providing a procedure for making decisions to fund abortion services on the basis of a vague concept of health. Allocation decisions, at least at the government level, generally represent a compromise among the demands of all interested parties. The respective merits of these claims to the resources are not a decisive consideration.

Although utilitarianism may be the most preferable theory of distributive justice for governments, it is not necessarily so for other decision-makers in the health care system: institutional authorities, professionals, and patients. In what follows, we will examine the allocation issues that face each of these groups and will indicate the role that justice plays in the resolution of these issues.

ALLOCATION BY GOVERNMENTS

Health care is one of the largest categories of government expenditure, in developed countries such as Canada. Since the delivery of health care is a provincial responsibility here, most government allocation decisions are made by provincial politicians and civil servants. At present, health care is the largest budget category in most provinces. For example, in 1992, the Ontario government allocated 32% out its budget to health; other social services received 21%, and education 17%.

In drawing up these budgets, politicians and civil servants are faced with several ethical questions. First of all, is the current proportion assigned to health care, as opposed to all other categories, adequate and fair? Second, how should the health care budget be apportioned according to: remuneration for physicians, nurses, and other health care workers; operating and capital expenses of hospitals, clinics, rehabilitation and chronic care facilities, and other institutions; drugs; research; new equipment and services; and so on? Third, which of these expenses are to be met from public funds, and which are to be charged to individual patients? Fourth, how much consultation with interested parties, for example health care professionals, patient organizations, and taxpayers, should take place before making these allocation decisions? The way in which these issues are dealt with by public officials tells us a great deal about the concept of justice that is operative in Canadian society.

Justice in Government Allocation Decisions

Most politicians and civil servants would claim, if asked, that when making decisions about the allocation of health care resources, they generally follow the utilitarian principle of justice — act so as to maximize the overall welfare of society. They attempt to give health care as much of the general budget as possible, without depriving society of its other basic needs (education, social services, transportation, police, fire fighting, defence, etc.). They claim that the present distribution of the health care budget is basically fair. If the income of physicians is much greater than that of nurses and other health care professionals, this is necessary to prevent physicians from seeking employment elsewhere, thereby depriving society of their essential services. If far more research funds are being directed to AIDS than to mental health, it is because AIDS is a fatal disease and easily transmissible. National health insurance itself is a good example of utilitarian justice, insofar as it provides everybody with the same level of health care, no matter what their income.

When the Canadian health care system is examined more closely, however, it appears that justice does not always direct the decisions of policy makers at the government level. There are important discrepancies between the quality of care available to different groups of patients. For example, those in need of acute care generally have access to very high quality services, although there are often long waiting lines for elective procedures. Those requiring chronic care, however, especially psychiatric patients, usually receive a bare minimum of professional attention (Sutherland, 1988, 186). Furthermore, despite equal access to the system, there is a great disparity between the health status of wealthy Canadians and that of the poor. Much of this difference can be attributed to the fact of poverty itself, which gives rise to nutritional problems, stress due to unemployment, and many other factors that impinge on one's health (Sutherland, 1988, 30-33). Moreover, national health insurance in Canada does not pay for all health expenses; drugs, both prescription and non-prescription, dental care, eyeglasses, and nursing home accommodation have to be paid from supplementary insurance plans, or from one's own pocket. All this is to say that the allocation of health resources cannot be limited to the health care budgets of the federal and provincial governments, but must take into account social services, labour, and employment sectors.

Since poverty is one of the principal factors in illness, programmes to reduce poverty, such as a full employment strategy, low-cost housing, and child support, along with remedial measures such as shelters for abused women and children, can contribute more than any medical measures to the health of Canadians. Other elements of "healthy public policy" include higher occupational health and safety standards and programmes to protect and improve the environment. Such preventive programmes would probably reduce the overall cost of health care in the long run, but to get them started, they will require additional funds. These could be taken either from other areas of the national and provincial budgets, such as defence or, if necessary, from components of the health care budget that benefit relatively few people, often those who can look after themselves (Childress, 1981).

The first task for governments, when allocating health care resources, is to avoid waste. Many medical services that were once commonplace have been shown to be either useless or actually harmful. Even now, an estimated 80% of medical treatments, including surgical procedures, have never been scientifically evaluated to determine whether they are effective (Rachlis, 1989, 10). A major task for governments is to sponsor evaluation research, in order to (a) identify useless, harmful, and inappropriate treatments, (b) determine the effectiveness of treatments, and (c) define appropriate indications for each effective treatment. One of the best ways to obtain this information is through controlled clinical trials, as discussed in Chapter 13. The information from these trials enables governments to distinguish (1) treatments that are highly beneficial from (2) those that provide only marginal improvements in patients and (3) treatments that provide no improvement at all. (Recall the discussion of contrast media in Chapters 3 and 4, for an indication of the problems in determining the cost-effectiveness of treatments.) Depending on cost considerations, governments can then provide funding for the first category of treatments, and perhaps some in the second category. All those in the third category would be deinsured.

Setting Priorities

Even if all waste were to be eliminated from the health care system, there would still be a large gap between demand and supply. Most medical services offer at least some benefit to those patients who receive them, and there are long lineups for some services in short supply. Government officials must, therefore, decide which ones are to be made available, and in what quality and quantity, knowing full well that these decisions are tragic: they will result in pain and suffering, and even death, for some patients; results that different decisions might prevent. Governments need to define and implement health care priorities based on justice.

One suggestion for such a set of priorities has been put forth by the American bioethicist, Daniel Callahan:

The primary goal of the health care system should be to provide those general measures of public health and basic medical care most likely to benefit the common health of the population as a whole, and to ensure that every person in the society receives care, comfort, and support in the face of illness, aging, decline, and death.

The secondary goal of the system should be — within the limits of a reasonable level of health care expenditures in relationship to other societal needs — to pursue a basic understanding of the causes of illness and death, and to aspire to the cure of those illnesses that bring premature death and thwart common human aspirations.

The emphasis of the primary goal falls upon societal health needs and the common individual need for caring in the face of sickness. The emphasis of the secondary goal falls on the pursuit of the cure of those forms of illness most likely to express individual differences and to thwart individual need. (Callahan, 1990, 187-188)

If Callahan's priorities were to be adopted, then health care practice and research would be directed away from extending life for terminally ill patients, and even healthy elderly persons, in favour of preventive health care, basic medical services, and palliative care. Some of his proposals, especially those concerning the elderly (see Chapter 12), have generated considerable controversy (Barry, 1991), but he has performed a very useful service in demonstrating one way of setting ethical priorities for allocating health care resources.

Democratic Decision-Making

It is a basic principle of democracy that all citizens should have an opportunity to participate in the establishment of public policies. The most common method of this participation is through the election of representatives, who will incorporate the preferences of their constituents into the government decision-making process. Since there are many competing interests within a pluralist society such as Canada, the role of the politician, and especially the cabinet, is to serve as a broker among interest groups, in order to produce policies that will satisfy the most powerful among them, while not completely alienating the others.

Until recently, most government health-care funding decisions were made with little input from ordinary citizens. As long as the economy was expanding, all sectors of the health care system were able to benefit from increased resources, and there were relatively few complaints about where the funds were going. With the dawn of rationing in the 1980s, however, came competition among these sectors for the limited available funds. Moreover, most health interest groups, whether professionals such as doctors or nurses, institutions, or patient organizations, demanded input into government funding decisions, in order to ensure that they would not be disadvantaged.

One response of Canadian governments to these demands has been to establish public commissions to make recommendations about the future of health care. These commissions have held public hearings, and invited written briefs from individuals and groups wishing to influence their recommendations. Despite this apparent openness to public participation, however, governments tend to prefer making major decisions in secret and then announcing them as "done deals." This strategy is not always successful. The Québec Bill 120, *Loi sur les services de santé et les services sociaux*, which was based on the recommendations of a Commission of Inquiry into Health and Social Services, met with widespread public opposition when first introduced in December 1990, and the government was forced to make many amendments to the law before it was adopted in August 1991.

One novel approach to public participation in health care decision-making, which has aroused considerable interest in Canada and elsewhere, was instituted in the American state of Oregon in the 1980s. The Oregon Health Decisions programme was established in 1982, to increase public awareness and build consensus on such bioethical issues as (a) what relative priority should be given to curative versus preventive medical services, and (b) how can community values influence a policy of rationing among these services. Widespread consultation on these issues took place, by means of public meetings, telephone polls, and three "Citizens Health Care Parliaments." Participants were asked to state the values that are most important for health care; prevention and quality of life were mentioned most frequently (Nelson, 1992, 108).

In 1989, Oregon adopted the *Basic Health Services Act*, which applies the recommendations of the consultation process to the allocation of public health resources. The purpose of the act was to provide universal access to basic medical care for all currently uninsured Oregon residents, while restricting insured services to what the State can afford to provide. To achieve this goal, the Oregon Health Services Commission divided all medical services into three categories: essential, very important, and valuable to certain individuals, and then ranked those within each category. Each of these services was to be costed, and then a cutoff point within this list was established, which depended on funds allocated to the programme in any one year. All citizens would have access to these services, but those who can afford supplementary insurance coverage, or who can pay their own medical bills, would still be able to obtain additional services.

The Oregon plan has been widely criticized, for singling out poor people for health care rationing. Its defenders argue that most poor people in Oregon would be better off under this plan than before and, in any case, the plan was just the first step towards a system of setting priorities for health services for the vast majority of Oregon's citizens (Dougherty, 1991). The plan did not receive the exemption from legislation it needed from the U.S. president, however, and is currently under revision. The relevance of this proposal for Canada is not in the degree of coverage provided, since health insurance in Canada is universal, but in the explicit list of services that were, and were not, to be available, and in the public consultation process that was used to develop this list. Some such process may well appeal to Canadians as preferable to the present decision-making system, in which ordinary citizens have very little input into health care policies.

ALLOCATION BY HEALTH CARE INSTITUTIONS

Once governments determine how much money is to be allocated to health care, it is up to health care institutions to decide how their share of the funds is to be spent. In Canada, most hospitals receive a global (generally unrestricted) operating budget from the provincial government each year, and have a considerable amount of discretion in determining how they spend these funds. Hospital authorities are therefore faced with many allocation decisions, such as what services to provide, which categories of patients to treat, and what equipment and drugs to purchase.

The utilitarian concept of justice usually operates at the institutional level as well, although, unlike governments, health care institutions usually have clearly established limits to their responsibilities for patients. Each institution serves a particular constituency, which is defined either geographically or by patient type (children, cancer patients, etc.). Institutions are not required to care for patients outside that constituency, because the government has established a system of primary (clinics and local general hospitals), secondary (regional general hospitals), and tertiary (specialized hospitals and institutes) institutions, in which citizens can receive appropriate medical care, according to where they live and what disease they have.

When institutions, because of limited funds, cannot meet the needs of all their patients, for example CAT scans and other high-tech diagnostic tests, heart surgery, or organ transplantation, most attempt to ensure that all needy patients will have equal access to the services, through a fair system of rationing distribution (usually a waiting line). Such a procedure reflects the utilitarian concept of justice, since it serves the interests of the majority of patients rather than giving special consideration to a minority (as would the merit approach, for example).

However, as at the government level, there are exceptions to utilitarianism in the allocation of institutional health care resources. In many hospitals, decisions about which services to provide (e.g., transplantation versus palliative care) are often made on the basis of their fund-raising potential or the hospital's reputation, rather than an overall assessment of patient need. Likewise, certain groups of patients (e.g., the chronically ill elderly) may receive a minimum of nursing and rehabilitative care, in comparison to patients who can be restored to good health, such as many cardiac patients.

At present, those who require acute treatment usually receive very good care in our hospitals. However, those with chronic diseases, especially psychiatric ones, fare much less well, and these diseases affect the poor much more than others. This is not just an institutional allocation problem, since government health ministries are generally responsible for targeting certain diseases as deserving special financial resources. However, individual institutions, especially those that receive a global budget from the government, have a considerable amount of discretion in the funding of programmes and services.

There is, of course, a strong ethical argument in favour of meeting the life-and-death needs of a few before the chronic needs of the many. However, it would hardly be fair to neglect the latter, simply because their situation is not as well publicized and/or politicized as is that of, for example, children needing organ transplants. Institutions have an obligation to resist pressures to provide some groups of patients with inadequate treatment, just because their diseases are not as "interesting" to the staff, to the community, or to potential benefactors of the hospital.

ALLOCATION BY HEALTH CARE PROFESSIONALS

Some of the most acute ethical dilemmas in resource allocation occur within the relationship between health care professionals, especially physicians, and individual patients. Physicians are responsible for initiating an estimated 80% of health care consumption, through tests, prescription of drugs, referral to other physicians, and hospitalization, and they have considerable discretion to decide whether or not their patients should have access to these resources.

A type of allocation decision that many physicians must make is the choice between two or more patients who are in need of the same scarce resource, for example emergency staff attention, the one remaining intensive care unit bed, organs for transplantation, radiological tests, and certain very expensive drugs. Physicians who exercise control over these resources must decide which patients will have access to them and which will not, knowing full well that those who are denied may suffer, and even die, as a result.

Some physicians face an additional conflict in allocating resources, in that they play a role in formulating general policies that affect their own patients, among others. This conflict occurs in hospitals and other institutions where physicians hold administrative positions, or serve on committees where policies are recommended or determined. Although many physicians attempt to detach themselves from their preoccupation with their own patients, in order to consider the general welfare of all patients or of the institution, others may try to advance the cause of their patients regardless of the needs of others. For example, in order to ensure that a particular patient receives a transplant, where access to organs is based on medical need, a physician may declare that the patient's medical condition is critical, when it may be no worse than that of any other patient.

The principal resource that nurses are called upon to ration is their own time. Budget cutbacks for nursing services have resulted in a significant reduction in the amount of nursing care available to all but the most acutely ill patients. Nurses often have to decide which call to answer, when two or more patients are requesting assistance at the same time.

At the professional level, the utilitarian concept of justice is a matter of considerable dispute. There is fundamental disagreement among Canadian physicians, with regard to their role in implementing a just distribution of health care resources. Some feel that their primary, if not exclusive, responsibility is to their own patients, and they neither can nor should take into account the needs of others, when deciding how to treat their patients. Other physicians reject this view, and attempt to ensure a just distribution of resources among all needy patients, not just their own. They prefer one of two alternatives: (a) a cooperative arrangement among physicians, to determine which patients are most needy and will, therefore, have first call on the scarce resources; or (b) a fair set of regulations, established by the hospital administration or government, which individual physicians will not be able to circumvent (Williams, 1991).

When physicians have to decide which of two or more patients should have access to a single resource that they both need, such as the one remaining bed in the intensive care unit, they may have recourse to a utilitarian criterion — which recipient will be likely to benefit society more, if restored to good health (for example, a young mother or an elderly widower). In the early days of kidney dialysis, when the number of machines was limited and the alternative to treatment was death, such "social worth" criteria were used. However, they were widely criticized as unfair, and are generally discredited (Fox, 1974). Nowadays, a combination of medical need and first-come first-served is the rule, although some physicians and nurses may still, consciously or unconsciously, discriminate against "unworthy" or "difficult" patients, when allocating scarce resources.

All patients should be treated fairly, in this case by individual health care professionals. Although doctors or nurses have a primary obligation to their own patients, they must not allow their patients to benefit at the expense of others, for example, by jumping waiting lines or by undergoing expensive tests of dubious benefit. Since our health care system exerts very little control over physician-patient interactions, the responsibility for conserving scarce health resources falls to both these parties, but especially to physicians, since they are the ones with direct access to most of the resources.

Just as the poor and otherwise disadvantaged have a special need for the health care resources of society in general, and of health care institutions, so too do individual physicians, nurses, social workers, and other health care professionals have a particular responsibility to these patients. This responsibility can be exercised in two ways: (a) by ensuring that the poor are treated no less well than any other patients; and (b) by working in locations or on diseases that affect the poor more than others. There are many opportunities for such work in psychiatric institutions, inner-city clinics, and northern and native settlements. If the needs of these patients are to be met, it will require the cooperation of individuals at all levels of the health care system, especially the policy makers who designate funds for special programmes for the poor, and the health care practitioners who provide the needed services.

THE PATIENT'S ROLE

The recipients of health care services also have an important role to play in allocation decisions. Unreasonable demands on the health care system (for example, recourse to hospital emergency rooms for routine medical care, consultations with three or more specialists for the same problem, family insistence on aggressive treatment for dying relatives) lead to increasing shortages of resources for patients who are truly in need of them. The Canadian health care system does not strongly discourage such patient-initiated wastage of resources.

Many individuals would agree in theory with the need to conserve scarce health care resources, but they do not want anything less than the best for themselves. As long as this attitude prevails, it will be difficult to achieve a just distribution of resources. Canadians have become used to the idea that their health care system provides unrestricted access to hospitals and physicians, at no cost to themselves. They see no particular responsibility for themselves to conserve these resources, since they are there to be used.

It is clear, however, that unreasonable patient demand is responsible for much overuse of health services. Perhaps an even greater strain on the system results from the so-called lifestyle diseases, especially heart and respiratory conditions due to work-related stress, smoking, excessive alcohol consumption, lack of exercise, or improper diet (Sutherland, 1988, 40-42). It would be unfair to penalize individuals who suffer from these diseases, since some of them have a genetic component, and others result from social deprivation or from addictions that may be beyond the control of the individuals concerned. Nevertheless, we all have a responsibility to prevent the development of these diseases, to the best of our ability. Our reward will, of course, be better personal health, as well as the realization that we are not using resources needed by others.

The inappropriate use of health care resources by patients is not always their preference. Indeed, two Canadian physicians have argued that patients often receive expensive and ultimately futile treatment, which they have not requested, and which they probably do not want. These authors calculate that most such treatments are administered to terminally ill patients who are no longer competent to make their own medical decisions. If these patients were asked in advance whether or not they would want to receive such treatments, many of them would probably say no. By respecting their wishes, huge sums could be saved for application elsewhere in the health system (Singer, 1992). We will return to this topic of advance directives in Chapter 16.

THE INTERNATIONAL DIMENSION

Beyond the government level of allocation decisions discussed above, lies the international horizon. Canadians are part of the global human family, and it can be argued that we have a responsibility to share our health resources with individuals in other countries, especially the poorest. This topic is seldom discussed in the context of bioethics, which tends to limit the application of justice within national boundaries. However, obligations to other people do not stop at national borders, but extend throughout the world. Canadians have long recognized this interrelatedness by funding health-related development projects overseas, and by contributing to the World Health Organization's programmes. However, these actions have generally been considered as charitable (gratuitous) acts, rather than as ones required by justice.

If we focus attention on standards of care, we must ask what the principles of distributive justice demand, when they are directed to the human community across the planet. The right to health care means at least a claim in justice to a fair share, and to a decent standard, of health, medical, and hospital services. Everyone recognizes that this standard cannot be identical in all places, nor identical at all times in the same place. Historical and geographical differences are part of the human condition. Yet, some disparities in the shares people enjoy within local communities, and within nations, are clearly recognizable as so unfair that the inequities are *morally intolerable*.

Clearly, there are terrible international inequities marking the shares of food, hospital care, and medicines that people receive within the global community. But how do we perceive these inequities? How do we judge them? Simply as facts, tragic indeed, but still as facts deriving from presumably unchangeable behavioural laws, based on national interests, that govern the relationships between nations? Are we really capable of perceiving and judging these inequities as *morally* intolerable? As wrongs we must right? Are we capable of seeing these inequities as totally incompatible with the relationships we in the developed world should have to people in developing countries?

The 1980 report of the North-South Commission, chaired by the late W. Brandt, former Chancellor of West Germany, repeatedly stresses its cardinal premise that the survival of humankind is a global challenge, an imperative powerful enough to create a bond of global solidarity (Nord-Sud Kommission, 1980). But we have not yet grown up into a mature consciousness of global community, and we remain wishy-washy, indeed even doubtful, about the extent of our moral imperative to work for the survival of others, and for assuring them standards of sustenance that are essential for human dignity.

Our liberal democratic societies of the developed world, if the late C.B. Macpherson's analysis is correct, harbour an inherent contradiction between two freedoms. *Liberal* "can mean freedom of the stronger to do down the weaker by following market rules; or it can mean equal effective freedom of all to use and develop their capacities. The latter freedom is inconsistent with the former." (Macpherson, 1977, 1) Capitalistic market freedom supersedes, when it does not outrightly contradict, the effective freedom of all for self-development.

Democracy has been judged, in the Macpherson analysis, to be little more than a market mechanism for registering the desires of people as they are, or as they are seen to be by power elites, within the economic market. Democracy has failed to be a transforming principle, advancing people towards what they might be or might wish to be. A dominant ethos perpetuates the image of human beings as consumers, as maximizers of their own satisfactions, and of the benefits and utilities that flow to them from society. Society, in this ethos, is little more than a collection of individuals constantly seeking power and possession over, and at the expense of, each other (Macpherson, 1977, 77-92). If R. Descartes grounded human existence in the power of thought, "Cogito, ergo sum," this prevailing ethos grounds human existence in the power of possession, "Habeo, ergo sum." (Smith, 1989) It is unlikely that international inequities, even terribly tragic inequities, will be seen as *morally* intolerable, when perceptions, judgments, and policies are shaped by an ethos that presents human beings as maximizers of their own consumer interests in a society that requires an equilibrium of inequality. A global ethic will require an epochal change in consciousness, a change that will lead to a preference for community over affluence (Macpherson, 1977, 91). But a new consciousness cannot arise within human beings, only on the force of interpretations and sermons. The consciousness of human global solidarity, with its implication that human beings *do* have a claim on us *just because they are human*, needs to be realized in particular endeavors before it expands to become the ethos and the foundation for a new global ethics.

CONCLUSION

The allocation of health care resources promises to be one of the most important bioethical issues of the 1990s, and beyond. It will affect the provision of care at all levels of the health system, and will pose challenges to all those who work in the system, as well as to all patients. It is most important that allocation decisions not be made according to political or economic considerations alone. As we have seen, they are fundamentally questions of justice and, therefore, ethical issues. This does not mean, however, that they can be solved simply by the application of some preconceived concept of justice. The resolution of allocation issues, at whatever level of the health care system they arise, requires consideration of many different types of information from many different sources. The task of bioethics as public ethics is to arrive at practical solutions to allocation problems, in which justice is honoured to the greatest extent possible.

REFERENCES

Barry R.L. and **Bradley G.V.**, eds. *Set No Limits: A Rebuttal to Daniel Callahan's Proposal to Limit Health Care for the Elderly.* Urbana and Chicago: University of Illinois Press, 1991.

Callahan D. *What Kind of Life: The Limits of Medical Progress.* New York: Simon and Schuster, 1990.

Childress J.F. "Priorities in the Allocation of Health Care Resources." In: E.E. Shelp, ed. *Justice and Health Care.* Dodrecht/Boston: D. Reidel, 1981, 139-150.

Daniels N. *Just Health Care.* Cambridge: Cambridge University Press, 1985, 59-85.

Dougherty C.J. "Setting Health Care Priorities: Oregon's Next Steps." *Hastings Center Report* 1991;21/3:1-10.

Evans R.G. "'We'll Take Care of It for You': Health Care in the Canadian Community." *Daedalus* 1988;117/4:171-172.

Fox R.C. and **Swazey J.P.** *The Courage to Fail: A Social View of Organ Transplants.* Chicago: University of Chicago Press, 1974, 240-279.

Kilbourn W. "The Peaceable Kingdom Still." *Daedalus* 1988;117/4:1-29.

Macpherson C.B. *The Life and Times of Liberal Democracy.* Oxford: Oxford University Press, 1977.

McGregor M. "Technology and the Allocation of Resources." *The New England Journal of Medicine* 1989;320/2:118-120.

Nelson R.M. and **Drought T.** "Justice and the Moral Acceptability of Rationing Medical Care: The Oregon Experiment." *The Journal of Medicine and Philosophy* 1992;17/1:97-117.

Nord-Sud Kommission *Das Überleben Sichern.* Köln: Kiepenheuer, 1980.

Office of Health Economics (London) "Special Report. Scarce Resources in Health Care." *Milbank Memorial Fund Quarterly* 1979;57:265-287.

Rachlis M. and **Kushner C.** *Second Opinion: What's Wrong with Canada's Health Care System and How to Fix It.* Toronto: Collins, 1989.

Singer P.A. and **Lowy F.H.** "Rationing, Patient Preferences, and Cost of Care at the End of Life." *Archives of Internal Medicine* 1992;152:478-480.

Smith C. "The Legacy of U.S. Interests." *The Globe and Mail* (Toronto), March 4, 1989:C-17.

Sterba J.P. "Recent Work on Alternative Conceptions of Justice." *American Philosophical Quarterly* 1986;23:1-22.

Sutherland R.W. and **Fulton M.J.** *Health Care in Canada: A Description and Analysis of Canadian Health Services.* Ottawa: The Health Group, 1988.

Williams J.R. and **Beresford E.B.** "Physicians, Ethics and the Allocation of Health Care Resources." *Annals of the Royal College of Physicians and Surgeons of Canada* 1991;24:305-309.

PART 4

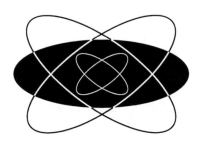

AT THE END
OF LIFE

15

WHEN THE DEATH OF SOME MEANS LIFE FOR OTHERS: RANSPLANTATION ETHICS

INTRODUCTION

Human organ transplantation is one of the great accomplishments of modern medical technology. Many thousands of individuals would now be dead, if they had not been able to exchange their diseased hearts, lungs, or livers for healthy ones from other human beings. Countless others have experienced dramatic improvements in the quality of their lives, thanks to the receipt of a kidney or cornea. Many types of transplantation that once were risky experiments are now routine medical procedures, and greatly preferable to alternative therapies.

There is, however, a down-side to transplantation, which means that this procedure is not always an unmixed blessing. In this chapter, we will examine some of the ethical dilemmas that confront the different participants in transplantation: the recipients, the organ donors, the transplant team of health professionals, and those responsible for public policies in matters of health care. These issues arise in each of the three subdivisions of bioethics: research, clinical, and public. However, the main focus of this chapter will be on the public dimension. Our discussion of these issues will begin with a brief history of transplantation.

HISTORY

The first successful transplant of a human organ took place in 1954, in Boston, U.S.A.. The organ was a kidney; it came from a living donor, and was transplanted to the donor's identical twin. Earlier attempts to transfer kidneys from donors unrelated to the recipients were unsuccessful, because the immune systems of the recipients rejected the organs.

During the 1960s and 1970s, medical researchers were able to develop new drugs to deal with the problem of rejection. The most effective of these drugs is cyclosporin, and together with improved surgical techniques and more experience in caring for transplanted patients, it has contributed greatly to the success rates of this procedure.

The development of anti-rejection drugs made it possible to transplant organs from living donors who were not related to the recipients, as well as organs taken from newly dead persons. The recourse to non-living donors meant that not just paired organs such as kidneys could be transplanted, but also organs such as hearts and livers. Although the first attempts at heart transplantation, in the late 1960s, were usually unsuccessful, largely because the problem of rejection had not been solved, this procedure is now fairly routine, and often results in many years of good health for persons who would otherwise die rapidly.

During the 1980s, rapid advances were made in liver transplantation, and this procedure is now more common in Canada than heart transplantation. Similar progress is occurring with lungs, and serious efforts are underway to increase the success rates of pancreas and kidney/pancreas procedures.

In order to retrieve cadaver (that is, a dead person's) organs for transplantation, two conditions must be fulfilled: (1) the donor must be dead, and (2) the organs must be alive. In practice, this means that the organs have to be removed very soon after death occurs, and therefore it is important to determine, as precisely as possible, the moment of death. Until the 1960s, the usual criteria for determining that a person had died were the permanent cessation of breathing and heartbeat. By the time such a determination could be made, however, the organs of the dead person were often unusable for transplantation. With the development of artificial means of life support, such as respirators and cardiac machines, it became possible to maintain the organs in relatively good condition, even while the patient was dying. However, the use of these machines to sustain the usual signs of life, breathing and heartbeat, meant that the traditional criteria for determining death were no longer adequate. In the late 1960s, the concept of "brain death" emerged, as a new and more adequate criterion for decisions regarding both the cessation of life-support treatment and the removal of organs for transplantation.

BRAIN DEATH

Dying is a complex process. The human body is composed of millions of individual cells, each of which comes into being, and eventually dies, without necessarily affecting the living status of the whole person. Even when the person has been declared dead by conventional standards, many cells continue to live for hours, or even days. There is, therefore, no one "moment of death" for the whole human body. Nevertheless, it is necessary to establish a working definition of death, in order to know when to stop medical treatment, to begin preparations for burial, and to remove organs for transplantation. The Canadian Medical Association has adopted this approach, as has the Law Reform Commission of Canada, in its report to Parliament, *Criteria for the Determination of Death*, and its Working Paper, *Procurement and Transfer of Human Tissues and Organs* (Canadian Medical Association, 1987A; Law Reform Commission, 1981; Law Reform Commission, 1992).

In 1968, a group of physicians at the Harvard Medical School published a set of criteria for determining when a person's brain has become so damaged that it can no longer sustain the principal conditions of human life, breathing and heartbeat. The criteria were derived from observation of hundreds of patients who had no discernible brain activity for a certain length of time, before their death was confirmed by traditional means of respiration and heartbeat. The concept of brain death that this document set forth has become widely accepted as an alternative means of determining death, when breathing and heartbeat are being sustained artificially.

The current medical and legal understanding of brain death in most countries, including Canada, stipulates that all brain functions, including those of the brain stem responsible for spontaneous breathing, must have ceased before death can be certified. Thus, patients who are in a permanent vegetative state and who will most likely never regain consciousness, but whose brain stems still function, are not yet dead. An alternative view of brain death, which is held by some philosophers, considers that the permanent loss of the "higher" functions of the brain, those that control consciousness, is sufficient to declare a patient dead. They argue that human persons are defined by their capacity for reason and judgment, both of which require consciousness. When this has permanently disappeared, what remains is not a human person but a radically different type of being. It may be still alive, but it should not be treated like a living human person (Veatch, 1976).

The acceptance of brain death has greatly facilitated the use of cadaver organs for transplantation. However, the controversy between the two understandings of brain death has obvious implications for the supply of organs. In Canada, and most other countries where transplantation is practised, organs cannot be removed until all the donor's brain functions have ceased. A rigorous set of criteria for determining whether this has occurred has been developed by the Canadian Congress of Neurological Sciences, and adopted by the Canadian Medical Association (Canadian Medical Association, 1987A). Proponents of the less restrictive concept of brain death argue that the supply of organs could be significantly increased if their concept were to be adopted, since there are thousands of potential donors who are dead by their criteria, but not by those of the CMA. As yet, their arguments have not been accepted by those in charge of transplantation.

CURRENT STATUS OF TRANSPLANTATION

In Canada, organ transplantation is a widely practised medical procedure, fully funded by provincial health insurance plans. In Table 15-1, you will find some recent statistics on the number of transplant procedures conducted in this country, in the year ending December 31, 1991, along with the numbers of patients on the waiting list for each organ, at the end of that year.

TABLE 15-1

	Organ Transplants	Waiting list at end of year
kidney (adult)	785	1557
kidney (child)	39	49
heart	144	78
liver (adult)	136*	51
liver (child)	38*	13
single lung	27	27
double lung	31	25
heart/lung	10	4
pancreas	1	1
kidney/pancreas	5	1

* age of recipient unknown in 47 cases of liver transplantation

Source: Canadian Organ Replacement Register

It is clear from these figures that the average waiting time for a transplant can be more than one year. Many of those in need of new organs do not survive that long. The waiting lists would be even longer except that some physicians do not enter patients on the list, because the chances of obtaining a suitable organ in time are too remote. Moreover, as new techniques are introduced that improve the success rates of certain types of transplantation, there is a rush to get on the list, and soon the demand far exceeds the supply of organs, or the capacity of transplant centres to perform the operation.

The shortage of replacement organs is the major reason for the gap between demand and supply in transplantation. Despite considerable efforts at public education, acquisition of organs seems to have levelled off in Canada, and in less than one third of deaths where organs could be retrieved for transplantation is this actually done. Increasing the supply is one of the greatest challenges faced by those involved in transplantation today.

OBTAINING ORGANS

Numerous proposals have been made for increasing the supply of organs for transplantation. These include:

- greater use of living donors;
- payment for organs;
- increased efforts to obtain consent for the removal of organs.

Each of these presents particular ethical difficulties, which will be analysed and evaluated in what follows. Where appropriate, reference will be made to the World Health Organization (WHO) *Guiding Principles on Human Organ Transplantation*, which were adopted by the World Health Assembly, the governing body of the WHO, on May 13, 1991 (Dickens, 1991), and to the Law Reform Commission of Canada Working Paper, *Procurement and Transfer of Human Tissues and Organs* (1992).

Living Donors

The use of organs from living donors is ethically problematic, since such procedures involve physical risks to the donors, with benefits for them that, at most, are psychological and emotional. However, in some countries, living donors have long been the major source of kidneys for transplantation. Even in Canada, where there is a strong preference for cadaveric organs, some 122 of the 785 adult kidneys and 9 of the 39 child kidneys transplanted in 1991 were from living donors. In 1989, the first transplant of part of a liver from a living donor, in this case the parent of the recipient, was performed in the U.S.A.. This operation was judged to be medically feasible, because the liver is capable of regenerating itself. The following year, the first living-donor lung transplant was performed, also in the U.S.A.. This procedure involved a lobe of the donor's lung, which, it was hoped, would enable the recipient to survive without seriously impairing the lung activity of the donor.

If there were an adequate supply of cadaveric organs for transplantation, then it would be unethical to use living donors, because of the risks involved.

However, this is not the case at present, and to prohibit organs from living donors would further reduce the already inadequate supply.

The options for using living donors include accepting any willing compatible donor, or imposing conditions on such donations. The principal arguments in favour of the first approach are that it respects the freedom of individuals (in this case, the donors) to control their lives, and allows them the satisfaction of helping desperately ill persons, usually members of their own families. However, this approach can also encourage reckless behaviour, either by the transplant team or the donors.

Since the arguments for a total prohibition of the donation of organs from living individuals are not fully persuasive, it is preferable to establish strict conditions for this practice. These should include the lack of a suitable cadaver organ, the exclusion of donors at greater-than-average risk (either medical or psychosocial), and adequately informed and freely given consent on the part of the donor. Where such consent is impossible to obtain, for example from infants or mentally incompetent persons, they should not be considered as potential donors of nonregenerative organs such as kidneys, although in certain extreme circumstances they may supply tissues such as bone marrow. The Law Reform Commission of Canada recommends that any organ and tissue donation from an incompetent subject be authorized by an independent third party such as a court, review board, or ombudsman (Law Reform Commission, 1992, 174-175). This rule is already set out in section 20 of the Québec *Civil Code* which, in the case of a child, requires both the consent of the person having parental authority over the child and the authorization of a Superior Court judge. The WHO *Guiding Principles* would further restrict living donors to those who are related to the recipients of their organs genetically or, perhaps, by marriage.

Anencephalic Newborns

In recent years, the controversy about the use of living organ donors has focused on the shortage of replacement organs for critically ill newborn babies. The need for such organs has grown rapidly, as transplantation techniques have been improved for this group of patients. However, the gap between the supply of, and the demand for, such organs is no less serious than for adults. Brain death is especially difficult to determine in infants, and the organs are often unusable by the time a definitive declaration of death has been made. To help solve this problem, some transplant specialists and ethicists have suggested that anencephalic infants, those born with a large part of the brain, that controls consciousness, missing, be considered dead at birth, and their organs removed at the first possible opportunity. They argue that these babies will die within one or two weeks in any case, and since they have no capacity for consciousness, they will not be harmed by having their lives terminated prematurely.

This view has engendered strong opposition from many quarters. It is argued that the number of organs that could be retrieved from anencephalics is so small that it is not worth the risks involved in changing the definition of brain death. And, if one class of human beings can be arbitrarily defined as dead, the same can happen to others, such as those in a permanent vegetative state, and severely mentally retarded or mentally ill persons (Canadian Paediatric Society, 1990). On the basis of arguments such as these, the Law Reform Commission of Canada has recommended that the definition of death as "the irreversible cessation of all brain functions," which it proposed in 1981, should not be modified to facilitate organ procurement from anencephalic infants (Law Reform Commission, 1992, 176).

An alternate approach to the use of anencephalic newborns as organ donors has been developed at St. Joseph's Hospital in London, Ontario. As soon as newborns experience difficulty in maintaining spontaneous breathing, they would be put on a respirator. By this means, the organs can be preserved in good condition for transplantation until the infants meet the standard criteria of brain death. This approach presents both practical problems, in determining the moment of death, and ethical problems, such as whether the infant is simply being used for the benefit of others (Dickens, 1988).

Organ Sales

In recent years, there have been many proposals for the remuneration of donors or their families, as an incentive to supply organs for transplantation. The transfer could take place during the lifetime of the donor (for paired organs such as kidneys), or at death.

In Canada, one suggestion for legalizing and promoting the sale of organs has been made by Aidan Vining, a Simon Fraser University business administration professor. Individuals would be offered a direct cash payment, a tax credit, or some other incentive, if they authorized the removal of their organs following death. The price to be paid would depend on the supply and demand at the time of the sale. The federal government would regulate the process, to ensure quality control and a fair allocation of the organs (Anon, 1984).

An alternative proposal has been advanced, in his private capacity, by Gilbert Sharpe, who is legal counsel for the Ontario Ministry of Health. Although he sees many practical difficulties in the implementation of a market system for human organs, he believes that the sale of organs should be permitted in some cases. It should take place within the Canadian medicare system, which would establish rates and make the payments. Only living donors would be included in the plan. For competent sellers of nonregenerative organs, such as kidneys, the following provisions should apply: "Likelihood of significant benefit to the person into whose body the transplant is about to be done, minimal risk of harm to the health of the donor, and the great urgency of the situation, together with a host of other protections — consent of family, independent counsel, review committees, court appeals and so on." (Sharpe, 1985, 31) Even more stringent protection would be provided for non-competent donors.

These proposals for the sale of organs have not generally been well received. George J. Annas claims that, in the United States, "there has been almost universal revulsion at the notion of a market in organs that would inevitably lead to the poor selling their body parts to the rich." (Annas, 1984, 22) On October 2, 1984, the U.S. Congress passed the *Organ Procurement and Transplantation Act*, which banned the buying and selling of human organs. In 1989, the Uniform Law Conference of Canada, which attempts to harmonize the laws of the different provinces and territories, developed a *Uniform Human Tissue Donation Act*, which includes an outright prohibition of buying and selling human organs (Law Reform Commission, 1992, 207). The Law Reform Commission has recommended that such commerce in organs be made a *Criminal Code* offence. The Canadian Medical Association, the Council of the Transplantation Society, and the World Medical Association, among other professional groups, have also condemned such commercial transactions in human organs. The WHO *Guiding Principles* include the following clauses:

- The human body and its parts cannot be the subject of commercial transactions. Accordingly, giving or receiving payment (including any other compensation or reward) for organs should be prohibited.

- Advertising the need for or availability of organs, with a view to offering or seeking payment, should be prohibited.

- It should also be prohibited for physicians and other health professionals to engage in organ transplantation procedures if they have reason to believe that the organs concerned have been the subject of commercial transactions.

- It should be prohibited for any person or facility involved in organ transplantation procedures to receive any payment that exceeds a justifiable fee for the services rendered. (Dickens, 1991)

The controversy about organ sales is fundamentally ethical in nature, in that it involves disagreements about moral values and principles, as well as the more fundamental question of what kind of society is most desirable. The proponents of the market system appeal to individual freedom and autonomy, especially one's right to control and dispose of one's own body, and to the beneficial results of increasing the supply of organs for transplantation. Their opponents contend that individual autonomy can and must be limited in certain circumstances; in this case, the poor need to be protected from the coercive temptation to sell their organs for profit. Some critics of organ sales also emphasize the value of altruism, and its incompatibility with the profit motive. And many abhor the idea of setting a price on human life.

The free-market ideology is radically individualistic and essentially economic — society functions best when each individual is given the maximum freedom to pursue his or her economic self-interest. The chief benefits of this system, in the eyes of its proponents, are the maximization of individual freedom and economic efficiency. In such a system, the sale of organs should be treated the same way as sales of personal services, although some special forms of regulation may be required, to prevent abuse.

Opponents of organ sales are generally dissatisfied with this individualistic approach to political economy. They consider the social nature of human beings to be equal, if not prior, to their individuality. Therefore, individual rights and freedoms must be balanced against social responsibilities and the needs of others. Even if their approach could be shown to be less efficient than the unrestrained free market, its proponents regard this as a small price to pay for a society that values social justice over unfettered individual autonomy. This line of reasoning leads to the rejection of the sale of organs, and to a call for legislation to prevent it. At the same time, it stresses the need for greater efforts to promote the voluntary donation of organs for transplantation.

Informed Consent

One of the major barriers to increasing the supply of donated organs is the difficulty of obtaining the consent of potential donors and/or their next of kin. Although polls have shown that a majority of Canadians are willing to donate their organs when they die, they are less willing to donate those of their deceased family members. In any case, they are often not even asked to do so.

Four different policies have been suggested for obtaining consent for organ retrieval:

- "strong presumed consent," whereby the law would grant physicians complete authority to remove usable organs, regardless of the wishes of the deceased or family members (also known as "routine salvaging");
- "weak presumed consent," whereby organs could be removed, unless the deceased or family members explicitly object (also known as "opting out");
- "strong required request," whereby all citizens would be asked to indicate their willingness to participate in organ donation (also known as "opting in");
- "weak required request," whereby family members would always be asked to approve organ removal from their dying, or newly dead, next of kin (also known as "recorded consideration" or "routine inquiry").

Although the first of these policies is potentially the most effective way of increasing the supply of organs, it is also the most objectionable from the standpoint of ethics. It goes against one of the most fundamental of human rights, the right to control one's own body. At controversy is the extent to which one can exercise this right posthumously.

The policy of "weak presumed consent" has been officially adopted by France and several other European countries. While allowing individuals and family members the freedom either to donate or not to donate organs, it does require those who object to this practice to take the initiative to register their refusal. Some ethicists question whether a failure to take such a step can really be equated with consent. Indeed, doctors in France rarely take advantage of their legal freedom to remove organs without consulting the next of kin, apparently because they believe that such action would be unethical.

There is widespread agreement among ethicists that "strong required request" is the best way to obtain informed and free consent for organ donation. It is directed to the individual who is most affected by the removal of the organ(s), the potential donor, and it provides reliable evidence that this individual has made an informed decision in favour of organ donation. This approach has been adopted in most, if not all, Canadian provinces and territories, where individuals are asked to indicate, on their driver's licences, their willingness to donate their organs at death. The Law Reform Commission of Canada considers this approach to be the preferred model for public policy (Law Reform Commission, 1992, 177). Although this approach is presently thought to be incapable of meeting the demand for organs, it does safeguard control over the disposition of one's body. There are some questions as to whether the supply is inadequate, or only the rate of recovery of organs so donated.

One interesting variation on the "strong required request" approach has been proposed by two Toronto physicians, Irwin Kleinman and Frederick H. Lowy. They suggest that an organ donation registry be established, which would enrol volunteers 18 years of age and above. These individuals would agree to permit all usable organs to be taken for transplantation at the time of their death. In return, they would have priority for receiving organs made available by the programme, should they ever have need of a transplant. The authors contend that this programme would increase the supply of organs, while respecting donor autonomy and satisfying the requirements of justice and altruism (Kleinman, 1989).

Even when individuals have declared their willingness to donate their organs, the removal of these organs is seldom done without the authorization of the next of kin. There are several reasons why such authorization is often not even sought. Many health care professionals feel that grieving relatives should not be burdened with the decision to donate organs. The medical staff are often busy with other seriously ill patients, and are reluctant to continue aggressive treatment of a dead person, when the only ones to benefit from this care will be patients unknown to them. Even when asked, family members may be uncertain whether the deceased would have wanted to donate organs, and may refuse to approve removal on that basis.

Despite these difficulties, several Canadian hospitals have instituted "strong required request" policies. This approach has been endorsed by the Canadian Medical Association, which encourages hospital staff to record in the dying patient's chart that they considered the possibility of organ donation (Canadian Medical Association, 1987B). The Law Reform Commission of Canada also supports this approach (Law Reform Commission, 1992, 178). In order for this policy to be effective, educational programmes for hospital staff are required, which will teach them to approach the next of kin of potential donors in a respectful and noncoercive manner. These programmes should also help the staff come to terms with their own feelings about death, which often prevent them from dealing openly with these matters (Youngner, 1985).

THE EXPERIMENTAL TRANSPLANTATION OF BRAIN CELLS FROM ABORTED HUMAN FETUSES

Up to this point, our discussion of transplantation has focused on human *organs*, such as hearts, kidneys, and livers. It is important to note, however, that other bodily tissues, and even cells, can be transplanted from one individual to another. Bone marrow transplantation is a proven treatment for certain forms of cancer. Some other types of tissue and cell transplantation are still at the experimental stage. One such procedure, which has generated widespread ethical debate, is the use of brain cells from deliberately aborted human fetuses. Spontaneously aborted fetuses are an unreliable source of cells for transplantation because such fetuses are often irretrievable; they often would not contain tissues at a stage of development sufficient for transplantation; or they carry genetic abnormalities that would rule out use of their cells or tissues for transplantation purposes.

After years of animal and human experiments, the accumulation of evidence indicates that transplantation cells from the brains of aborted human fetuses may offer some chance of improving control of Parkinson's disease symptoms, or even of stopping the progression of Parkinson's disease.

The underlying causes of Parkinson's disease are currently unknown, and no effective cure is available. The disease symptoms occur when certain brain cells (neurons) degenerate and fail to produce normal amounts of a neurochemical substance, called dopamine. The symptoms are devastating, and include rigidity of arms and legs, shaking of the extremities, loss of facial expression, and difficulty speaking. The symptoms get progressively worse, as the neurons continue to degenerate and the disease advances. A drug, levodopa, used now for years, helps to stabilize Parkinsonian patients, and controls these symptoms for a while. Eventually, however, the side effects of the drug increase and its efficacy wears off. Patients become very handicapped and cannot carry out life's daily activities (Mardsen, 1990).

Swedish medical scientists published a report, in February 1990, on what appears to be a successful transplantation effort (Lindvall, 1990). They transplanted dopamine neurons from four aborted human fetuses (aged 8 to 9 weeks) into the brain of a 49-year-old man suffering from advanced Parkinson's disease. The patient experienced noticeable relief of symptoms at examination, two months after the operation.

The Swedish scientists drew the following conclusions from this transplantation experiment:

- that human fetal neurons can survive, grow, and restore production and storage of dopamine in the brain of a patient with Parkinson's disease;

- that the transplanted fetal neurons lead to improvement in the symptoms of the Parkinsonian patients;

- that only time will show if the transplanted fetal neurons survive and function permanently;

- that additional research is necessary, to settle important unanswered questions (Lindvall, 1990, 576-577; Mardsen, 1990, 952).

The Human Fetal Tissue Transplantation Research Panel of the National Institute of Health (NIH), in the United States, identified ten key ethical questions raised by transplantation of neurons from aborted human fetuses in the experimental treatment of Parkinsonian patients (The Human Fetal Tissue Transplantation Research Panel, 1988, 1-16). In one fashion or another, nine of the questions touch upon the link between deliberate abortion and the availability of fetal brain cells for these transplantation experiments in the treatment of Parkinson's disease.

Acceptability in Principle

We *first* consider whether *transplantation use of brain cells from aborted human fetuses is acceptable in principle*. Some believe that deliberate abortion is morally acceptable, and see no ethical objection to using neuronal tissue from aborted fetuses for transplantation purposes. A second position is based upon the immorality of abortion, and asserts that the transplantation use of tissue from aborted fetuses necessarily involves complicity in the immoral act of abortion, and may even encourage future abortions. The Research Panel found it *morally possible to separate abortion from the subsequent use of tissues from aborted fetuses*. This moral distinction is based on two considerations: first, that abortion under many circumstances is legally permitted; second, that guidelines can be established to prevent transplantation plans from exercising any influence on the decision for abortion, or on the timing and mode of abortion (The Human Fetal Tissue Transplantation Research Panel, 1988, 1-2).

If transplantation use of neuronal cells from aborted human fetuses is acceptable in principle, as the NIH Research Panel and others argue, such use would be ethically unacceptable if the abortion were performed for the sake of doing the transplantation. So, and this is our *second* consideration, *conditions of ethical acceptability* have to be established.

Conditions for Ethical Acceptability

The following conditions are *ethically necessary*, for the ethical acceptability of using neuronal cells from aborted human fetuses for transplantation purposes:

- Though transplantation of fetal brain cells would be unlikely or impossible without induced abortion, the abortions must not be performed for the purposes of the clinical trial.

- The investigators must take care that the needs of this trial, and the putative needs of Parkinson's patients for human fetal dopaminergic cells, not be adduced to influence in any way a woman's decision to abort her fetus.

- The procedures used for the abortion (mode and timing) should be determined solely on the basis of the woman's needs, and should not be modified to satisfy any requirements of the trial.

- Some Parkinson's patients in the trial may have strong objections, based on their personal moral views or on the moral positions of the church or religion to which they belong. They should be informed about the trial in a way that gives them the freedom to object to the use of fetal tissue in the experimental treatment of their condition, if they so desire.

- Women undergoing induced abortion should not be allowed to specify which Parkinson's patient in the trial will receive the cells of her fetus.

- Money, gifts, or privileges should not be given by anyone to anyone, in connection with the retrieval of human fetal dopaminergic cells for the purposes of this trial.

- Obviously, and lastly, the aborted fetus has to be dead. A fetus born alive, after an abortion attempt, is no longer a fetus. It is a baby, and legally and ethically has to be treated as such.

A debate has arisen around the question of whether consent for the transplantation use of her aborted fetus's neuronal cells should be sought from the woman who is requesting the abortion (Burtchaell, 1988; Freedman, 1988; Robertson, 1988; Burtchaell, 1989).

A Cause for Possible Future Concern

A more difficult ethical question will probably arise, if current trials eventually demonstrate that transplantation of human fetal dopaminergic cells effectively produces major therapeutic benefit for Parkinson's patients; even more so, if similar transplantation of other fetal neuronal cells is demonstrated to offer significant improvement in other neurologically based, high-morbidity and high-mortality diseases, including Alzheimer's disease and Huntington's disease.

The possible forthcoming ethical question may be phrased as follows: if we allow transplantation use of cells, tissues, and organs taken from fetuses aborted for reasons having nothing to do with transplantation, how can we assure that we will not succumb to pressure to abort fetuses precisely for transplantation purposes?

This pressure could become more than fictional or imagined if neuronal transplantation of fetal neuronal cells proves successful, and if demand for fetal neuronal cells exceeds the "normal" abortion supply. A gap between demand and supply often creates a market. Can we effectively resist possible future pressure for acceptance of abortion for transplantation purposes, as well as possible future pressure for commercializing the process? A counterquestion from feminist bioethicists is whether we demean women, even to suppose that a woman would consider abortion to supply or sell fetal tissues.

Do we proceed now with "normal" abortion fetal-cell retrieval for transplantation, and cross the other bridge if we come to it? Or do we block the transplantation use of "normal" abortion fetal cells now, because we fear that we will be unable to halt future acquiescence to a possible societal demand or offer, that fetuses be aborted precisely for transplantation purposes? If fetuses can be aborted for transplantation, may they be conceived in order to be aborted to supply transplantable tissues, as so-called "designer fetuses"?

There is a reasonable, but fragile, answer to this question. Fear that people may, in the future, abort human fetuses precisely for transplantation purposes *should not now* block the experimental use of fetal dopamine-producing cells for transplantation into Parkinson's patients. Aborting fetuses to obtain their organs for others should always remain unethical, and procedures should be strengthened to prevent this from happening. The answer is fragile, however, because it is quite uncertain that we will ever be able effectively to enforce this prohibition, especially in a country where abortion is legally permitted for a wide variety of reasons at just about any time in pregnancy, other perhaps than the weeks immediately preceding birth.

DISTRIBUTING ORGANS

Since the demand for all organs for transplantation far exceeds the supply, transplant units have had to develop methods for determining which patients should have priority. Among the alternative methods are the following:

- random selection, such as by a lottery,
- first-come, first-served,
- severity of medical need,
- probability of success,
- social need or worth,
- some combination of these.

Each of these alternatives can be argued for on ethical grounds. Conversely, each one has certain drawbacks. The lottery and first-come, first-served approaches are scrupulously fair in one sense, but, when applied to all potential recipients, they do not take account of numerous ethically relevant factors, such as the severity of the patient's condition and the chances of success. Medical need is an appropriate criterion for any medical procedure, but it is often difficult to distinguish degrees of need, especially with a condition that is invariably fatal. Social need is even more arbitrary to assess, and is generally rejected by ethicists as a criterion for the selection of organ recipients (Annas, 1985). However, it is not always clear whether an aspect of the patient's condition is social or medical. For example, should a candidate for liver transplantation, whose own liver has been destroyed by alcohol abuse, be rejected if the transplant team is not convinced that he can control his drinking habit? Or should a heavy smoker be excluded from the waiting list for a lung transplant? These questions are subjects of vigorous debate among medical specialists and ethicists at the present time, and so far no consensus has been achieved. Part of the difficulty is in determining whether addiction to alcohol or tobacco is to be regarded as a moral or personal failing, a socially-conditioned behavioural characteristic, or a morally neutral disease or disability that should not attract a discriminatory response.

In Canada, the methods of allocation can vary from one transplant centre to another, but most give priority to urgent medical need. This may provide organs to patients with the worst prospects of survival. Where the need is less immediate, patients are entered on a waiting list and are usually allocated organs as they become available, in accordance with blood and tissue compatibility. It is possible that social need or worth factors influence physicians when they enter patients on the waiting list, but there is no evidence for this.

No matter which of these criteria is employed for selecting organ recipients, there remains the further question of who should be eligible for consideration. Hospitals could decide to perform transplants only for their own patients. Provinces could restrict reimbursement for transplant expenses to their own residents. The Canadian government could implement a quota system for potential recipients from other countries. At present, there is little discussion of these issues, and Canadian transplant centres participate in organ exchange programmes that attempt to ensure equitable distribution throughout the country.

However, as the demand for organs increases, not just in Canada but around the world, this question of eligibility for access to transplantation services will have to be resolved.

ALTERNATIVES TO TRANSPLANTATION

The shortage of organs and the difficulty of allocating them fairly are not the only ethical issues in transplantation. A more fundamental issue is whether the costs of this service are justified, in view of other demands on society's limited health care budgets.

Organ transplantation is a very expensive procedure, and is a popular target for those who wish to reduce expenditures on health care. However, it has been demonstrated that a kidney transplant is considerably less costly than the alternative form of treatment, dialysis, and the same is true for some other types of transplantation. Nonetheless, it must be admitted that patients who undergo transplantation receive an extraordinarily large share of public health care funds. And if the supply of organs does increase, so will the demand for money to provide transplantation services.

There are three different policies that can be adopted for dealing with this problem:

- provide transplantation for all eligible patients for whom organs can be found, no matter what the cost;
- allocate these therapies to some patients, but not to others;
- discontinue these procedures, so that no one with organ failure will be treated at public expense.

Were health care resources unlimited, the first option would obviously be preferable. However, in the present situation, the adoption of this policy would mean that funds would be even more restricted than at present, for all other aspects of health care, especially the less glamorous areas of community and occupational health.

It may well be that, if given the chance to decide, the Canadian public would be willing to accept lower standards of general health care, in order to release funds for expensive life-or-death therapies such as transplantation, which benefit a relatively small number of individuals. On the other hand, they may come to the opposite conclusion. Both decisions would be ethically defensible, and both are in effect in different parts of the world. In Canada, there is no forum for the public examination of such policies and their alternatives. Decisions about the allocation of health care resources are made by physicians, health administrators, and government officials, rather than by the public or legislative assemblies. The present Canadian policy is to provide transplant services for some patients but not for others, according to the pattern described above. This is also a defensible approach, since the health care resources of this country are considerable, but not unlimited. As long as there are other needs not being met, however, the allocation of large sums to transplant services needs to be justified more explicitly than is now the case.

Another alternative to transplantation of human organs is the development and use of artificial and animal organs. Considerable progress has been made on artificial joints, such as the hip, and certain animal tissues are routinely implanted into humans (e.g., heart valves from pigs). However, the use of entire organs from an animal or of artificial organs in humans is quite another matter. Two widely publicized attempts to transplant the hearts of baboons into humans were utter failures, and despite great efforts to develop an artificial heart, all that has been achieved is a device that can keep a person alive temporarily, until a donated organ becomes available. Indeed, it is questionable whether any human organ can be replaced permanently by a manufactured substitute. The heart, for example, is much more than a simple pump; it produces various secretions that play an important role in regulating different bodily functions. In consequence, it may be unethical to allocate large amounts of public funds to the development of artificial and animal replacement organs, when the same funds could be used more profitably for other purposes.

Since transplantation is essentially a curative procedure, any discussion of alternatives must include prevention of the underlying diseases. Although many cases of organ failure are eminently preventable, by refraining from smoking, overeating, and excessive consumption of alcohol, others are genetically determined, or otherwise beyond the control of the persons so affected. The overall need for transplantation, as well as for other health services, could certainly be reduced by preventive measures. However, it is very much a matter of debate at present whether patients with "self-inflicted" diseases should be denied treatment, or whether they have the same right to health care resources as anyone else. In any case, preventive health will never entirely eliminate the need for organ transplantation, and so the ethical problems associated with this procedure will always be with us.

CONCLUSION

In this chapter, we have dealt primarily with the public dimension of bioethics. We have seen that human organ transplantation raises many of the types of conflicts discussed in Chapter 2, especially conflicts on the level of ethos, morality, and ethics. Unlike some of the issues discussed in previous chapters, however, these conflicts have produced very little public controversy in Canada. There have been no court cases, few legislative initiatives, and no public demonstrations involving transplantation. It seems to have been regarded as a private rather than a public matter, to be considered within the confines of the hospital, professional associations, and the physician-patient relationship.

This relative calm is unlikely to persist. The conflicts related to transplantation have the potential to produce serious public discord. If the gap between supply and need increases, as it likely will, if only because of financial restraints, dissatisfied patients and their families may well become more vocal in their demands for expansion of these life-saving services. If the present altruistic system of organ donation does not improve the supply of organs, there may be pressure for a "presumed consent" policy. These public conflicts could spill over into the realm of clinical ethics, as individual patients become more demanding for access to transplantation.

If public authorities are compelled to address these conflicts, the relationship of bioethics and law, as discussed in Chapter 3, will be put to the test. Is legislation needed to resolve these conflicts? If so, what form should it take? What role should be assigned to courts to resolve disputes? We have seen how these questions have been dealt with in relation to abortion and sterilization. We can only hope that lawmakers will review the experience with these issues, before attempting to formulate public policy in relation to transplantation.

REFERENCES

Annas G.J. "Life, Liberty and the Pursuit of Organ Sales." *Hastings Center Report* 1984;14/1:22-23.

Annas G.J. "The Prostitute, the Playboy, and the Poet: Rationing Schemes for Organ Transplantation." *American Journal of Public Health* 1985;75/2:187-189.

Anon. "Future Market in Human Organs Suggested." *The Globe and Mail* (Toronto), September 1, 1984:28.

Burtchaell J.T. "The Use of Aborted Fetal Tissue in Research: A Rebuttal." *IRB: A Review of Human Subjects Research* 1989;11:9-12.

Burtchaell J.T. "University Policy on Experimental Use of Aborted Fetal Tissue." *IRB: A Review of Human Subjects Research* 1988;10:7-12.

Canadian Medical Association "Guidelines for the Diagnosis of Brain Death." *Canadian Medical Association Journal* 1987A;136:200A-B.

Canadian Medical Association "Organ Donation." *Canadian Medical Association Journal* 1987B;136:752A-B.

Canadian Paediatric Society, Bioethics Committee "Transplantation of Organs from Newborns with Anencephaly." *Canadian Medical Association Journal 1990;142/7:715-717.*

Dickens B.M. "The Anencephalic Organ Donor and the Law." *Transplantation/Implantation Today* 1988;5:42-46.

Dickens B.M. "WHO Guiding Principles on Human Organ Transplantation." *Transplantation/Implantation Today* 1991;8:12-18.

Freedman B. "The Ethics of Using Human Fetal Tissue." *IRB: A Review of Human Subjects Research* 1988;10:1-4.

Kleinman I. and **Lowy F.H.** "Cadaveric Organ Donation: Ethical Considerations for a New Approach." *Canadian Medical Association Journal* 1989;141:107-110.

Law Reform Commission of Canada *Procurement and Transfer of Human Tissues and Organs*. Working Paper 66. Ottawa: Ministry of Supply and Services, 1992.

Law Reform Commission of Canada *Report on Criteria for the Determination of Death*. Ottawa: LRCC, 1981.

Lindvall O. et al. "Grafts of Fetal Dopamine Neurons Survive and Improve Motor Function in Parkinson's Disease." *Science* 1990;247:574-577.

Mardsen C.D. "Parkinson's Disease." *Lancet* 1990;335:948-952.

Robertson J.A. "Fetal Tissue Transplant Research Is Ethical." *IRB: A Review of Human Subjects Research* 1988;10:5-8.

Sharpe G. "Commerce in Tissue and Organs." *Health Law in Canada* 1985;6/2:27-31, 44.

The Human Fetal Tissue Transplantation Research Panel *Report*. Vol. I. Washington, DC: The National Institute of Health, 1988.

Veatch R.M. *Death, Dying, and the Biological Revolution*. New Haven: Yale University Press, 1976:21-76.

Youngner S.J. et al. "Psychosocial and Ethical Implications of Organ Retrieval." *The New England Journal of Medicine* 1985;313/5:321-323.

16

WHEN LIFE-PROLONGING TREATMENT IS QUESTIONABLE: THE ETHICS OF WITHHOLDING AND WITHDRAWING TREATMENT

Deciding when to withhold or withdraw life-prolonging treatment is one of the most difficult bioethical issues faced by health care professionals, family members and, above all, by patients themselves. Of all the issues treated in this book, no other one, with the possible exception of abortion, has generated as much professional, legal, ethical, and public controversy and commentary. Numerous court cases have dealt with this issue, and an enormous and ever-increasing literature reflects the views of doctors, nurses, theologians, philosophers, lawyers, economists, and others on the many questions raised by advances in life-prolonging technology.

Saving lives always has been, and will ever remain, a central goal of clinical practice. However, until fairly recently, doctors and hospitals were quite powerless in the face of life-threatening illness and trauma. Because little could be done to save life, little had to be decided. The situation began to change around the time of the Second World War. New drugs and surgical techniques, respirators, dialysis machines and other vital-organ support and monitoring technology, specialized intensive care units, and the number of hospitals equipped to offer new life-prolonging care proliferated after the end of the War, and up to the present day.

People used to be born and to die in the home. Today, people usually die in hospitals and institutions, places equipped with complex technology capable of prolonging life, frequently only biological life, when a return of sick people to health and vitality is no longer possible. Dying today calls for decisions. The initiation and continuation of intensive care procedures often result in little more than the prolongation of a person's dying; or in the prolongation of life that is, for the sick person, only marginally bearable or definitely miserable. Doctors, nurses, and families, often pressed by lucid suffering patients, are increasingly forced to ask whether administering treatment "to the bitter end" and for extension of life at all costs, particularly at costs of suffering that the patient cannot bear, is the right thing to do.

Movements, commissions, working groups, a voluminous clinical ethics literature, and numerous court cases have, over the past two decades, championed "dying with dignity," in opposition to technical prolongations of life when a patient's organism, though still minimally functional, can no longer support or permit the exercise of self-fulfilling personal control over life's events. The kinds of decisions that have to be taken with, and often on behalf of, the seriously ill are not purely technical. These decisions become an intrinsic component of the dying process. Depending on which decisions are taken, and on how they are reached, some people will have the chance to die well, as masters of their dying, not alone and not lonely. Others may die before their time, without a chance to live through their dying. Others may die too late, reduced to impersonal biological systems that have to be tended. Some may die uninformed and unenlightened, caught in the act of playing scene two when the drama is about to close. Still others may die, who could have lived.

Decisions with such consequences call upon the deepest beliefs and values of people, and they are, understandably, often the centre of conflicts on the level of ethos and morality, as discussed in Chapter 2. Most of the time, the conflicts and uncertainties raised by such decisions are resolved at the bedside. The resolution is obtained by careful attention to, and respect for, the patient's body and biography, as the norm of clinical ethics that should govern decision-making about life-prolonging treatment. At times, however, the uncertainties and conflicts have resisted resolution at the bedside, and hospitals, doctors, families, and patients themselves have turned to the courts for clarification and guidance.

Many of the difficult issues associated with life-prolongation dilemmas were described forcefully in video presentations of two cases, one fictional, the other real, made in the 1970s and used extensively in courses on ethics for medical and nursing students. The first section of the chapter describes these two video-presented cases, and will serve as a preparation for the following section, where we review some of the most important decisions taken by courts in the U.S. and Canada over the last twenty years, on the issues of life-prolonging treatment. Third, we shall examine the major concepts used in ethical reasoning to formulate judgments about initiating or discontinuing life-prolonging measures. The difficulties encountered by doctors, nurses, and families, when lucid and competent patients refuse life-prolonging treatment, are quite different from those faced when there is a need to make decisions on behalf of patients who cannot formulate or express their own wishes. In later sections, we concentrate on these differences, and on the approaches generally taken to reach decisions for these different categories of patients. The chapter then closes with a review of a selection of guidelines proposed for prolongation-of-life decision-making.

MUST PATIENTS LIVE AT ALL COSTS?

The dominant model of the patient-physician relationship today is based upon shared decision-making, as discussed in Chapter 5. Though we now find insistence on life-prolonging treatment of terminally ill, or of severely and irreversibly damaged patients to be inappropriate, and even intolerable, we need to keep in mind that this practice was not uncommon several years ago, when doctors generally decided what was best for their patients. Patients were often not involved at all in life-or-death decisions taken on their behalf, and when patients did attempt to oppose a doctor's "save life at all costs" ethic, they usually met with firm and effective resistance. The combination of "doctor knows best" medical paternalism, with a rigid physician adherence to the "save life at all costs" ethic, led to acute personal suffering for some patients, and this is illustrated in the video presentation of two cases, the first real, the second fictional, that we now consider.

Dax's Case: Please Let Me Die!

In the summer of 1973, Donald Cowart, a twenty-five-year-old Texan, was critically burned in a freak gas explosion. His first reaction was to ask for a gun to kill himself, but instead he was rushed to hospital for emergency treatment. Burns covered over 65% of his body, he was blind and had lost the use of his hands. For more than a year he underwent repeated surgical procedures, and daily treatment that was extraordinarily painful. Throughout this period, he constantly demanded that the treatment be stopped and that he be allowed to die, but his doctors would not comply. They believed that treatment was in his best interests, and they were able to override his refusal by having him declared incompetent because of his suffering, and having his mother authorize treatment on his behalf.

Cowart's condition eventually improved to the point where he could be discharged from the hospital. Although it took many years to get his life in order, and he attempted suicide once, he did graduate from law school, establish a successful law practice, and marry. However, he remains, to this day, an outspoken advocate of a patient's right to make decisions regarding his or her medical treatment, and he still contends that his demand to refuse treatment should have been respected.

The case of Dax Cowart (as he now calls himself) has become one of the most famous examples of (not) withholding life-prolonging medical treatment, as a result of a video entitled *Please Let Me Die*, which was produced by one of his doctors in 1974, and a longer film, which was released in 1985 under the title, *Dax's Case*. A book of essays that comment on this case from various perspectives has also been produced (Kliever, 1989). Together, these works present a powerful argument for the right to refuse treatment, but they also raise numerous questions about how far this right extends, and what are its limits.

The Quadriplegic Sculptor: Whose Life Is It Anyway?

Brian Clarke's play, *Whose Life Is It Anyway?* presented in video form and later the subject of an American film, was also produced in French as a play with the French title, *Quelle vie*, in Montréal's Théâtre du nouveau monde in 1980. We here use the French names for the characters in this play.

Brian Clarke's play is a story about a former sculptor now confined to bed as an incurable quadriplegic, after a road accident and successful life-saving medical treatment. But the life that has been saved now needs to be maintained. Joncas, the former sculptor, wishes to die. He has alternatives, but not many. He can live only with uninterrupted medical and nursing care. He cannot feed himself or attend to any of his basic bodily functions. He will never be able to do so again. He will have to be fed and catheterized, or he will die. He can only live in a hospital or in an institution for constant care. The hospital is his new placenta, the catheter his umbilical line to life.

Joncas grows into the realization that this kind of life is, for him, not worth the effort. About this realization, at least, he *can* do something. He demands to be released from hospital, or at least from life-prolonging treatment, fully conscious that he will die. He is opposed. He is told by his physician, Dr. Emery, that he cannot take this kind of decision and, at any rate, that he is too depressed to really know what he is doing, too depressed to take such a decision rationally. Joncas is in the hospital's power. He cannot move, and those who saved his life now refuse to release him from their care. Who rightfully has power over this life that has been saved?

In the play, the judge, who comes to hold court in the hospital and decide the case, finds himself before an exceptional case and an exceptional man, not a depressed, irrational person. The judge decides that Joncas has power over his own life; not the hospital, not the doctor. The judge supports Joncas's refusal of a life-prolonging treatment that keeps his brain alive and simultaneously helpless to execute its own commands and creations.

At the time the play was produced in Montréal, an ethicist, a lawyer, and a psychiatrist were each asked to write a commentary on the play for the *McGill Law Journal* (Roy, 1981). The trends of thought in these commentaries will appear again in the jurisprudence we shall examine that deals with cessation of life-prolonging treatment.

The psychiatrist, in his commentary on the play, disagrees with the judge's decision. Emphasizing the relative and fluctuating character of human liberty, the psychiatrist asks whether Joncas's present demand to have treatment stopped and to be allowed to die would be his desire three or more months from now if he is forced to accept treatment and to live. The psychiatrist, though for reasons quite different from those of Dr. Emery in the play, believes life-prolonging treatment should be forced upon Joncas, but he does not specify for how long.

The ethicist and the lawyer in their commentaries mutually defend the following ideas: that self-determination is a fundamental principle in both ethics and law; that refusal of life-prolonging treatment may be a justifiable exercise of liberty, and cannot be generally or automatically labelled as irrational and suicidal; that refusal of life-prolonging treatment, when the life prolonged is intolerable for the patient, is equivalent neither to suicide nor to euthanasia.

The psychiatrist's commentary focuses attention on the difficulties of expert psychiatric testimony, when a case goes beyond objective scientific data and elicits the psychiatrist's personal and subjective views or judgment. That is when psychiatrists tend to differ. However, when the persons differing in their necessarily subjective views about whether life-prolonging treatment is in the patient's best interest are precisely a lucid, nonpathologically depressed patient and his doctor, clinical ethics and legal thought, insofar as they are represented in these two commentaries, join in affirming that it is the patient's will that should prevail.

We should not read too much out of this play and its commentaries. Yet, this play did challenge and crystallize a great deal of thought on cessation-of-treatment issues in legal, ethical, and medical circles in the early 1980s in Canada. That thought subsequently came to the fore and to expression in numerous day-to-day real-life cases in Canadian hospitals, and in several of these cases that went to Canadian courts.

COURT DECISIONS: A REFLECTION OF EVOLVING ATTITUDES AND THOUGHT

There has been a remarkable evolution in North America over the last twenty years, both in attitude and thought, regarding legal and ethical obligations to sustain life by all technological means available. In a major shift of attitude, people have come to place great emphasis on quality of life, as a balance to a rigid insistence that life must always be sustained for as long as possible because life is sacred. Relatives, doctors and nurses, and the courts have come to recognize that life, in circumstances of unrelievable pain, suffering, and loss of function, can be a fate worse than death itself.

A major shift in thought was away from concern about the "ordinary" or "extraordinary" character of the measures employed to prolong life, to concern about whether life-prolonging measures, regardless of their being innovative and complex or routine and simple, are consistent with the clinical and personal goals of each patient. The dominant consensus today is that the distinction between "ordinary" and "extraordinary" means can no longer serve as a criterion for clinical-ethical decisions, or for public policy on withholding or discontinuing life-prolonging measures. The guiding view now is that there is no intrinsic ethical or legal difference between various life-prolonging measures, such as cardiopulmonary resuscitation, respiratory support, chemotherapy, hemodialysis, medications such as vasopressors or antibiotics, and the provision of assisted nutrition and hydration (Task Force, 1990). The real issue is whether any intervention, regardless of its being a measure of basic or advanced life support, is proportionate to the goals of each individual patient. When informed patients freely refuse such care, their refusal should be respected. However, were patients in a health care system such as that of Canada to demand rare and costly care, difficult decisions would have to be made as to whether a patient's goals exceed societal means.

These two major shifts in attitude and thought have been underway for over twenty years, and societal consensus on these changes crystallized only slowly and in connection with a multiplicity of specific issues. Many of these issues were at stake in the selection of court decisions, predominantly from the U. S. and Canada, that we now consider. Arguments presented in some of the earlier court cases, and in commentaries upon the court decisions, at times used the "ordinary-extraordinary means" distinction that has now been superseded.

The Quinlan Case — 1975-1976 — U.S.A.

One of the best known American court cases dealing with withdrawal of life support was that of Karen Ann Quinlan, who, on April 15, 1975, lost consciousness after taking a combination of alcohol and a tranquillizer. When it appeared that she would never recover from her persistent vegetative state (a condition marked by sleep-wake cycles and an inability to perceive or respond to communication), her parents asked that she be removed from her respirator and be allowed to die. They argued that, in the circumstances, respirator support was extraordinary treatment and, therefore, not mandatory. Hospital officials and doctors refused to honour this request, believing that such an action would be tantamount to euthanasia, which they felt to be both illegal and immoral. The Quinlans then sought a court order to support their position. A judge of the Superior Court of New Jersey, the state where the Quinlans lived, refused this request, on the grounds that a court should not interfere with a doctor's decision to act in the patient's best interests. This ruling was appealed to the Supreme Court of New Jersey. On March 3, 1976, this Court overturned the first judgment and authorized the withdrawal of the respirator if, in the opinion of the patient's physicians, supported by a hospital ethics committee and her own wishes reliably expressed by someone familiar with them, there was no reasonable possibility of her ever recovering consciousness. Karen was skilfully weaned off reliance on the respirator but, contrary to all expectations, the patient did not die. Instead, she survived in her persistent vegetative state for another thirteen years, sustained by artificial feeding through a tube, but with no other special medical care. Her parents never requested that the feeding be stopped.

One of the decisive factors in the Karen Ann Quinlan case was the presentation of reliable evidence that she would not have wanted to be kept alive in a persistent vegetative state. Although she had not signed a document to this effect, she had discussed the matter with others. The final court decision was based, therefore, not only on her best interests, but also on her own wishes.

The Saikewicz Case — 1976-1977 — U.S.A.

Joseph Saikewicz was profoundly mentally retarded all his life. He had an extremely low I.Q. and a mental age corresponding to that of a three-year-old child. He lived nearly all his life in state institutions and, in 1976, he was in the Belchertown State School in Massachusetts, where he had lived since 1928.

In the Spring of 1976, doctors found that Mr. Saikewicz, then aged 67, was afflicted with an incurable form of cancer called myeloblastic monocytic leukemia. This disease is marked by internal bleeding, severe anemia, and susceptibility to infections. At that time, chemotherapy offered a small chance of very temporary benefit: prolongation of life from several months to a year in about 50% or less of cases. The guardian for Mr. Saikewicz, appointed in May 1976, decided that this treatment would not be in Mr. Saikewicz's best interests, because he would not understand what was happening to him during the months of pain and discomfort he would experience due to the chemotherapy. In May, the Probate Court supported the decision not to start chemotherapy for Mr. Saikewicz, but this court judgment was then referred to the Supreme Court of Massachusetts.

The Supreme Court, in its opinion delivered in November 1977 (over a year after Mr. Saikewicz's death without having received chemotherapy), stated that a *competent* adult in a terminal condition like that of Mr. Saikewicz could refuse treatment, in this case, chemotherapy, that would only extend life briefly and would amount to little more than a prolongation of dying. One may think today that this was not a very controversial or daring position, and that it was hardly relevant to Mr. Saikewicz, since he had been incompetent all his life to take any decisions on his own behalf. Yet, with this position, the court was making new law in Massachusetts in 1977, and was also preparing its decision regarding Mr. Saikewicz, because, as William Curran pointed out, a guardian for an incompetent person could not do for the person what the person, if competent, could not legally do for himself (Curran, 1978, 499). By finding that a competent person could refuse treatment, the court opened the way for the guardian of an incompetent person to refuse treatment on his or her behalf.

The court, then, accepted that decisions to refuse life-prolonging treatment could be taken on behalf of incompetent persons. It was on the issue of who should make such decisions that the court caused great consternation and provoked much critical commentary. The Massachusetts Supreme Court expressed the view that all decisions on behalf of incompetent persons, regarding withholding or withdrawing life-prolonging treatment, must be authorized by a Probate Court. This view, had it held sway, would have enormously complicated decision-making on behalf of terminally ill incompetent persons. But this view was not to hold sway.

The Dinnerstein Case — 1978 — U.S.A.

When Mrs. Shirley Dinnerstein's son and daughter agreed with their mother's doctor that Mrs. Dinnerstein, given her bad heart condition and her state of advanced Alzheimer's disease, should not, in the case of cardiac arrest, be resuscitated, and that a "no code" order to that effect was justified, the matter was referred to the Probate Court of Norfolk County in Massachusetts. This was in keeping with the ruling, a year before, of the Massachusetts Supreme Court in the Saikewicz case.

The Norfolk County Probate Court referred this case to the Massachusetts Appeal Court, and this court, in its June 30, 1978, decision, ruled that "no code" orders for irreversibly terminally ill, incompetent patients do not require prior judicial review and approval.

The Appeal Court acknowledged that it is within the competence of the medical profession to decide, in the light of the family's wishes and the patient's condition, what treatments are or are not in keeping with peaceful dying. This decision interpreted the Supreme Court's Saikewicz case ruling about the need of Probate Court authorization as applying only to situations in which life-prolonging treatments have a chance of bringing about cure or stabilization of the condition being treated (Schram, 1978, 875).

The Dawson Case — 1983 — Canada

Stephen Dawson, born in 1976, contracted spinal meningitis a few months after birth, and suffered severe brain damage as a result. A shunt had to be implanted in his brain, to draw off excess cerebrospinal fluid. When Stephen was nearly seven, this shunt blocked and Stephen's parents refused their permission for corrective surgery, because they believed their child, given his incapacities and mental retardation, was not living a happy life and had no real future.

When Stephen's case went to the Provincial Court of British Columbia, the judge ruled that, when treatment only serves to prolong an incurable condition, the decision to initiate or withhold such treatment belongs to the family. Stephen's case then went for rehearing with fresh evidence to the Supreme Court of British Columbia, and Judge McKenzie, reaching a different conclusion from the earlier Provincial Court finding, drew attention to three crucial considerations.

The first centred on the description of the kind of life Stephen was leading. Descriptions of Stephen as retarded, blind, deaf, partially paralyzed, and afflicted with cerebral palsy had to be balanced by the testimony of those, who, in caring for Stephen, recognized that he could be a happy little fellow, able to enjoy and respond to affection and play. The Provincial Court concentrated on the first part of the description, and viewed the proposed corrective surgery as possibly cruel and unjust treatment. The Supreme Court, not so certain that Stephen experienced his life as a burden and as an intolerable suffering, ordered the corrective surgery to be performed.

However, two other crucial considerations influenced Mr. Justice McKenzie's decision. First, without corrective surgery, Stephen might very well not die rapidly, but continue to live for an indeterminate time. Second, Stephen's condition might then turn out to be even more impoverished and agonizing that it would be if surgery were performed.

The Stephen Dawson case carries the lesson that it is ethically crucial to be very careful about descriptions of patients that serve as the basis for life-death decisions. It is tragically wrong to decide a patient's fate on the basis of a description that does not match the real person.

The second lesson coming from the McKenzie decision is that it would be as wrong to conclude that all handicapped persons now have to be given life-prolonging treatment right to the bitter end, as it would be wrong to refuse such treatment on the bias that a handicapped life is not worth living.

The Couture-Jacquet Case — 1986 — Canada

In February 1986, the Québec Court of Appeal upheld the right of family members to refuse life-prolonging chemotherapy for their terminally ill children. Carole Couture-Jacquet was a three-year-old girl, suffering from a rare form of pelvic cancer. Her mother and grandmother had previously given permission for three twelve-week sessions of chemotherapy treatment at the Montréal Children's Hospital. The treatment had produced various side effects, including vomiting, constant nausea, loss of hair, loss of 50% of kidney functioning, and significant hearing impairment. Her physicians recommended a further course of chemotherapy, which offered an estimated 10% to 20% chance of cure. Without the treatment, her life expectancy was approximately six weeks.

After considering this information, Carole's mother and grandmother refused permission for the treatment. The Montréal Children's Hospital then applied to the Québec Superior Court for an order to allow the treatment, and the order was granted. The patient's mother and grandmother appealed this decision to the Québec Court of Appeal. This court agreed with the family members, judging that the low estimated success rate of the treatment did not justify its distressing side effects. This judgment is noteworthy for its sensitive use of proportionality reasoning. Liberating Carole from the chemotherapy's continuing, and even increasingly, distressful side effects was seen as more important than taking the treatment's estimated 10% to 20% chance of arresting progression of the tumor for a limited time.

The Cruzan Case — 1990 — U.S.A.

In June, 1990, the U. S. Supreme Court rejected the request of the parents of Nancy Cruzan, a thirty-three-year-old woman who had been in a persistent vegetative state for seven years, to remove the feeding tube that was keeping her alive. Although the court affirmed the right of competent persons to refuse medical treatment, and included artificial feeding and hydration within the definition of medical treatment, it ruled that the State of Missouri, where the Cruzans lived, had the authority to require "clear and convincing evidence" that an incompetent patient would not have wanted such treatment. The Supreme Court of Missouri had earlier ruled that there was no such evidence in Nancy's case; for example, she had not written a living will. In November 1990, the Cruzans returned to court with additional testimony from Nancy's physician and three friends that she would not have wanted to be kept alive in such a state. The judge agreed, and shortly afterwards her feeding tube was withdrawn. She died on December 26, 1990.

In nearly all cases involving life-sustaining issues, courts in the U. S. have placed great emphasis on the principle of self-determination. Decisions to discontinue life-prolonging treatment, such as respirator support or assisted nutrition, on behalf of incompetent patients are legally problematical in the United States when these patients have failed to express their wishes about life-prolonging treatments when they were lucid.

The 1985 ruling of the New Jersey Supreme Court in the case of Mrs. Claire Conroy illustrates this situation. When Mrs. Conroy's only relative, her nephew and legal guardian, requested from a trial court in 1983 that his aunt's feeding tube be removed, the court's permission to have the tube withdrawn was stayed while its decision went into appeal. Mrs. Conroy died a month later with her feeding tube still in place.

Two years later, the New Jersey Supreme Court rejected the distinction between ordinary and extraordinary means, and stated that artificial feeding is like other life-sustaining treatments. Decisions about such treatments should be based on the proportionality principle; that is, upon an estimate of whether the burdens outweigh the benefits for the patient.

This seems straightforward and reasonable. However, the New Jersey Supreme Court then complicated matters considerably when it outlined the procedures to be followed in estimating that the burdens of treatment outweigh the benefits for incompetent patients. The court rejected the idea that this estimate should be made jointly by physicians and families, and proposed a very burdensome process involving a court-appointed guardian, the State Office of the Ombudsman, and two appointed physicians not affiliated with the incompetent patient's institution or attending doctor.

Such a procedure is remarkably unnecessary, and has been qualified as both unrealistic and profoundly disturbing (Lo, 1986).

The Malette Case — 1979-1990 — Canada

On March 30, 1990, the Ontario Court of Appeal released its judgment in the case of *Malette v. Shulman.* The case originated in June 1979, when Mrs. Malette, a Jehovah's Witness, was given a blood transfusion by Dr. David Shulman after she had been seriously injured in an automobile accident, and suffered blood loss that the physician thought might endanger her life. A nurse had advised Dr. Shulman before transfusion that Mrs. Malette carried a signed (but not dated or witnessed) card that stated (in French): "As one of Jehovah's Witnesses with firm religious convictions, I request that no blood or blood products be administered to me under any circumstances." After her recovery, Mrs. Malette sued Dr. Shulman, the hospital, its Executive Director, and four nurses for negligence, alleging that the blood transfusion had been medically unnecessary, and for battery, meaning unauthorized touching, alleging that the transfusion was performed without her consent. When the case came to trial, Mr. Justice Donnelly of the Ontario Supreme Court dismissed the action for negligence, but awarded damages of $20,000 against Dr. Shulman for battery, having decided that the card continued to represent Mrs. Malette's true wishes.

In a unanimous decision, the Ontario Court of Appeal upheld the judgment of the lower court. Basing its decision on the doctrine of informed consent, the court stated: "A doctor is not free to disregard a patient's advance instructions any more than he would be free to disregard instructions given at the time of the emergency... The principles of self-determination and individual autonomy compel the conclusion that the patient may reject blood transfusions even if harmful consequences may result and even if the decision is generally regarded as foolhardy... To transfuse a Jehovah's Witness in the face of her explicit instructions to the contrary would ... violate her right to control her own body and show disrespect for the religious values by which she has chosen to live her life." The court concluded that the card carried by Mrs. Malette, even though undated, constituted a valid expression of her prevailing wishes concerning medical treatment, and that Dr. Shulman did not have reasonable grounds to doubt that this was the case. The award of $20,000 was upheld.

The Cases of Nancy B. and R. Corbeil — 1992 — Canada

An ethical consensus has grown in Canada, over the last fifteen years, in support of the view that physicians are quite justified in withholding or discontinuing treatments that do little more than prolong a patient's dying and suffering. However, physicians, nurses, hospital administrators, and others have, at the same time, demonstrated a reluctance to disconnect a respirator from conscious and lucid patients, particularly when the prognosis is for continued life for a considerable period of time. The case of Nancy B. illustrates this situation. There is similar reluctance among health care professionals to collaborate with patients, for example, quadriplegics, who refuse nourishment, because they want to die soon. This is the situation in the case of Robert Corbeil.

In the case of Nancy B., already discussed extensively in Chapter 3, Judge Dufour, in his decision rendered in January 1992, clarified two points of law in support of his judgment that Nancy B.'s refusal of respirator treatment should be honoured. First, a doctor's act of disconnecting a respirator, in response to her patient's informed and voluntary request, cannot be said to be either an unreasonable act or an act of criminal negligence. Secondly, disconnection of a respirator, in the circumstances of Nancy B.'s case, in no way amounts to either homicide or to aiding suicide.

Not long after the decision in the Nancy B. case, another Québec judge had to deal with a request by a patient to be allowed to starve himself to death. Robert Corbeil was a thirty-five-year-old father of two children; he had been seriously injured in an all-terrain-vehicle accident in May 1990, and was permanently paralyzed from the neck down. He could, however, breathe on his own, and was perfectly lucid. When he was informed, in September 1991, that his handicap would be permanent, he decided that he wanted to die. Given his condition, the only means of death available to him was to stop eating. Since he was living in a long-term-care institution, the administrators of the institution requested court authorization to respect the patient's wishes, in order to protect themselves from possible recrimination.

In deciding the case, Judge Gontran Rouleau of the Québec Superior Court declared that Mr. Corbeil had the right to refuse to eat and to be fed, even if he would die as a result. There was no evidence that the patient was incompetent to make this decision. Furthermore, the judge ruled that the patient should not be transferred against his wishes to another institution, such as a hospital, where he might be given life-prolonging treatment. Instead, the personnel at the long-term institution were ordered to provide comfort care, to make his death as easy as possible.

Judge Rouleau's decision emphasizes two important legal and ethical consider-ations. First, the relevant question is whether a patient is sufficiently conscious, lucid, and balanced to take a decision on his own behalf. It is quite irrelevant that others find his decision to be unreasonable. Second, it is the patient, no one else, who can decide whether his life is so devoid of quality as to be unbearable.

Since this decision was rendered, and as of this writing, Mr. Corbeil seems to have regained a desire to live, has started to eat again, and even seems prepared to go to other institutions, where he could receive rehabilitation therapy.

LESSONS FROM THE COURT CASES

Court cases dealing with life-prolongation issues have been much more numer-ous in the U. S. than in Canada, over the last twenty years. This may have been influenced by the consideration that patients in the U.S. may fear heavy medical bills for care, and hospitals run for profit may favour prolonging treatment rather than having empty beds. A review of all the twists and turns of thought reflected in the U.S. court decisions would surpass the purpose and space of this chapter.

If we focus attention on the Canadian cases, the judicial decisions rendered in the cases of Couture-Jacquet, Nancy B., and Robert Corbeil confirm and reflect the direction of numerous day-to-day practical judgments of clinical ethics in Canada, on issues of life-prolongation treatment. This trend is away from a rigid "prolong-life-at-all-costs" ethics, towards an ethic based primarily upon the dignity and quality of life, particularly as determined by patients them-selves, rather than on the duration of life taken as an absolute value.

Moreover, the decisions of Judges Dufour and Rouleau implicitly endorse the former Canadian Law Reform Commission's recommendations, presented in Chapter 3, that ambiguous sections of the *Criminal Code of Canada* should be clarified, so that they cannot be interpreted as obliging physicians either to treat patients against their informed and voluntary refusals, or to initiate or continue treatments that are therapeutically futile and not in patients' best interests.

THREE GUIDING CONCEPTS

As is evident in the previous section, the right of patients, or their surrogates, to refuse life-prolonging medical treatment has become established in law. Nevertheless, deciding when to exercise this right is still one of the major prob-lems in clinical ethics. Attempts to clarify this issue have been hindered by conceptual and semantic disagreements. Therefore, before proceeding to discuss when withholding and withdrawing of treatment is appropriate, and who should make such decisions, we will establish working definitions of some of the key terms in the debate: dying with dignity, futility and proportionality.

Dying with Dignity

This expression is used to signify practices as diverse as palliative care and active euthanasia. Because of its ambiguity, some authors reject the term altogether (Lynch, 1982). However, because it is so widely used, we prefer to retain the expression, while assigning it a precise meaning.

In a *first* sense, dying with dignity means dying without a frantic technical fuss and bother to squeeze out a few more moments or hours of biological life, when the important thing is to live out one's last moments as fully, consciously, and courageously as possible. Helping people to die with dignity means recognizing that biological life is not an absolute, not the highest value. It means recognizing that a moment arrives when technological attempts to prolong biological life may interfere with higher personal values, and should give way to other forms of care.

Second, dying with dignity means dying without that twisting, racking pain that totally ties up a person's consciousness, and leaves him or her free for nothing and no one else. Methods exist today to control pain, while maintaining patient consciousness. Yet, a wide gap still exists between what can be done and what is, in fact, achieved. Many patients still suffer high enough levels of pain to make pain the dominant experience during their final period of life. This process is degrading, particularly so when it can be, but is not, avoided, because of the ignorance or insensitivity of caregivers or others.

Third, dying with dignity means dying in surroundings that are worthy of a human being who is about to live what should be one's "finest hour." When our bodies, which mirror the world to us, are in a phase of final collapse, we are not helped to rise to the pitch of our dignity if we are placed in sterile rooms, devoid of art and all the objects that carry the rich memories of our lives. Matters are worse if our last days of consciousness and relationship with those who contributed to the meaning of our lives are dominated by the intrusive apparatus of life-prolonging technology. The environment of a dying patient should clearly say: the technical drama of medicine has receded to the background, to give way to the central human drama, the drama in which genuine communication between a dying person and family and friends is the only last thing that really matters.

Human beings are too unique, too varied, and too complex to fit into one simple model of what dying with dignity means. There is good reason to be very critical of the ideology that there is only one right way to die. There are many ways to die with dignity. Resigned acceptance of imminent death is no more an expression of human dignity than is Dylan Thomas's admonition to "not go gentle into that good night" and to "rage, rage against the dying of the light."

Futility

There is widespread agreement today that physicians are not obligated to offer, and patients are not obligated to undergo, treatments that are futile, i.e., that have no hope of success. However, there is much confusion and controversy about the meaning of futility.

The futility of potential intervention is to be judged in terms of the clinical goals for each individual patient. The central question is: will the intervention benefit the patient as a whole? Antibiotics will reverse a pneumonia in a persistent-vegetative-state patient. Because this effect can be achieved, some physicians believe antibiotic therapy *in this situation* is not futile, and hence obligatory. However, what is the goal of treatment for this patient in a persistent vegetative state? If the clinical goal is to return the patient to even a minimum of intellectual and relational capacity, then the treatment is indeed futile and non-obligatory, because it can never serve attainment of this goal.

It is essential to distinguish, and even separate, two components in the concept of futility: the component of physiological effect and the component of benefit (Schneiderman, 1990). Some treatments are futile because they cannot produce a desired physiological effect for a particular patient, or a particular category of patients. For example, the probability of chemotherapeutically halting a metastatic process may, on the basis of clinical trial results or on the basis of accumulated clinical experience, be virtually nil. Other treatments may be futile because they are useless in attaining the clinical goals of care, even if they can have the effect of prolonging biological life. If the goal of clinical treatment is to restore a sick person to a measure of independent life, then treatments are futile if they only prolong a dying process, or preserve the patient in a permanent state of unconsciousness, or tether the patient indefinitely to life-support machines in an intensive care unit.

Consideration of each individual patient in his or her body and biography, the total patient, is the key to the proper use of futility as a criterion for withholding or withdrawing life-prolonging treatment. Prolonging a dying process may be justifiable, if the patient and family need that extra time to achieve important personal goals. One man in an irreversible and advanced stage of leukemia returned to hospital, time and again, for blood transfusions. Some members of the clinical team accused others of overly aggressive therapy, until the man returned to hospital once more, this time to die. He explained that, though he knew the treatments would never cure him, they at least gave him the time to complete the porch he was building around the house for his wife. In a quite different situation, a physician aggressively maintained life support for a severely brain-damaged teenager, so that his mother and father could synchronize their schedules of grief. The father, unrealistically expecting his son's return to conscious life, was accusing his more realistic wife of giving up hope, of abandoning their son. The marriage and the equilibrium of the surviving nine-year-old brother were in danger. The physician worked carefully and sensitively with the father who, five months later, came to hospital with his wife and son. He apologized to his wife in the presence of the doctor, and both parents requested that no further efforts whatsoever be made to prolong the biological shell of their child. Efforts to extend the life of a nonsalvageable patient, though futile for the patient, can be justified, within reasonable limits, if they contribute to the healing of an endangered family life.

Proportionality

The distinction between extraordinary and ordinary medical treatment, in classifying the elements of decision-making about withholding or withdrawing life-prolonging treatment, is no longer widely used. In its place is the distinction between proportionate and disproportionate treatment. The proportionality rule, succinctly stated, affirms that life-prolonging treatments are contraindicated when they cause more suffering than benefit (Cassem, 1980). Patients should be allowed to die, when the only treatments that could prolong life cause a burden of suffering that exceeds the joys and opportunities for personal fulfilment that extended life could ever offer. One of the Law Reform Commission of Canada's suggested amendments to the *Criminal Code of Canada* states that physicians are not bound to administer treatments that are therapeutically useless and not in the best interests of patients (Law Reform Commission, 1983). The Vatican *Declaration on Euthanasia* proposes that it is ethically justifiable to discontinue the use of advanced life-prolonging techniques, when the results fall short of expectations. Direct appeal is made to the proportionality rule, when this document draws attention to the fact that patient, family, and medical staff may judge that certain techniques impose on the patient strain or suffering out of proportion to the benefits that he or she may gain from such interventions (Vatican, 1980).

The notion of proportionality has become a cornerstone of medical ethics. The Canadian Paediatric Society, for example, states four conditions under which withholding or withdrawing of life-prolonging treatment would be ethically justifiable. The first two conditions deal with futile treatment, and with prolongation of the dying process when death is imminent. The last two conditions rest on the notion of proportionality. Life-prolonging treatments may be abandoned when other forms of treatment will allow a greater degree of caring and comfort, or when the prolongation of life will cause the patient intolerable and intractable pain and suffering (Canadian Paediatric Society, 1986).

WHEN PATIENTS ARE COMPETENT

There is a widespread legal consensus that competent patients have the right to refuse medical treatment, for whatever reasons they find compelling. Most ethicists would agree that this is a wise social policy, given the requirements of public ethics in a pluralistic society such as Canada. However, at the level of clinical ethics — making treatment decisions for specific patients — it is generally held that the ethical right to refuse treatment is not unlimited. There are certain medical conditions for which it is appropriate to refuse certain types of treatments; for other combinations of conditions and treatments, refusal might be quite unjustified. Some examples follow.

Terminal Illness

The easiest type of treatment-refusal decision to justify is when the patient is suffering from a terminal illness, such as advanced cancer, and the proposed treatment can, at best, extend life a short while. Since such treatments often involve discomfort for patients, these individuals are fully justified in concluding that the advantages of treatment, especially a longer life, are outweighed by the disadvantages. There is little controversy on this matter in medical, legal, ethical, and religious circles. The following statement of the Roman Catholic Church reflects this widespread consensus:

> When inevitable death is imminent in spite of the means used, it is permitted in conscience to take the decision to refuse forms of treatment that would only secure a precarious and burdensome prolongation of life, so long as the normal care due to the sick person in similar cases is not interrupted. (Vatican, 1980, 10)

Similar positions may be found in the consensus report of the Task Force on Ethics of the Society of Critical Care Medicine and in the Appleton Consensus on international guidelines for decisions to forego medical treatment (Task Force, 1990; The Appleton Consensus, 1989).

Non-Terminal Illness

Considerably more problematic, from the standpoint of clinical ethics, is the situation of patients such as Nancy B. and Robert Corbeil, who are suffering from a serious illness or disability, which may indeed be incurable, but which is not likely to result in death in the near future (say, within one year). According to the method of clinical ethics outlined in Chapter 2, there are no universal rules to be applied in these cases. Instead, each patient needs to consider the burdens and benefits of continuing treatment, in the light of his or her values, preferences, strengths, and responsibilities. What may be right, even obligatory, for one person may be wrong for another with the same medical condition. The

Roman Catholic Church document quoted above offers some useful advice about the criteria that should be considered when making such decisions:

> In any case, it will be possible to make a correct judgment as to the means by studying the type of treatment to be used, its degree of complexity or risk, its cost and the possibilities of using it, and comparing these elements with the result that can be expected, taking into account the state of the sick person and his or her physical and moral resources. (Vatican, 1980, 8-9)

No matter what criteria are employed, the ultimate decision-maker must be the patient. Others can advise, counsel and even attempt to persuade (but not coerce), but in the end they should support the patient in whatever decision he or she makes.

Religious Reasons

For some people, a crucial factor in deciding whether a proposed treatment should be refused is their religious faith. Perhaps the best-known example of this is the opposition of Jehovah's Witnesses to blood transfusions. These individuals cite Biblical passages as the basis of this prohibition, e.g., Genesis 9:4: "Only flesh with its soul — its blood — you must not eat," and Acts 15: 28f: "Keep abstaining from things sacrificed to idols and from blood." They are willing to die rather than receive a blood transfusion.

The legal doctrine of informed consent is generally interpreted as giving competent adult Jehovah's Witnesses the right to refuse blood transfusions, no matter how routine this treatment is for other patients. As noted above, the court decision in Ontario in the case of *Malette v. Shulman* recognized the further right of Jehovah's Witnesses to make advance directives in this matter.

Another example of religious influence on treatment decisions is the Orthodox Jewish belief that life is precious and should be preserved as long as possible. In the words of a noted Jewish scholar:

> There is an emphatic stress on the importance of human life. Therefore, to prolong a human life even for a short while is a good deed. Though death is inevitable, it is seen as an event to be opposed. (Siegel, 1978, 249)

The Jewish reluctance to withhold or withdraw life-prolonging treatment, even when death is imminent, is a further indication of how people's views differ on this matter and, consequently, how difficult it is to make general rules. In a pluralistic society such as Canada, the best policy is probably one that allows the exercise of individual conscience in treatment decisions, at least for competent adults. At the same time, it may be necessary to enact certain provisions to protect the interests of those who cannot make their own decisions, such as children and adults who have lost, or who never had, the capacity of rational thought.

WHEN PATIENTS ARE NO LONGER COMPETENT

There comes a time, in the lives of many individuals, when they can no longer make medical decisions for themselves, even such basic ones as whether or not to undergo life-prolonging medical treatment. Their incompetency may be a result of advanced senility, coma, or persistent vegetative status. Treatment decisions for these patients have to be made by others, according to specific criteria.

The principal criterion for such decisions is the probable desires of these patients, if they were still capable of rational thought. Those who knew the patients well can suggest how they would have wanted to be treated, in a situation of terminal illness or incapacity. This is known as the "substituted judgment" approach, and was essentially the one used in the Karen Ann Quinlan and Nancy Cruzan cases.

If patients have not adequately expressed their wishes about how they would want to be treated, or if relatives and friends give contradictory accounts of these wishes, then another criterion for treatment decisions must be invoked. This is known as the "best interests" test, since the treatment option chosen is the one that would seem to be best for the patient. However, it is often difficult to determine what actually is best for any particular patient. There are no less than four different ways to approach this issue, namely:

- treat every patient aggressively, until it is certain that treatment is no longer needed, either because the medical problems are cured or because the patient is dead;
- withhold treatment, if the medical condition of the patient is so severe that there is little or no doubt that he or she would be better off dead;
- withhold treatment when the quality of life of the patient will likely be very low, because of serious physical and/or mental handicaps and the inability or unwillingness of family members and/or society to provide necessary care;
- withhold treatment at the family's request, no matter what their reasons.

Each of these options has its supporters, and each is backed by ethical arguments. The *first* is based on the belief that life is intrinsically valuable, and patients, no matter how unwell, should be given every chance to live. As is evident from the case of Karen Ann Quinlan, doctors can make mistakes about the expected outcome of certain medical conditions. Where there is any uncertainty about the patient's chances of survival, according to this option, every effort should be made to prolong life.

The other three options reject such attempts to extend life by all possible means. It has been demonstrated, over and over again, that the vast majority of patients with certain types of conditions will either die within a short time or will survive with severe handicaps. The few exceptions to this rule should not be used to justify treating all the others, since not only will the treatment most likely do them no good, but it can cause them, and their families, actual harm.

If the first option is rejected, a choice must be made among the other three. The *second*, which focuses on the medical condition of the patient, is the most "objective," in that it attempts to exclude variable factors, such as the capacity of the family to provide care and the availability of social support services. This option works well for patients whose prognosis is clearly dismal, but it is not so adequate for those with less certain prognoses.

The *third* alternative, which is based on an assessment of the patient's likely quality of life, is attractive because the patient is not the only one involved in the situation. Children, siblings, and society in general are also affected by decisions about the survival of very ill patients, and should perhaps have a say in this matter. At the same time, the more elements that are introduced as criteria for decisions about treatment, the more difficult such decisions become. Quality of life is an expression that is used very loosely, and it may not always be suitable for deciding which patients should be given a chance to live.

The *fourth* option, letting family members decide, avoids the issue of appropriate criteria or, rather, turns it over to the family to determine for themselves. It is argued that they are the ones most knowledgeable about the potential quality of life of the patient, and will be the most affected if the patient survives. On the other hand, they may be in a difficult emotional state when faced with a decision whether or not treatment should be initiated or terminated and, as well, they might possibly give inordinate weight to their own interests, rather than those of the patient.

Even when it is clear which of these general approaches is to be used to make treatment decisions about incompetent patients, such decisions will necessarily vary according to the condition of the patients and the treatments that are suggested. To this extent, these decisions are comparable to those that have to be made by competent patients, as described above. However, the most important criterion for determining treatment options for incompetent patients is not their terminal or non-terminal condition, but rather whether their loss of decision-making capacity is temporary or permanent.

Permanent Loss of Competence

The vast majority of patients in a persistent vegetative state, or those suffering from advanced senility of the Alzheimer's type, will never regain consciousness. It is uncertain if they have any feelings at all, even hunger and thirst. Their quality of life is so low as to be practically nonexistent, and it is questionable whether it is in their interest to continue living.

Many other permanently incompetent patients are less severely affected in their physical and mental functions. They may be conscious, mobile, and capable of enjoying certain experiences and activities. Their quality of life is significant, and it is clearly in their interest to continue living, as long as they can maintain their present level of functioning.

Decisions about withholding or withdrawing life-prolonging treatment must take into account the condition of the patient. Those who will never regain consciousness should normally not receive any form of treatment other than food, liquids, and hygienic care, especially if they are terminally ill. Even if they are not terminally ill, there is widespread agreement that other medical interventions, even antibiotics for infections, are not required, unless the patients clearly indicated beforehand that they would want to receive such treatments. There is a growing body of opinion that even food and nutrition may be withheld from persistently unconscious patients, as occurred in the case of Nancy Cruzan.

The other group of incompetent patients, those who can still enjoy life to a certain extent, have a stronger interest in life-prolonging treatments, especially if they are not terminally ill. In situations of terminal illness, it is generally acceptable to withhold aggressive treatments and allow comfortable death to occur. However, where there is a reasonable chance of recovery from a serious illness, even aggressive therapy such as cardiopulmonary resuscitation might be justified. Factors that have to be taken into account in such decisions include the likelihood of full recovery, or of recovery in a reduced state (for example, partial paralysis after a stroke) and the pain and discomfort associated with the treatment. Each case is different, and the pros and cons of treatment must be weighed carefully in order to decide whether treatment is really in the best interests of the patient.

Temporary Loss of Competence

In cases where there is a good chance that medical treatment can restore the patient's decision-making competence, then normally the treatment should be undertaken. Once competency is restored, patients can make their own decisions about future treatment. They may wish that they had been allowed to die, as did Donald Cowart, but unless they clearly express such a desire in advance, health care professionals are bound to act as if patients want all appropriate treatment.

If, on the other hand, prospects for recovery of anything approaching normal health are very doubtful, then the decision whether or not to treat becomes much more difficult. Emergency room staff are faced with these decisions frequently; their problem is compounded by the uncertain prognosis for many critically ill patients, and the need to undertake treatment immediately if there is to be any chance of recovery. Since their job is to heal, they usually do everything they can to treat the patient, as long as they feel there is some chance of success and there is no evidence, such as an advance directive, that the patient would not want to be treated.

PATIENTS WHO HAVE NEVER BEEN COMPETENT

This category of patients includes infants and severely mentally disabled individuals of all ages. The employment of the substituted judgment approach is not possible for them, since their present or previous wishes cannot be known. Treatment decisions must be made on the basis of their best interests and potential quality of life.

As a general rule, these patients should be treated in the same fashion as patients who were once competent, but are now permanently incompetent and whose treatment preferences are not known. When they are suffering from a terminal illness, they should be kept comfortable and fed, but no medical interventions should be initiated to prolong their dying. When they are afflicted by a life-threatening but curable illness, decisions are much more difficult. In addition to the likely outcome of the treatment and the pain and discomfort it will entail, it is necessary to take into account the patient's psychological reaction to the treatment, which may be quite different from that of a competent person. Once again, it is clear that treatment decisions must be made on the basis of the details of the case, which vary from one patient to another.

CHILDREN

When is a young person sufficiently autonomous to share decision-making with parents and physicians, in circumstances where the decision is about withholding or withdrawing life-prolonging treatment? Leikin has proposed that a person, irrespective of age, is competent to consent to foregoing such treatment if he or she has experienced an illness for some time, understands the illness and the benefits and burdens of its treatment, has the ability to reason about the illness and treatment, has previously been involved in treatment decisions, and, most importantly, understands the personal meaning and finality of death (Leikin, 1989). Some adolescents do have these abilities. They have shared, and even directed, decisions for or against being allowed to die. Whether pre-adolescents have these abilities is an unresolved question.

Physicians should work closely with parents, to determine the extent of a young person's maturity and ability to share in such decisions. Young people in middle and late adolescence may be quite capable of understanding the gravity of their illness and the relative imminence of their death, but they may also experience the threat of separation from their parents most acutely at this time. That experience may well increase their need to depend upon their parents for the critical decisions that have to be made about their treatment. Exaggerated and unrealistic assumptions about an adolescent's independence are not components of respect for autonomy. There is no substitute here for a case-by-case assessment of each gravely ill adolescent's strengths and vulnerabilities (Baylis, 1993).

DECIDING FOR OTHERS

Decisions about initiating and withdrawing treatment for incompetent patients are often very difficult, and can be quite conflictual. If, as generally happens, several doctors are involved in the case, they may disagree among themselves about what should be done. If they favour aggressive treatment, the nurses might be opposed because of the suffering they see in the patient. Family members may disagree with the medical team. Finally, even when all these participants are of one mind, they might be opposed by the hospital administration, by the courts, or by provincial legislatures, which have enacted child welfare laws. These laws provide that the province may intervene, when a child is in need of protection because parents fail to provide, or refuse, reasonably indicated medical care. The federal *Criminal Code* also requires parents to provide "necessaries of life," but courts usually defer to medical evidence as to what is, in fact, necessary.

In North America, the primary decision-making authority in cases involving children is usually assigned to the parents. The Canadian Paediatric Society statement takes this position, but it also stipulates several exceptions to the general rule:

- when parents are incompetent to make decisions for themselves;
- when there are unresolvable differences between the parents; or
- when they have clearly relinquished responsibility for the child; in such cases the identification of a legal guardian should precede any decisions regarding withholding treatment.

Even when the parents are clearly competent to make the decision, if the physician involved feels that they are not acting in the best interests of the child, a court can be asked to decide the matter (Canadian Paediatric Society, 1986).

Robert Weir, a specialist in the ethical problems of incompetent patients, answers the question of who should decide by setting forth four qualifications for the role of decision-maker: relevant knowledge and information, impartiality, emotional stability, and consistency. Since no individual is likely to possess all these qualifications, he proposes a serial ordering of decision-makers: (i) parents or other family members, (ii) attending physician, (iii) ethics committee, and (iv) the courts. In cases of disagreement between the family and the physician, either party may appeal to the ethics committee and, if necessary, to the courts (Weir, 1984, 255-271).

In Canada, recourse to the courts has been relatively infrequent, except in cases involving Jehovah's Witnesses. Although competent adult Witnesses have the legal right to refuse treatment, they may not do so on behalf of their children. Canadian doctors and hospital authorities routinely seek, and are granted, authorization by the courts under child welfare legislation to administer blood transfusions to the children of Witnesses, if this treatment is felt to be in the children's best interests.

In all but a few cases, however, recourse to the courts is neither desirable nor necessary. Decisions about whether or not to treat permanently incompetent patients are primarily ethical in nature, and should be dealt with according to the methods of clinical ethics. But provincial human rights codes provide for nondiscrimination against the physically and mentally disabled. Ideally, all interested parties will participate in the decision-making process and will have, as their principal focus, the best interests of the patient. If the parties cannot agree among themselves, an ethics consultant or committee may help them to resolve their differences. Once the ethical decision is made, the medical management of the case is the responsibility of the physicians and nurses involved in the case. Even when it has been decided to withhold or withdraw aggressive treatment, caregivers have an important role to play, in administering palliative care to relieve any pain that the patient might experience, and in helping family members deal with their grief.

ADVANCE DIRECTIVES

An advance directive is a statement about how a person would want to be treated, in situations where he or she is not capable of expressing desires. It can take various forms: an oral statement to family members, friends, or a doctor; a written document, such as a living will; or a durable power of attorney, whereby another person is chosen to make decisions on the patient's behalf, when the latter is no longer capable of doing so.

Advance directives became popular in the U. S., beginning in the late 1960s; they were heavily promoted by patient advocacy groups, such as Concern for Dying and the Society for the Right to Die. Under pressure from these groups, many American states passed laws guaranteeing the right of patients to have their wishes regarding medical treatment respected. The first state to pass "living will" legislation was California, in 1976. This law gave terminally ill persons the right to authorize, by advance directive, the withdrawal of life-prolonging procedures when death is believed imminent. By 1991, at least forty-two of the fifty American states had such laws in place (Society for the Right to Die, 1991). Although these laws vary in many ways, they are all intended to provide for withdrawal of such procedures as mechanically assisted breathing and blood circulation, for patients who will die within a short time if these procedures are terminated. In such cases, there is relatively little controversy nowadays about honouring a patient's request to cease treatment. Having won this battle, the right-to-die movement is now lobbying for what it calls "second generation" treatment-refusal legislation, which would have the following features:

- it should not be restricted to the terminally ill, but should apply to all competent adults and mature minors;
- it should not limit the types of treatment an individual can refuse, but should apply to all medical interventions;
- it should permit individuals to designate another person to act on their behalf, and set forth the criteria under which the designated person is to make decisions;
- it should require health care providers to follow the patient's wishes, and provide sanctions for those who do not do so;
- it should require health care providers to continue to provide palliative care to patients who refuse other interventions (Legal Advisors Committee, 1983).

In Canada, interest in passing legislation to legitimize advance directives has developed only recently. As of 1992, only two provinces, Québec and Nova Scotia, had adopted such legislation, although at least two others, Manitoba and Ontario, were considering similar proposals.

Despite their immediate appeal, as is evidenced by the large number of individuals who have made living wills, advance directives do have drawbacks. Unless they are very detailed about the exact types of treatment to be refused for every possible type of life-threatening illness, it may be quite difficult to interpret the wishes of a person who needs a certain treatment, but is unable to make the decision at the time. Competent patients have the great advantage of knowing their medical problems and the various treatment options, as well as how they feel about living and dying at the moment of decision.

Another problem with advance directives is that doctors are often uncertain whether aggressive medical treatment can restore a patient to full health. Victims of automobile accidents, for example, who will die without immediate treatment, may be capable of complete recovery or, on the other hand, may survive in a persistent vegetative state or with severe handicaps. The presence of a living will may influence doctors to withhold treatment from someone who could be completely cured, especially if they could be sued for not following the patient's instructions. On the other hand, the first instinct of doctors is to cure the sick, where possible. Thus, living wills can cause enormous difficulties for doctors, when faced with unconscious patients who need immediate emergency care.

Despite these and other difficulties, advance directives are generally endorsed by medical, legal, and ethical experts, as a useful means of determining how an incompetent patient should be treated (Singer, 1992). The Canadian Medical Association has recommended that, on request, doctors assist patients in executing such directives, and follow them unless there are reasonable grounds for not doing so (Canadian Medical Association, 1992).

Patients should realize, however, that advance directives are limited in their scope, and should be supplemented by, for example, ongoing discussions with family members and health professionals about their treatment preferences.

GUIDELINES

Although every patient is unique, this does not mean that there is no place for general policies and guidelines for withholding and withdrawing life-prolonging treatment. As we have seen, there is widespread legal and ethical agreement on some aspects of this issue. In order to help patients, families, and doctors to make these decisions, and to ensure that there will be some consistency in the resolution of similar cases, numerous health care institutions have formulated policies and guidelines for terminating treatment.

Many of these documents concentrate on just one type of treatment, cardiopulmonary resuscitation (CPR). As a result, they are known as DNR (do not resuscitate) policies. A study of such policies in U.S. hospitals has revealed the following common themes:

- DNR policies should be documented in the written medical record of the patient.
- DNR orders should specify the exact nature of the treatment to be withheld.
- Patients, when they are able, and families should participate in DNR decisions. Their involvement and wishes should be documented in the medical record.
- Decisions to withhold CPR should be discussed with other staff, including nurses.
- DNR status should be reviewed on a regular basis.
- DNR is not equivalent to medical or psychological abandonment of patients (Youngner, 1987, 25).

An example of such a policy, which is further restricted to terminally ill patients, has been adopted by the Canadian Medical Association, the Canadian Nurses Association and the Canadian Hospital Association (Canadian Medical Association, 1984). It has been used by many Canadian hospitals, as a basis for more detailed guidelines designed to serve the particular patient population of each institution.

A more comprehensive approach to these issues has been taken by the Hastings Center, an American bioethics research institute. The Center has prepared a volume entitled *Guidelines on the Termination of Life-Sustaining Treatment and the Care of the Dying*, which covers all aspects of the subject of this chapter (The Hastings Center, 1987). A third set of guidelines for non-treatment decisions was produced in 1988, at an international conference in Appleton, Wisconsin. The document is entitled *Suggested International Guidelines for Decisions to Forgo Medical Treatment* (The Appleton Consensus, 1989).

CONCLUSION

None of us can escape the question of how we would want to be treated, when we are afflicted with a life-threatening or terminal condition. Moreover, many of us will have to make such decisions for others, whether family members, loved ones, or patients. Because they can result in death, these decisions are among the most difficult concerns of clinical ethics. Fortunately, there has developed a widespread consensus on many of the legal and ethical aspects of the issue, so that those making the decisions can benefit from the collective wisdom and experience of many other patients, caregivers, ethicists, and jurists. The method of clinical ethics and of public policy ethics, as indicated at the end of Chapter 2, is based upon prudential deliberation of the many (*une phronesis à plusieurs*).

REFERENCES

Baylis F. and **McBurney C.**, eds., *In the Case of Children: Paediatric Ethics in a Canadian Context*. Toronto: The Hospital for Sick Children, Bioethics Department, 1993.

Canadian Medical Association, Canadian Nurses Association and **Canadian Hospital Association** *Joint Statement on Terminal Illness*. Ottawa, 1984.

Canadian Medical Association "Advance Directives for Resuscitation and Other Life-Saving or Sustaining Measures." *Canadian Medical Association Journal* 1992;146/6:1072A.

Canadian Paediatric Society, Bioethics Committee "Treatment Decisions for Infants and Children." *Canadian Medical Association Journal* 1986;135:447-448.

Cassem N. "When Illness Is Judged Irreversible: Imperative and Elective Treatments." *Man and Medicine* 1980;5:154-166.

Curran W.J. "Law-Medicine Notes. The Saikewicz Decision." *The New England Journal of Medicine* 1978; 298:499-500.

Kliever L.D., ed. *Dax's Case: Essays in Medical Ethics and Human Meaning*. Dallas, TX: Southern Methodist University Press, 1989.

Law Reform Commission of Canada *Euthanasia, Aiding Suicide and Cessation of Treatment*. Report #20. Ottawa: Ministry of Supply and Services Canada, 1983.

Legal Advisors Committee of Concern for Dying "The Right to Refuse Treatment: A Model Act." *American Journal of Public Health* 1983;73:918-921.

Leikin S.A. "A Proposal Concerning Decisions to Forgo Life-Sustaining Treatment for Young People." *Journal of Pediatrics* 1989;115:17-22.

Lo B. and **Dornbrand L.** "The Case of Claire Conroy: Will Administrative Review Safeguard Incompetent Patients?" *Annals of Internal Medicine* 1986;104:869-873.

Lynch A. "Death without Dignity." *Annals of the Royal College of Physicians and Surgeons of Canada* 1982;15/2:117-122.

Roy D.J., Baudouin J.L. and **Dongier M.** "Theatre Reviews." *McGill Law Journal* 1981;26:1068-1083.

Schneiderman L.J., Jacker N.S. and **Jonsen A.R.** "Medical Futility: Its Meanings and Ethical Implications." *Annals of Internal Medicine* 1990;112/12:949-954.

Schram R.B., Kane J.C. and **Roble D.T.** "Law-Medicine Notes. 'No Code' Orders: Clarification in the Aftermath of Saikewicz." *The New England Journal of Medicine* 1978;299:875-878.

Siegel S. "Death: Post-Biblical Jewish Tradition." In: W.T. Reich, ed. *Encyclopedia of Bioethics*. Vol. I. New York: The Free Press, 1978, 246-249.

Singer P.A. et al. "Advance Directives: Are They an Advance?" *Canadian Medical Association Journal* 1992;146:2, 127-134.

Society for the Right to Die *Refusal of Treatment Legislation*. New York: Society for the Right to Die, 1991.

Task Force on Ethics of the Society of Critical Care Medicine "Consensus Report on the Ethics of Foregoing Life-Sustaining Treatments in the Critically Ill." *Critical Care Medicine* 1990;18/12:1435-1439.

The Appleton Consensus "Suggested International Guidelines for Decisions to Forgo Medical Treatment." *Journal of Medical Ethics* 1989;15/3:129-136.

The Hastings Center *Guidelines on the Termination of Life-Sustaining Treatment and the Care of the Dying*. Briarcliff Manor, NY: The Hastings Center, 1987.

Vatican Congregation for the Doctrine of the Faith *Declaration on Euthanasia*. June 26, 1980:1-12.

Weir R.F. *Selective Nontreatment of Handicapped Newborns*. New York and Oxford: Oxford University Press, 1984.

Youngner S.J. "Do-Not-Resuscitate Orders: No Longer Secret, but Still a Problem." *Hastings Center Report* 1987;17/1:24-33.

17

WHEN PEOPLE ASK FOR DEATH: THE ETHICS OF EUTHANASIA

In his story about the death of Ivan Illyitch, Tolstoy asked: "And the mujiks [the peasants], how do the mujiks die?" If Philippe Ariès is correct (Ariès, 1974), the peasants died the way Solzhenitsyn describes the dying of older folk in the *Cancer Ward*: no puffing up of themselves, no fighting against death, no pretending they were not going to die, no stalling about squaring things away. They prepared themselves quietly and they departed easily, "as if they were just moving into a new house."

If that is how the mujiks died, it is not how many people today think they will die. People today fear loss of control, when the time comes to die. They fear, as an editorial in the science journal *Nature* states, a "twilight life tethered to feeding tubes or respirators." (Editorial, 1991)

Of course, as the previous chapter demonstrated, resistance has grown, over the last twenty years, against technological zeal to prolong life at all costs and to the bitter biological end. There is, today, a solidly entrenched consensus, both in clinical ethics and in law, in favour of allowing people to die in peace and dignity. Some physicians still seem to be unaware of this, and some particular cases will always provoke agonizing discussion, but the trend in North America against senseless tethering of people to life-prolonging technology is generally serene and probably irreversible.

However, liberation from enslavement to life-prolonging technology is, for some people, not quite enough. Chapter 3 introduced the story of a young man in the terminal stages of AIDS. This young man had a head full of projects, and wanted to live. Yet, knowing he would inevitably die soon from AIDS, he asked for sufficient drugs, and instructions on how to use them, so that he could time his death to occur before he wasted away and lost his mental competence. And that is what he did.

There is a similar story in the recent medical literature. Diane, a married woman with a husband, a college-age son, a business, and her artistic work, was diagnosed as having acute myelomonocylic leukemia (a cancer of cells in the blood). She rejected the chemotherapy option. The side effects and the roughly 25% chance of long-term survival were not for her. What Diane feared most, according to Dr. Quill, her physician, was increasing discomfort, dependence, and hard choices between pain and sedation. Diane made it clear to her family and to Dr. Quill that, when the time came, she wanted to advance her death in the least painful way possible. Dr. Quill thought this made sense, aware as he was of Diane's desire for independence, and of her wish to stay in control. He consequently referred her to the Hemlock Society for information about suicide, and made sure Diane knew how to use the barbiturates for sleep, as well as the amount needed to bring about her own death. This is what Diane did — she advanced her own death — when bone pain, weakness, fatigue, and fevers began to assume control of her life (Quill, 1991).

Diane's story, the story of the young man with AIDS, and other similar stories challenge us to clarify what and how we think about the requests of sick people for rapid, painless death. Some are able to administer such death, rapid and painless death, to themselves. Others are not capable of doing this. So we have to clarify what and how we think about the involvement of doctors in the administration of death. People have been thinking, writing, and proposing legislation about euthanasia for a long time, but the term means quite different things to different people, so the first section of this chapter specifies the definitions and distinctions we shall use in this book. The current controversy on euthanasia, destined perhaps to be the most hotly debated bioethical issue of the 1990s, takes up many of the concerns, ideas, arguments, and legal proposals presented at various periods throughout this century. So the second section situates the current euthanasia controversy in its historical context. We then turn to the two key issues of this chapter. Is euthanasia or assisting sick people in euthanasia ever ethically justifiable? Our focus here is in clinical ethics, as discussed in Chapter 2. Should euthanasia or assistance in euthanasia be legalized or decriminalized? With this question, we enter the domain of public policy ethics and law. Subsequent sections present the reasoning and arguments advanced for and against affirmative answers to these two central questions. Though they are related, each of these questions requires its own analysis. An affirmative answer to the first question — yes, euthanasia is ethically justifiable in certain circumstances — would not necessarily entail the affirmation that euthanasia should be legalized. On the other hand, the fact that many people claim euthanasia to be unjustifiable in any and all circumstances would not necessarily require that it should continue to be treated as a crime under law. Whether it should is precisely what is under debate today.

EUTHANASIA: WHAT ARE WE TALKING ABOUT?

Every discussion of euthanasia is bedevilled by the many different understandings of the term, as used in popular, academic, and professional discourse. It is very difficult for opponents and proponents of euthanasia to agree on a definition of the term.

Defining Euthanasia: Three Difficulties

There are at least three reasons for this difficulty. The *first* derives from the fact that definitions of euthanasia are frequently shaped, often inadvertently, by the moral stances people have already adopted on the issue. Those in favour of euthanasia may, in defining the term, speak of it as a "deliverance," or as "helping people to die a peaceful, dignified death," or as "aid-in-dying," and who could possibly be against that? Those against euthanasia may, in defining the term, speak of it as "killing," or as "destruction of life," and who could possibly be in favour of that? These kinds of definitions signal a moral stance, and are really opening moves in a moral debate. They do not contribute much to the logical task of distinguishing euthanasia from other acts, from which it is both conceptually and clinically different.

The *second* difficulty in achieving consensus on the meaning of euthanasia resides in the fact that people involved in the controversy are really constructing quite different kinds of definitions. Some want to include under "euthanasia" acts that they believe to be morally equivalent, even if they are conceptually and clinically different. For example, some see no moral distinction between withholding life-prolonging treatment, discontinuing such treatment, controlling pain adequately, and administering death rapidly and painlessly, So, they speak of passive and active euthanasia. Others prefer to reserve the term "euthanasia" for the act of administering death rapidly and painlessly. Some hold this preference because they are convinced there is a moral difference between this act and the above-mentioned acts of withholding or discontinuing life-prolonging treatments, or of administering drugs needed to control pain. Others prefer the restricted meaning of euthanasia simply to facilitate ethical and legal discussion, and to avoid confusion.

Third, agreement on the meaning of euthanasia is difficult, because the term is not historically neutral. Those who believe that euthanasia is ethically justifiable and should be legalized want the understanding of the term, as used today, to be freed from any connection to the programme of the Nazi doctors. Some who oppose euthanasia believe that decoupling euthanasia today from euthanasia as practised under Hitler's Reich may well lead to uncivilized abuses, similar to those committed by some doctors in the Nazi period (Lifton, 1986).

Euthanasia: A Working Definition

We are not above the difficulties just described, nor are we immunized against them, as we set about now to clarify how the term "euthanasia" will be understood in this chapter. We will, accordingly, not simply stipulate, but also offer reasons for the distinctions and definitions we think are needed to present and analyze answers given to the chapter's two central questions, about the ethical justifiability of euthanasia and about the wisdom of legalizing euthanasia. What are we talking about, when we ask these two questions?

Euthanasia, in this chapter and book, means: the deliberate, rapid, and painless termination of life of a person afflicted with incurable and progressive disease.

In this definition we assume:

- that termination of life in this way, of a sick person in these circumstances, will be compassion-motivated. However, since motivation is often difficult to ascertain reliably, we do not include "merciful" or "compassion-motivated" in the definition;

- that termination of life will be of persons afflicted with a condition or disease that is inexorably drawing them towards death, even if that death may be far from imminent;

- that rapid, painless termination of life will usually be achieved by parenteral (by injection) or oral administration of a lethal dose of a drug or of a combination of drugs;

- that euthanasia may be either self-administered or administered by someone else, usually a physician.

We shall qualify *euthanasia* as *voluntary* or as *nonvoluntary*, depending on whether the sick person has or has not requested and given full consent (informed, comprehending, and voluntary) to termination of his or her life. We assume that *nonvoluntary* euthanasia would be considered, if at all, only for patients who never were, or are now no longer, capable of requesting or consenting to termination of their lives. We assume, with voluntary euthanasia, that the sick person's request for termination of life does not arise from a pathological and treatable depression.

Assisted euthanasia refers to self-administered euthanasia, when the sick person desiring to advance his or her death requires help from others, usually physicians or health care professionals, in obtaining lethal dosages of drugs and instructions on how to use these effectively.

The Distinction Between Euthanasia and Suicide

We draw attention to the *distinction* we are making *between suicide and voluntary euthanasia*. The distinction rests upon the presence or absence of an incurable and progressive disease or condition that is inexorably, that is, independently of one's will, drawing a sick person towards death. When faced with imminent or inevitable death from disease, a person's request for euthanasia may be quite compatible with a strong desire to live. This was the case with the young man with AIDS, mentioned earlier. He wanted to live, but he could not bear the degradations of bodily wasting and loss of mental competence that he foresaw he would have to live through, before his inevitable death arrived. So he advanced his death. We reserve the term *suicide* for persons' termination of their own lives, when they are not afflicted with a disease or condition that is drawing them inexorably towards death. We note that, though suicide is generally and correctly assumed to be the expression of a pathological state of mind, usually depression, some knowledgeable and experienced professionals admit that suicide, in some circumstances, can be quite rational (Motto, 1981; Narveson, 1986).

Euthanasia Is Different From Allowing to Die and From Controlling Pain

Central to the controversy on euthanasia is the fact that some people acknowledge, and others deny, the reality and the ethical sense of the *distinction between euthanasia and withholding or discontinuing life-prolonging treatment* (Gillon, 1988). Some claim that this distinction has no ethical sense whatsoever, and simply masks the hypocrisy of those who do not have the courage to act decisively on behalf of the suffering and the dying (Rachels, 1986).

We maintain that the distinction between euthanasia, as we have defined the term, and withholding or discontinuing life-prolonging treatment is clinically, ethically, and legally essential, and that the distinction is logically defensible.

The logical defence of this distinction rests upon two assumptions that we can formulate, but not fully discuss, in this chapter. The *first* assumption is that doctors do not possess *carte blanche* authority to intervene into the bodies and lives of sick people. Quite the contrary! Each intervention has to be justified. When treatments, including life-prolonging treatments, have been started and are doing harm rather than good, it is continuance, not discontinuance of the treatment that needs justification.

In the course of illness, a moment arrives when it is no longer possible to restore health, function, or consciousness, when it is also no longer possible to reverse a dying process. The most that even the aggressive use of sophisticated technology can achieve is to prolong that dying process, to stop that dying person from dying now, or soon. It is in these situations that we correctly speak of withholding or withdrawing interventions that are not stabilizing a person's life, but only prolonging a person's dying. It is in these situations that we speak correctly of *allowing a person to die*. As the mother of a young man in persistent vegetative state said, when she asked the doctor to stop artificial feeding of her son: "Doctor, please let my son complete his death."

The *second* assumption is that doctors are quite justified in using every proportionate means at their disposition, to relieve suffering due to the pain and symptoms of disease. Administering medication in dosages and in frequencies needed effectively to relieve pain and symptoms, is logically and clinically a quite different act from the act of administering death rapidly and painlessly. It is in part because of a failure to grasp this distinction that some doctors, fearful of legal liability for hastening death, have gone just so far, and not far enough, in their use of medications to control patients' pain and symptoms.

The issue, at this moment, is not whether euthanasia is ever ethically or legally justifiable. The issue is whether the use of the right amount of medication to control pain and symptoms is logically, clinically, and legally an act different from the act of terminating a patient's life rapidly and painlessly. We maintain that there is a real difference between these two acts, and that recognition of this difference is necessary to permit coherent debate on the possible ethical and legal justifiability of euthanasia. Some, as we shall see, claim that euthanasia or assisting euthanasia is justifiable in circumstances where it is deemed to be necessary, such as when methods of pain and symptom control fail to offer patients the relief they desire.

Distinctions Not Used in This Book

Many articles and books on euthanasia distinguish active from passive euthanasia. Equivalent distinctions, such as direct and indirect euthanasia, or euthanasia by act and euthanasia by omission, are also used to create two categories of euthanasia.

We prefer not to use these distinctions in this book, because they lead to confusion and distract attention from the currently central ethical and legal controversy about the acceptability of rapidly and painlessly administering death.

These distinctions lead to confusion, because the category of passive euthanasia (or indirect euthanasia or euthanasia by omission) encompasses two kinds of decisions and acts that are logically and clinically different: acts of withholding or discontinuing treatments that *can reverse* a disease process leading to death (for example, withholding surgery from infants afflicted with an intestinal blockage); and acts of withholding or discontinuing treatments that *cannot reverse* a disease process leading to death but can only prolong the dying process (for example, respirator support, chemotherapy, and assisted nutrition for conditions like those discussed in the previous chapter).

The kinds of acts encompassed by the category of withholding or discontinuing life-prolonging treatment are the centre of a particular kind of ethical and legal controversy, which has been underway within hospitals and the courts for at least two decades. A high degree of ethical and legal consensus has been attained on this controversy, as discussed in the previous chapter, and we do not want to confuse that controversy with the currently renewed conflict of views about whether administering death painlessly and rapidly should be legalized, or is ever ethically justifiable.

So we reserve the term *euthanasia* for the (compassion-motivated) rapid and painless termination of life, of persons afflicted with diseases or conditions that are drawing them inexorably to death, even if death is not imminent. When euthanasia is used in this sense, there is no doubt that the administration of death is what is intended and attempted. Whether euthanasia in this sense should ever be acceptable in ethics or in law is at the centre of the current controversy, upon which we focus attention in this chapter.

Limitations on the Validity of our Distinctions

The two distinctions we have made, between euthanasia and allowing to die (by withholding or discontinuing life-prolonging treatment), and between euthanasia and the effective relief of pain and symptoms do not hold true in some circumstances, and become very blurred in others.

The expression "allowing to die," as distinguished from euthanasia, really only makes sense in the cases of persons who are dying; in the cases, that is, of persons afflicted with a disease that is inexorably drawing them to death, even if that death is not imminent. The assumption is that clinical interventions are powerless to reverse the disease process. If treatments do exist that could reverse the progression to death of a potentially lethal disease or condition, we are not allowing patients with such a disease or condition to die when we withhold or discontinue such treatments. We are provoking their death by inaction. In these situations, exemplified in the refusal to correct a Downs syndrome child's intestinal blockage by feasible surgery, the distinction between euthanasia and withholding treatment breaks down quite completely. In both cases, death is administered: by an act of lethal injection in the case of euthanasia, and by inaction in the case of withholding feasible life-saving surgery.

Second, methods do exist today to control pain while maintaining consciousness in patients afflicted with advanced disease. Sometimes, though, pain is so constant and pervasive that patients can be relieved only by dosages and combinations of medication that either make them extremely drowsy or sink them into a deep sleep. Though there is controversy about how often such intense pain occurs, many people find the distinction between induction of heavy drowsiness or unconsciousness and euthanasia to be thin, and logically not very compelling.

EUTHANASIA IN THIS CENTURY

Nearly all the aspects of euthanasia currently under discussion in the 1990s have appeared in this century's earlier debate on the subject. Yet, it would be naïve and intellectually misguided to think that we could simply lift euthanasia proposals and arguments out of their historical context and compare them, as though the social, political, and medical particularities of each period had no influence at all on euthanasia reasoning and practice. We are not today, nearly fifty years after the Second World War, in the same situation as were people who advocated and opposed euthanasia from the 1920s to the 1940s, the first period of intense activity on euthanasia in this century. One critical difference is that we can refer back to, and learn from, their experiences and the consequences of their actions. Shaping today's decisions and policies in the light of the experiences and actions of our predecessors, or the activation of our memory of history, is an integral phase of method in ethics and law. It is for this reason, and not to attempt invalid comparisons of the sort mentioned above, that we now review, even if all too briefly, the major periods in the history of euthanasia in his century.

Euthanasia: 1920-1945

In 1873, two English journals, the *Fortnightly Review* and the *Spectator*, disagreed on an issue that would come up repeatedly throughout this century's waves of controversy over euthanasia. The *Fortnightly Review* argued that only voluntary euthanasia could be justified. Highly critical of this restriction, the *Spectator* claimed that those often in greatest need of euthanasia are incapable of giving consent. This debate foreshadowed controversies over euthanasia that would occur in Germany, England, and the United States from the 1920s up to the end of the Second World War, and that are occurring again today.

A climate of opinion favourable to euthanasia, and open advocacy of the practice, were evident in Germany prior to Hitler's ascendancy to political power. As early as 1920, the jurist Karl Binding and the psychiatrist Alfred Hoche published a book under the title, *The Permission to Destroy Life Unworthy of Life* (Binding, 1920). Both authors were distinguished university professors; Binding at Leipzig and Hoche at Freiburg.

This book included the incurably ill, but also mentally ill persons, the feeble-minded, and retarded and physically deformed children in the category of lives unworthy of life. The authors endorsed both voluntary and nonvoluntary euthanasia, and proposed a controlled juridical process to govern the practice. Applications for euthanasia would have to be evaluated by a panel, consisting of a general medical practitioner, a psychiatrist, and a lawyer. Emphasis was placed on compassion, on consistency of this practice with medical ethics, and on the economic burden society had to bear in the case of those for whom the book was proposing euthanasia.

The ideas of Binding and Hoche greatly influenced later German thinking on euthanasia, and their book is considered by many to mark the beginning of the euthanasia movement in Germany. A meeting of psychiatrists in Bavaria, in 1931, discussed euthanasia for persons with chronic illness. By 1936, euthanasia was openly enough accepted that the practice could be mentioned incidentally, and in a matter-of-fact way, in an article in an important German medical journal (Alexander, 1949, 39).

In 1941, a film was released as part of a media programme to persuade the German public of the acceptability of euthanasia. The film, *I Accuse* ("Ich klage an"), shows a physician injecting his wife with a lethal dose of a drug, in response to her desperate request that he do something to relieve her of the pain and suffering of her multiple sclerosis. However, by 1941, thousands upon thousands of patients with the most diverse conditions and illnesses, adults and children, were being put to death in the six major euthanasia stations in Germany (Northeim, Sonnenstein, Grafeneck, Bernburg, Brandenburg, and Hadamar). The pretense at medical diagnosis and prognosis had long been abandoned. There was no question of consent, and medical records were falsified to keep this mass euthanasia programme secret (Lifton, 1986; Mitscherlich, 1949). While public protest induced Hitler to slow down the euthanasia programme for adults, euthanasia of malformed and mentally retarded children continued until the end of the War. Some of the techniques developed for the euthanasia programme, such as exposure of patients to carbon monoxide gas, or to cyanide gas, were later used against the entire Jewish population of the German territories, as well as against other so-called racially impure groups, resulting in over six million deaths.

There was also a flurry of euthanasia discussion in England and in the U.S., during the 1930s. In 1931, Dr. Killick Millard chose euthanasia as the subject of his *Presidential Address* to the Society of Medical Officers of Health in England. He later published this address in a book that included the text of a proposed legislative bill in favour of voluntary euthanasia (Millard, 1931). The English Euthanasia Society, which became the Voluntary Euthanasia Society in 1969, was formed in 1935. This Society promoted the legalization of voluntary euthanasia, and pursued its objective with the 1936 *Voluntary Euthanasia Bill*, introduced by Lord Ponsonby into the House of Lords. This Bill was defeated by a 35-14 vote.

Proposals for legalizing euthanasia were being put forward in the U. S., during this same period. Senator John H. Comstock of Lancaster introduced the *Voluntary Euthanasia Bill* into the Nebraska Legislature in 1937. In the same year, an unsuccessful attempt was made to introduce a similar Bill, minus the Nebraska Bill's provision for limited nonvoluntary euthanasia, into the New York Legislature. In 1938, the Reverend Charles F. Potter founded the Euthanasia Society of America. In the following year, Dr. Foster Kennedy, recently elected President of the Society, advocated nonvoluntary euthanasia, particularly in cases of newborn defective babies. There are indications that the American Society at first envisioned the eventual legalization of nonvoluntary euthanasia as one of its objectives. The Society dropped this objective, following a 1941 poll of New York State medical opinion, which produced results unfavourable to nonvoluntary euthanasia.

Shortly after the Second World War, the military and medical crimes trials were held at Nuremberg. The revelation of horrendous crimes against humanity, perpetrated in Germany prior to and during the war, produced widespread revulsion against euthanasia, even when voluntary and for the purpose of relieving suffering.

Euthanasia: After the Second World War

While, in the wake of the Nuremberg trials, the World Medical Association condemned the practice of euthanasia in 1950, in England the House of Lords reopened debate on voluntary euthanasia legislation in 1952. In 1957, Professor Glanville Williams published his articulate, and still cited, brief in favour of euthanasia (Williams, 1957). This book, as well as *Euthanasia and the Right to Death*, edited by Reverend A.B. Downing (Downing, 1969), prepared the way for the *Voluntary Euthanasia Bill 1969*, which Lord Raylan introduced into the House of Lords. This bill was defeated by a 61-41 vote. In 1971, a special panel of the Board of Science and Education of the British Medical Association published a report, *The Problem of Euthanasia*, condemning voluntary euthanasia (Trowell, 1973, 151-158). The English Voluntary Euthanasia Society published a rejoinder, *Doctors and Euthanasia*, in the same year (Trowell, 1973, 159-171).

Voluntary Euthanasia Bills were also introduced into several state legislatures in the U.S. during this same period (Idaho, 1969; Montana, 1973; Oregon, 1973), but none was passed. However, a large number of U.S. state legislatures passed so-called "natural death" statutes, permitting refusal in advance of life-prolonging treatment when death is expected within a relatively short period. Many, both proponents and opponents of euthanasia, consider these statutes to be a step along the way to its legalization (Marker, 1989). Moreover, the decriminalization of attempted suicide, passed in Canada in 1973, tended to remove the legal stigma from voluntary, self-administered euthanasia.

Euthanasia: The Contemporary Period

In most Western countries, the practice of euthanasia is still illegal in the 1990s, no matter what good reasons one may have (for example, ending the suffering of terminally ill patients). The one major exception to this pattern is the Netherlands. Although euthanasia is still a criminal offence there, Dutch prosecuting lawyers, basing themselves on judgment of courts, have developed guidelines according to which doctors (and only doctors) who administer euthanasia will not be prosecuted. These guidelines, which have the support of the Royal Dutch Medical Association, stipulate that there must be an explicit and repeated request by a patient that leaves no reason for doubt concerning his or her desire to die; the mental or physical suffering of the patient must be very severe, with no prospect of relief; the patient's decision must be well-informed, free, and enduring; all options for other care have been exhausted or refused by the patient; and the doctor must consult another physician before acting (Sneiderman, 1992). The number of deaths by euthanasia in the Netherlands is estimated at between 5,000 and 10,000 each year (ten Have, 1992).

Although no other country has, as of this writing, followed the example of the Netherlands, the practice of helping patients to end their own lives (assisted euthanasia) is tolerated in some countries. This practice is illegal in Canada, but in Germany there is no legal prohibition of what the Germans call "aid-in-dying." If German patients are capable of exercising control over their actions, and act out of freely responsible choice, then physicians are permitted to provide them with lethal drugs. For patients who cannot find a physician willing to assist in their suicide, the German Society for Humane Dying provides its members with a booklet that contains instructions for administering lethal dosages of readily available prescription drugs (Battin, 1992).

In North America, pressure is growing to legalize assisted euthanasia. In November 1991, voters in Washington State took part in a referendum on death with dignity, which included a provision to legalize euthanasia. Despite public opinion polls that showed a two-thirds majority in favour of voluntary euthanasia, the proposal was defeated by 54% of voters. A similar proposal was defeated by California voters in November 1992, by an almost identical margin.

Until recently, there has been relatively little public discussion of euthanasia, or pressure for its legalization in Canada. The Canadian member of the World Federation of Right to Die Societies, Dying With Dignity, is small and has had very little influence on legislators, health care professionals, or the general public. The 1983 Report of the Law Reform Commission of Canada, *Euthanasia, Aiding Suicide and Cessation of Treatment*, made the following recommendations to the government:

- The Commission recommends against legalizing or decriminalizing voluntary euthanasia in any form and is in favour of continuing to treat it as culpable homicide.

- The Commission recommends that mercy killing not be made an offence separate from homicide and that there be no formal provision for special modes of sentencing for this type of homicide other than what is already provided for homicide.

- The Commission recommends that aiding suicide not be decriminalized ... (Law Reform Commission of Canada, 1983, 31)

In 1991, a Member of Parliament introduced a Private Member's Bill that opposed these recommendations, and would have legalized euthanasia in Canada. Bill C-261, an *Act to legalize the administration of euthanasia under certain conditions to persons who request it and who are suffering from an irremediable condition and respecting the withholding and cessation of treatment and to amend the Criminal Code*, received first reading on June 19, 1991. As the title indicates, the Bill had two purposes. The secondary aim was to entrench the right of individuals to refuse life-prolonging medical treatment, and to protect physicians who do not provide such treatment. The primary purpose of the Bill was the legalization of euthanasia.

Bill C-261 did not define euthanasia but, rather, suggested a process by which it could be administered. An individual who is suffering from an "irremediable condition" and is not less than eighteen years of age would be able to make a written application to a "referee in euthanasia" for a "euthanasia certificate." The referee, who would be appointed by the Attorney General, would interview an applicant and his/her physicians and, if satisfied that the applicant understands the nature and purpose of the application and has made it freely, would then issue a euthanasia certificate. The certificate could be presented to a qualified medical practitioner, who would administer euthanasia. Refusal to grant a certificate could be appealed to the Attorney General. The Bill included a sample application form and two medical certificate forms for transmission to the referee.

Bill C-261 was debated for its allotted time, but did not come to a vote. According to the rules of the House of Commons, it could not be discussed further during that session of Parliament. Given the general reluctance of Canadian legislators to deal with controversial bioethical issues, it is likely that the government will continue to follow the Law Reform Commission's advice, and not introduce changes to the present prohibition of euthanasia. However, since Canada is greatly influenced by what occurs in the U.S.A., if euthanasia is legalized in that country, there will probably be increased pressure here to at least consider changes in the current policy.

IS EUTHANASIA EVER ETHICALLY JUSTIFIABLE?

Related Questions

The film *Breaker Morant* demonstrated the thesis that, in war, situations arise that fall outside all existing rules. Similar situations seem to arise, from time to time, in caring for the terminally ill. If decisions to stop all life-prolonging treatments and to allow "nature to take its course" are morally and legally justifiable, should not society, as Dr. John Freeman asked twenty years ago, allow physicians to help nature take its course — quickly? (Freeman, 1972)

How is such a question to be answered? By measuring the proportion of benefits to harms? The focus then would be on the patient. If the patient is bound to die, given the irreversibility of a lethal disease and the rightness of a decision not to intervene to prolong life, of what good to the patient, family, or to anyone is an interim period of slow decline into death? Why should patients, families, and caregivers be bound passively to await death? But should the focus be only on the patient, when the balance of benefits to harms is considered?

Do we answer the question (about helping nature to take its course quickly) by considering long-term consequences? Here, the focus would be on the medical profession and society. Should a society give such power to doctors, or to any profession? There are many kinds of suffering, and there are sufferers of all ages. If we justify euthanasia for some patients on the grounds of mercy, is it possible to establish generally acceptable and nonarbitrary limits to the putative medical mandate to shorten "useless dying curves" by administering death? Do we try this as an experiment, and closely monitor what happens? Or do we, in the fear that "things might get out of hand," arbitrarily decree that no one, doctors included, is ever morally justified in terminating a patient's life?

Some, many perhaps, would argue that such a decree is not arbitrary at all. It is simply the expression of the most basic of all principles: that no human being has dominion over the life of another. Judges, philosophers, and religious leaders have reiterated this principle in various ways over the ages.

That fact, however, does not silence the questions. How do we know that this principle should hold, and should hold without exception? Even if one accepts that no human being has dominion over the life of another, do human beings not have dominion over their own lives? How can the constraint of the dominion principle be justified, when the act it prohibits, euthanasia, appears, in some circumstances, desirable from every empirical point of view and is, in fact, desired by everyone involved in a particular case? Is the authority of reason able to resolve this most important of our ethical questions, or does the prohibition of euthanasia rest, rather, on belief?

Conflicting Answers

Beliefs inevitably enter into any discussion of the ethics of euthanasia. Because people in pluralistic societies hold quite different and conflicting beliefs, the issue of euthanasia exhibits conflicts on the level of ethos, as mentioned in Chapter 2.

Theological Ethics

Those who say that euthanasia is ethically unjustifiable, in any and all circumstances, may ground this position in their beliefs about the origin and destiny of human life. If life is a gift of the Creator, then human beings do not possess dominion or sovereignty, either over the lives of others or over their own lives. On the basis of this or similarly conceived beliefs, no human being possesses unlimited autonomy over his or her life. The autonomy is limited by the divine plan for all human life. Within this plan, the gift of life is inalienable.

People who hold beliefs of this kind, however, may arrive at quite different theological conclusions about the ethics of euthanasia. There is controversy, even within theological ethics, about whether euthanasia is ever ethically justifiable. Some theologians hold that euthanasia is never justifiable, under any circumstances. Others argue that even if euthanasia is unacceptable *in principle* — and the principle is often the above-mentioned belief about the divine origin of life — it is impossible to claim absolutely that there are never circumstances in which euthanasia could be at least ethically tolerable *in fact*. Still others distinguish excusability or nonculpability from ethical acceptability. They admit that prolonged and intolerable pain, or the crushing experience of constantly observing people suffer such pain — the pressure of empathy — may free people requesting or practising euthanasia from all moral guilt. Yet, the act of euthanasia nevertheless remains ethically unjustifiable.

Medical Ethics

One may observe a similar plurality of views within professional ethics. Some physicians will reject euthanasia in all circumstances, because they believe such an act is against the fundamental meaning and purposes of medicine. It would be a fundamental contradiction for a healer and saver of life to administer death. This ethos is rooted in the Hippocratic tradition. In M. Mead's interpretation, it is the Hippocratic Oath and its prohibition of killing that permitted patients to trust physicians without reservation, and permitted physicians to practise the art and science of healing without being conscripted to administer death for social purposes (Mead, 1965, 131).

It is on the level of ethos, the level of interpretation of the constitutive meaning and purpose of medicine, that many physicians disagree about whether euthanasia, as a matter of medical ethics, is ever acceptable. One trend of interpretation, still the most dominant, emphasizes that medicine is dedicated to life, health, and healing, and that doctors, therefore, must never be involved in euthanasia. Were a society ever to accept euthanasia, this view would emphasize that persons other than doctors would have to be trained and authorized to administer death rapidly and painlessly. Doctors should never be involved in the administration of death (Trowell, 1973, 129-130). The trust of patients in their physicians and nurses is an essential factor in the healing process, but how could patients ever really trust their doctors, if patients knew they were involved in the administration of death?

Those who defend the ethical justifiability of physicians' involvement in assisting or administering euthanasia usually appeal to another element in the ethos of medicine, the physician's commitment to the relief of suffering. The assumption in this defence is that suffering, in some circumstances, is so intractable that death is the only practicable relief. There is some controversy about whether the suffering of some patients is so intense as to exceed the powers of relief of modern palliative medicine and palliative care. Some physicians claim they do encounter patients who so suffer, and that they are justified by the ethos of their profession in administering euthanasia in such circumstances.

Care and compassion motivate some physicians to administer euthanasia, when all other available means seem powerless to relieve intensely suffering patients. Thus did Dr. Nigel Cox in England recently inject two ampoules of potassium chloride into a 70-year-old woman, who had suffered for over twenty years from acute rheumatoid arthritis. Mrs. Lilian Boyes's pain was so intense that she could not bear to be touched. She refused all treatment other than painkillers and, when these were no longer having their desired effect, Mrs. Boyes asked Dr. Cox for a fatal injection. He at first refused, then later complied when Mrs. Boyes appeared not about to die rapidly on her own, but likely to continue to live perhaps for days or longer in intense pain (Lewis, 1992; Brahams, 1992).

Doctors who argue that euthanasia is justifiable, in some circumstances of extreme and grinding pain, also confront the issue of patient trust in physicians who would involve themselves in the administration of euthanasia. How, they wonder, can patients really trust physicians, if they know their physicians are forced to abandon them at their moment of greatest need? One physician has claimed that patients and families, mature enough to consider and request euthanasia, will not lose trust in a physician willing to follow them on such a personal path (Boisvert, 1988, 117).

Clinical Ethics

In Chapter 2, emphasis was placed on the patient, body and biography, as the norm of clinical ethics. Practical judgments, about what should or should not be done at any moment to help patients make therapeutic choices that best match their clinical needs and life plans, have to be reached in terms of the patients' clinical courses and their own choices about the treatments and sufferings they are able or unable to bear. This is what respect for the principle of autonomy requires.

We must now consider this principle, the principle of the patient as the norm of clinical ethics, in the context of extreme suffering, even if cases of such are rare, rather than frequent. Even if we assume, and it is correct to do so, that the modern methods of palliative medicine and palliative care are powerful enough to manage adequately most kinds of pain and symptoms, situations do seem to occur when the kind or intensity of suffering surpasses the power of palliative methods.

Chapter 3 alluded to one such situation, the case of the woman in the very terminal stage of throat cancer, who was not expected to live for more than a couple of days and who did not want to die during one of her frequent choking episodes. She did not want her last moments of consciousness to be of that special kind of panic and terror associated with choking. She vigorously nodded her agreement, for she could not speak, when her husband and sons asked the doctor to "put her to sleep" at a time they would indicate during the next couple of days.

The doctor refused to do this, because he saw euthanasia as the only route open to him for complying with their request. Unfortunately, the woman did die two days later, in a choking episode.

This woman was dying. Her death was inevitable and imminent. Her life was already out of the doctor's hands, and anyone else's hands, for that matter. Only the timing of her death was still in the doctor's control. Many would assert that this doctor, upon the woman's silent request and upon the explicit request of her caring family, would have been quite justified ethically in timing that death to occur in a period of tranquillity.

It is quite difficult, if not impossible, to assert in any absolute way that situations never do and never will occur in clinical practice, where advancing death seems to be the only way to give patients relief from certain kinds and intensities of suffering. However, if euthanasia or advancing death may, at times, be clinically and ethically justifiable, or at least ethically tolerable as the lesser of two evils, should euthanasia for that reason be legalized or decriminalized?

SHOULD EUTHANASIA BE LEGALIZED?

Since the Second World War, numerous proposals have outlined how euthanasia could or should be legally regulated, rather than legally banned. These proposals cover a spectrum, from relatively loose arrangements leaving control of euthanasia largely in the hands of doctors, to regulatory schemes favouring bureaucratically heavy systems of safeguards. A detailed analysis of these proposals would far exceed the space available for this chapter, and would also be tangential to our purpose in this section. We are setting out to weigh the reasons advanced for and against the legalization of euthanasia, and to formulate an answer to this section's title question. Though we cannot possibly offer a comprehensive discussion of *how* euthanasia should be regulated if it is to be decriminalized, we cannot avoid considering whether safeguards can be devised that are both adequate and practicable for the avoidance of abuse. This issue is central to any consideration of whether euthanasia should be legalized.

The Case for Legalizing Euthanasia

Most people who accept euthanasia as ethically justifiable, at least in some circumstances, claim that only voluntary euthanasia should be legalized. This means that only those persons who openly and stably desire to die should have death legally administered to them. This position appeals to the values of autonomy, liberty, self-determination, and freedom from suffering, values highly prized in Western societies. Why should those who have the professional knowledge and skills to administer death rapidly and painlessly not be given legal authorization to do so, for those suffering persons who want to advance their deaths, but cannot administer death to themselves because they lack the necessary knowledge, ability, or both? Those favouring legalization of voluntary euthanasia argue that there are no convincing reasons to withhold such legal authorization, and that there are solid grounds for granting such authorization to physicians.

One of the strongest arguments advanced to defend the legalization of voluntary euthanasia combines an advocacy of principle with an assumption of fact. The argument assumes that euthanasia frequently is the only way adequately to relieve intense suffering (a matter of fact) and that it is wrong in such circumstances not to honour patients' informed, lucid, and stable requests for rapid and painless death, as their chosen way of escape from such suffering (a matter of principle). However, if euthanasia is a crime under law, it is extremely difficult for physicians, who believe euthanasia to be ethically acceptable in specified circumstances, to honour a patient's request for euthanasia or for assistance in euthanasia. The physician faces the possibility of prosecution, conviction, imprisonment, removal from the medical register, and destruction of career. Certain features of this schematic summary of the case for legalization deserve amplification.

First, *regarding the principle of autonomy and self-determination*. Some who advocate the legalization of voluntary euthanasia take it, as a starting point, that the voluntary request for euthanasia is a liberty that does not have to be justified. Legal restrictions on this liberty are what require justification. From this point of view, the proper question is not why should people have a legal right to voluntary euthanasia. We should, rather, ask why should criminal law restrain the liberty of a patient and physician, by prohibiting them from doing what they want and choose to do (Morris, 1970, 255).

Moreover, any legal restriction on this liberty should not, in a pluralistic society, be equivalent to the imposition of the religious and moral beliefs of some people on others who hold quite different beliefs. The legal restriction, to be justified, would have to be shown to be a necessary protection of the common good, or the individual good and rights of others who may not desire euthanasia.

Some also emphasize that the request for euthanasia can be voluntary, even if the patient is no longer conscious or lucid enough, at the time euthanasia is to be administered, to confirm his or her earlier express request. Voluntariness is respected in such situations, provided euthanasia is administered under circumstances foreseen and agreed upon in the patient's earlier request, expressed in a living will or via a person whom the patient has appointed to speak in his or her behalf.

Voluntary euthanasia, lastly, requires at least two willing persons, a willing patient and a willing physician. The physician, however, acts in this matter not only as a private person with liberties and rights, but also as a professional, as a public person with obligations and responsibilities. We shall have to return to this point, when we consider the case against legalizing euthanasia.

Second, *regarding the principle of compassion*. The strongest argument brought forth, to defend the legalization of euthanasia, is based on the demands of compassion. Over twenty years ago, A. B. Downing, in advocating the legalization of euthanasia, emphasized that we shall probably never be able to eliminate totally from human experience the suffering that is both hard to bear and hard to behold. He buttressed this observation with the words of the former dean of St. Paul's Cathedral, the Very Reverend W. R. Matthews, who stated: "It seems to be an incontrovertible proposition that, when we are confronted with suffering which is wholly destructive in its consequences and, so far as we can see, could have no beneficial result, there is a *prima facie* duty to bring it to an end." (Downing, 1969, 23)

Though palliative medicine and palliative care have greatly reduced the burdens of pain and suffering in advanced disease, particularly in advanced stages of cancer, it is still quite true, as a recent *Lancet* editorial on the Dr. Nigel Cox case observed, that there is a long way to go before it will be possible to promise that no terminal state is so bad that it cannot be rendered pain-free, with dignity maintained by pharmacological or other means (Editorial, 1992).

There is even more, though, to this matter of compassion. We are all, in Western societies, far away from being able to offer adequate palliative and hospice care to all who might need and desire it. For others, it is not just a question of pain and symptom control that conditions their requests for euthanasia. Some people simply do not want to live for years in varying states of dementia, incapacity, or deep disability. If these persons request euthanasia as their only available escape from unbearable existence, should compassion not also reach out to them?

Moreover, some instances of unbearable existence are iatrogenic. They are the results of laudable attempts to halt the advance of disease and to prolong life. Many patients, now still alive and suffering, would likely have died much earlier in the course of their disease, had doctors not intervened with the full array of medical and surgical treatments, to slow down its advance. These patients gained time, but now, when no power can halt the progression of disease, some of them face a drawn-out course of existence and dying that is extremely difficult to live through.

These unhappy events are not an argument against intervening early in the course of disease, to halt its progress and to extend a patient's life. However, these distressing outcomes of the fight against disease, when they do occur, may well provoke some physicians to think along the lines of Dr. Benrubi's recent reflections:

> In effect, however, although we prolong life, we also prolong agony, and when the agony becomes unbearable we offer no help ...

> As physicians, we agree that we should try to give a patient the additional two years of life, but we refuse to help pay the ultimate price of those two years when it comes due. It is my contention that since we physicians brought the patient to the state she is in, we cannot abandon her by saying that euthanasia violates the purpose of our profession. (Benrubi, 1992, 197-198)

Third, *regarding regulation of euthanasia and safeguards against abuse.* Euthanasia should be legalized, some argue, because in contemporary society we really have only two choices. Either the legal prohibition of euthanasia is maintained, and euthanasia then remains underground and uncontrollable; or euthanasia is legalized, and is then practised in an open and controllable fashion. Many persons in favour of legalizing voluntary euthanasia insist that stringent procedural safeguards are necessary to prevent abuse, notably, the abuse of non-voluntary euthanasia.

The Netherlands is the one society in the Western world in which a middle approach to the regulation of euthanasia has been attempted. Euthanasia has not (yet) been legalized in the Netherlands, but an informal arrangement exists, according to which doctors will not be prosecuted if they respect five guidelines, already presented earlier in this chapter, in their administration of euthanasia.

This informal regulation of euthanasia in the Netherlands increasingly seems to be quite definitely inadequate for the prevention of abuse. The guidelines are vague; they are subject, in fact, to widely divergent interpretation by physicians practising euthanasia, or they are simply ignored (Gomez, 1991, 96-97). Under the informal regulatory arrangement currently in force in the Netherlands, there is, in the view of one Dutch advocate of legalized euthanasia, as reported by John Keown, almost total lack of control of how euthanasia is administered (Keown, 1992, 42). Some, of course, do not agree with these assessments, as may be seen by consulting the Remmelink Report (van der Maas, 1992).

If the one informal approach to the regulation of euthanasia with which we have experience in Western societies does not seem to be working well, should euthanasia, then, be legalized?

The Case Against Legalizing Euthanasia

Those who plead in favour of legalizing or decriminalizing euthanasia appeal to the values of autonomy, compassion, and honesty. Legal safeguards and procedures are required, to assure that only those persons who are suffering unbearably (compassion) and who desire (autonomy) their lives to be terminated rapidly and painlessly would be given euthanasia. The legal prohibition of voluntary euthanasia, so the argument continues, favours clandestine voluntary euthanasia, and such a practice militates against honesty and openness, essential conditions for maintaining an accountable profession and a democratic society.

Though many reasons can be brought forth to construct the case against legalizing euthanasia, we limit our attention, in this chapter, to the illusory character of the assumptions upon which the case in favour of legalization is based.

First, *regarding the voluntariness of euthanasia*. It is highly questionable that any society will be able to uphold the voluntary character of euthanasia, once euthanasia becomes a legally and socially acceptable option. *Voluntary* means freedom from coercion, pressure, undue inducement, and psychological and emotional manipulation. There is no law permitting voluntary euthanasia that could, even if implemented via complex procedures, protect conscious and vulnerable people against subtle manipulation to request socially acceptable administered death, when they would rather live and be cherished. The position in favour of legalizing voluntary euthanasia rests upon an assumption of ideal hospitals, doctors, nurses, and families. That assumption is often illusory, and when it is, in fact, an illusion, the voluntariness of euthanasia is in peril.

Second, *regarding safeguards against nonvoluntary euthanasia*. Those who propose legalization of euthanasia usually claim, but not always, that only voluntary euthanasia should be legally permitted. The assumption is that after legalization of voluntary euthanasia, societies in the Western world would be enduringly willing and able to withstand pressure for extension of euthanasia to those who never were able, or to those who have irreversibly lost the ability, to request or to consent to the termination of their lives.

There are good reasons to believe this assumption is illusory. There are many persons in hospitals, chronic care wards, and nursing homes across the land whose lives, by standards external to themselves and in the eyes of others, are hardly worth living. Many of these persons retain little more than the ability to sense and experience biological pain and comfort, gentleness of care, pleasing sound, human presence, and warmth. Some can hardly experience even these things, but their relatively strong bodies still cling to life.

It is naïve to imagine that social barriers against nonvoluntary euthanasia would not crumble, in a society that legalizes voluntary euthanasia on the basis of compassion. Should compassion not also extend to those who, in the eyes of others, are suffering the indignity of profound mental and physical handicaps, even if they are suffering no pain, but who cannot request euthanasia?

This naïvety is reinforced, when one adverts to the fact that insistence on *voluntary* euthanasia is, for some proponents of euthanasia in the Netherlands, little more than a strategic move towards a much more expanded administration of euthanasia. The 1985 report of the Netherlands State Commission on Euthanasia accepted euthanasia for comatose patients upon family request, when such patients continued to live despite discontinuance of life-prolonging treatments. Moreover, the Dutch Medical Association is reported to be preparing guidelines for euthanasia when persons, such as handicapped newborn children or comatose patients, cannot request or consent to the rapid and painless termination of their lives (de Wachter, 1992, 29). Some physicians in the Netherlands do not even consider such terminations of life to be euthanasia, because they consider that euthanasia, by definition, has to be voluntary. Some would consider the rapid and painless termination of life in these circumstances to be little more than normal medical practice (ten Have, 1992, 35).

Third, *regarding the control of pain and suffering*. The case for legalizing euthanasia appeals to compassion. Euthanasia, it is claimed, should be legalized, because it is inhumane to allow people to continue suffering when they request release by rapid and painless termination of life. The assumptions behind this claim are that patients *frequently* suffer agony from pain that is uncontrollable; and that administration of death is the only effective release from suffering that arises, not from unmanageable pain, but from the human condition.

However, it is simply wrong to assume that pain can be frequently managed only by killing the patient. The binary logic, dying with pain or euthanasia, may have held true in earlier periods, prior to the development of modern methods of palliative medicine and palliative care. That logic needs not hold true anywhere in the world today. For example, the World Health Organization guidelines for the relief of cancer pain have been shown to be effective in controlling pain adequately up to the time of death (Grond, 1991). These guidelines propose both the sequential use, and the skillful combination, of nonopioid and opioid pain medication.

Unfortunately, many doctors and nurses have not mastered the state-of-the-art knowledge and skills that offer adequate management of pain. Where the binary logic, dying with pain or euthanasia, would still hold true, the most reasonable solution would require rapid and widespread education of doctors and nurses in the methods of palliative medicine and palliative care. Legalization of euthanasia is an unjustifiable substitute for such education.

Suffering, as is widely recognized, involves more than the experience of pain. Each person is distinctive, individuated, profoundly different from everyone else. So, also, is each person's suffering. Memories, lost opportunities, guilts, dated moments of hurt and betrayal, the fragility of lovers and joys, loneliness, and unfulfilled dreams are all as unique as the days, times, places, and persons to which they are bound. Suffering of this existential sort is universally part of the human condition, and it can be unbearable for anyone isolated in loneliness. Euthanasia is no adequate answer to this kind of suffering. If such suffering cannot be borne alone, then the solution rests with mobilizing a community of caring persons around those who suffer deeply. Legalization of euthanasia is no civilized substitute for the formation of such communities of care.

Fourth, *regarding the protection of doctors against prosecution.* Some have argued that legalization of euthanasia is needed to protect well-meaning doctors against prosecution, when they administer euthanasia to suffering persons who, on their own initiative, truly request rapid termination of their lives.

The illusion here is in the assumption that a law can be devised, so clear in its conditions and implementation procedures, that professionals and family survivors will generally conclude that a euthanasia-administering doctor honoured the patient's true desires, and abided by all the conditions and procedures of the law. But that honouring and abiding are matters of fact. These are matters that are brought before courts of law, particularly by well-meaning, or even ill-meaning, persons who suspect a physician of insensitivity or negligence, or by families torn by dissension over the fact that death was administered to their relative.

It is quite naïve to imagine that a law permitting voluntary euthanasia would, in Canada, reduce the likelihood or frequency of doctors appearing before the courts to defend their administration of euthanasia. The more frequent these acts of euthanasia would become, the more likely it is that a law permitting voluntary euthanasia would be used as a legal opportunity for the pursuit of doctors by those who do not morally accept the law; or by those who doubt the law was respected in a particular case; or by some grieving family members who believe other family members were all too eager in supporting a loved one's request for euthanasia.

Fifth, *regarding slippage into insensitivity and abuse.* Proposals to legalize euthanasia harbour an illusion. That illusion docks in the bay of well-meaning simplicity, the simplicity of assuming that a society permitting voluntary euthanasia, and tolerating nonvoluntary euthanasia, could remain committed to high standards of care for vulnerable, poor, and marginalized people. The simplicity, and the naïvety, consists in the narrow focus on the particular situation in which one person, a physician, wants to do good for another person, a patient requesting release from unbearable suffering. It is naïve to imagine that a policy and a law permitting euthanasia will not lead to insensitive, inhumane, and intolerable abuse simply because those who designed the law were governed by pure motives and noble purposes (Fairbairn, 1988, 134).

This narrow and naïve focus of attention is blind to what Loren Graham, writing about eugenics and genetics in Russia and Germany during the 1920s, has called "second-order" links between changing values and the uses a society can make of a science or a policy. Second-order links are difficult to see. They depend upon existing, and changing, political and social situations, and upon the persuasiveness of current, and emerging, philosophies and ideologies, however flawed these may be (Graham, 1977). The abuses that a law permitting euthanasia could come to serve depend upon second-order links between such a law and currently latent, or later emergent, ideologies of human insensitivity.

When Karl Binding, a doctor of jurisprudence and philosophy, and Alfred Hoche, a doctor of medicine, published their book on euthanasia in 1920, they were, in all probability, unable to foresee the second-order links between their benevolent ideas on euthanasia and an emerging ideology that would lead, within less than twenty years, to the Nazi euthanasia programmes. But these links were eventually forged, and evidence at the Nuremberg trials established the influence this book exerted on those who designed and implemented the Nazi programmes.

Those who favour legalization of voluntary euthanasia believe it to be utterly unproven and quite unlikely that legalization of euthanasia will provoke a societal slide down the slippery slope to intolerable abuses. Admittedly, such a slide is not certain. The issue is whether we should try this social experiment.

Voluntary Euthanasia Should Not Be Legalized

At the end of this century, the signs in Western societies of overt discrimination, of latent racism, and of utilitarian insensitivity to vulnerable people are too prominent to justify insouciant attitudes regarding the legalization of euthanasia. The law prohibiting euthanasia, even voluntary euthanasia, should be maintained.

Yet, there is no law that can exactly match the infinite variety of human and clinical situations. In some situations, advancing death may seem to be the only adequate way of bringing patients their desired relief. We need not change our laws, to guarantee doctors immunity from prosecution in circumstances that seem to justify euthanasia. We need, rather, to perfect communication between patients, families, doctors, and clinical staff so that, when such circumstances arise, all together will know and come to agree on what is the right thing to do. It is not inconsistent to judge certain acts of hastening death to be ethically justifiable, or at least ethically tolerable, and yet simultaneously to maintain that laws should not be changed to grant doctors or anyone else advance legal authorization to administer euthanasia.

Some will raise the objection: but doctors will be uncertain and concerned that someone could still accuse them of murder. They will then administer ethically justifiable euthanasia, if they do at all, only in fear and trembling of the possible legal consequences they may have to endure.

Chaim Perelman, professor of law at the University of Brussels, has considered this situation. He draws attention to the fictions that juries and judges use, in exceptional circumstances, to avoid applying the law against persons who have committed acts against the law, but acts that are seen as ethically understandable and justifiable in the particular circumstances. The fiction in question consists in a jury "qualifying facts in a way contrary to reality, by declaring that the accused has not committed murder, and it does this to avoid applying the law." (Perelman, 1980, 41) In Perelman's view, this recourse to fiction "is better than providing expressly, in law, for the fact that euthanasia is a case for justification or excuse." (Perelman, 1980, 118) The "perjured jury" has an honoured place in the administration of justice but many legal systems do not have a jury system; for example, the Netherlands.

We share Perelman's belief that indulgent legislation in the matter of euthanasia would court the risk of grave abuse. We should all rally to protect those who, in rare circumstances, know how to exercise charismatic authority, the authority that consists in knowing what to do when all established ethical and legal rules fail to apply. We should not, however, give facile credence to those who would want to generalize that exercise of charismatic authority. It is sane, not inhumane, to surround those who would administer beneficent death with spotlights of vigilance. Fear and trembling in this matter is not a bad thing at all.

REFERENCES

Alexander L. "Medical Science Under Dictatorship." *The New England Journal of Medicine* 1949;241:39-47. The full reference for the German medical journal article is given in reference 2 of Dr. Alexander's article.

Ariès P. *Western Attitudes Toward Death: From the Middle Ages to the Present.* Baltimore and London: The John Hopkins University Press, 1974:1-25.

Battin M.P. "Assisted Suicide: Can We Learn from Germany?" *Hastings Center Report* 1992;22/2:44-51.

Benrubi G.I. "Euthanasia -The Need for Procedural Safeguards." *The New England Journal of Medicine* 1992;326:197-199.

Binding K. and **Hoche A.** *Die Freigabe der Vernichtung lebensunwerten Lebens: Ihr Mass und ihre Form.* Leipzig: F. Meiner, 1920. A new English translation of this book, under the title, "Permitting the Destruction of Unworthy Life," appeared in the journal *Issues in Law & Medicine* 1992;8/2:231-265.

Boisvert M. All Things Considered ... Then What?" *Journal of Palliative Care* 1988;4/1-2:115-118.

Brahams D. "Euthanasia: Doctor Convicted of Attempted Murder." *Lancet* 1992;340:782-783.

de Wachter M.A.M. "Euthanasia in the Netherlands." *Hastings Center Report* 1992;22/2:23-30.

Downing A.B. "Euthanasia: The Human Context." In: A.B. Downing, ed. *Euthanasia and the Right to Death*. London: Peter Owen, 1969:13-24.

Editorial "Final Exit: Euthanasia Guide Sells Out." *Nature* 1991;352:553.

Editorial "The Final Autonomy." *Lancet* 1992;340:757-758.

Fairbairn G.J. "Kuhse, Singer and Slippery Slopes." *Journal of Medical Ethics* 1988;14:132-134.

Freeman J. "Is There a Right to Die -Quickly?" *Journal of Pediatrics* 1972;80/5:904-905.

Gillon R. "Euthanasia, Withholding Life-Prolonging Treatment, and Moral Differences Between Killing and Letting Die." *Journal of Medical Ethics* 1988;14:115-117.

Gomez C.F. *Regulating Death: Euthanasia and the Case of the Netherlands*. New York: The Free Press, 1991.

Graham L.R. "Political Ideology and Genetic Theory: Russia and Germany in the 1920s." *Hastings Center Report* 1977;7/5:30-39.

Grond S. et al. "Validation of World Health Organization Guidelines for Cancer Pain Relief During the Last Days and Hours of Life." *Journal of Pain and Symptom Management* 1991;6/7:411-422.

Keown J. "On Regulating Death." *Hastings Center Report* 1992;22/2:39-43.

Law Reform Commission of Canada *Euthanasia, Aiding Suicide, and Cessation of Treatment*. Report #20. Ottawa: Ministry of Supply and Services Canada, 1983.

Lewis J. "Doctor Convicted of Mercy Killing." *Manchester Guardian* September 27, 1992:3.

Lifton R.J. *The Nazi Doctors. Medical Killing and the Psychology of Genocide*. New York: Basic Books, 1986.

Marker R.L. "The Ethical Values that Civil Law Must Respect in the Field of Euthanasia." *The Linacre Quarterly* August 1989:22-35.

Mead M. "From Black and White Magic to Modern Medicine." *22 Proceedings of the Rudolf Virchow Medical Society*, 1965.

Millard C.K. *Euthanasia*. London: C.W. Daniel, 1931.

Mitscherlich A. and **Mielke R.** *Doctors of Infamy. The Story of the Nazi Medical Crimes*. New York: Henry Schuman, 1949.

Morris A.A. "Voluntary Euthanasia." *Washington Law Review* 1970;45:239-271.

Motto J.A. "Rational Suicide and Medical Ethics." In: M.D. Basson, ed. *Rights and Responsibilities in Modern Medicine*. New York: Alan R. Liss, 1981:201-209.

Narveson J. "Moral Philosophy and Suicide." *Canadian Journal of Psychiatry* 1986;31: 104-107.

Perelman C. *Justice, Law and Argument.* Dordrecht, Boston, London: D. Reidel, 1980.

Quill T.E. "Death and Dignity. A Case of Individualized Decision Making." *The New England Journal of Medicine* 1991;324:691-694.

Rachels J. *The End of Life: Euthanasia and Morality.* New York: Oxford University Press, 1986.

Sneiderman B. "Euthanasia in the Netherlands: A Model for Canada?" *Humane Medicine* 1992;8/2:104-115.

ten Have H.A.M.J. and **Welie J.V.M.** "Euthanasia: Normal Medical Practice?" *Hastings Center Report* 1992;22/2:34-38.

Trowell H. *The Unfinished Debate on Euthanasia.* London: SCM Press, 1973.

van der Maas P.J., **van Delden J.J.M.** and **Pijnenborg L.** *Euthanasia and Other Medical Decisions Concerning the End of Life.* An investigation performed upon request of the Commission of Inquiry into the Medical Practice Concerning Euthanasia. Amsterdam: Elsevier, 1992.

Williams G. *The Sanctity of Life and the Criminal Law.* New York: Alfred A. Knopf, 1957.

P A R T 5

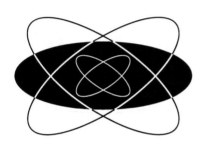

BIOETHICS:
ON THE
FRONTIERS

18

BIOETHICS ON THE FRONTIERS OF THE HUMAN GENOME PROJECT

SCIENCE, ETHICS, AND SOCIETY

The need for critical reflection and vigilance, over the uses made of new scientific knowledge and technology, is no less now at the end of this century than it was in the 1960s, when Salvador Luria, writing about genetic therapy and genetic engineering as future possibilities emerging from deep discoveries in molecular biology, called for leadership to awaken the public and government from complacent attachment to distorted priorities (Luria, 1969, 409).

Writing at mid-century, Peter Medawar saw the great glory, as well as the great threat of science, as linked to the trend that anything that is, in principle, possible, can be done, if the intention to do it is sufficiently resolute. Medawar then observed that, while scientists exalt in the glory of science, the reaction of ordinary people in the middle of the twentieth century is more often to cower at the threat of science (Medawar, 1990, 15).

In the 1990s, people are less likely to cower at the threat of science, and they are more awakened to the momentous events occurring in biological science and technology than they were in the 1960s. Scientists still do exult in the glory of science, and they sometimes speak of their work in metaphors suggesting a sacred mission, as when they describe the human genome project (to be discussed below) as a search for the "holy grail" (Kevles, 1992, viii; Gilbert, 1992, 83). Yet, scientists have also shown that they are capable of taking the initiative in drawing attention to the ethical implications of their work, as they did at the Gordon Conference in 1973, when the discovery of recombinant DNA was announced, and as they did when they met at Asilomar in 1975, to devise guidelines for work with recombinant DNA technology (about which more will be said later in this chapter); indeed, as they are still doing today (Suzuki and Knudtson, 1989).

Between the 1960s and the 1990s, a new method evolved, as mentioned at the end of Chapter 2, to identify and confront the ethical and social implications and dangers of new and powerful developments in biological science and technology. People recognize more clearly now than they did thirty years ago, that social control of scientific technologies destined to exert major social impact requires more than scientists' reflection on the ethical implications of their own work, as necessary and laudable as the ethical initiatives of scientists are. The new method of bioethics brings together people from many different walks of life and professions, to work with scientists in devising alternatives to the idea, mirrored in Medawar's statement above, that power is its own ethic. That collaboration inevitably involves tension, particularly so when the reductionist method of science (the attempt to understand wholes, likes organisms, in terms of their ever-smaller parts, the cells and genes), of itself necessary and valid, is held to be both the only valid scientific method and the preferred approach to understand and solve complex social problems, as well.

As thoughtful people have already realized, the availability of a complete map (location of the genes in the chromosomes) and sequence (order of the large molecules making up the gene) of the entire human genome, the twin objectives of the human genome project, will have wide and profound social significance. A complete *biological book* on humankind will enormously increase scientific ability to "read," "edit," and "rewrite" the genes upon which human structures and functions depend (National Research Council, 1988, 100).

The ethical challenge, over the coming decade, will be to mount a concerted effort of people throughout the world to specify the goals for which this new power should be used; and to mount observatories of vigilance, to prevent potential abuses of a power over life — over human, animal, and plant life — quite unlike any known before in history.

THE ASSUMPTIONS, OBJECTIVES, AND LIMITS OF THE CHAPTER

The Limits

The tools and methods of genetic engineering, deriving from the discovery and development of recombinant DNA technology over the last twenty years, have a wide range of applications (Murrell, 1989). It is the use of genetic engineering, for example, in the construction of transgenic mice (mice in which genes from other species, for example, human genes, have been inserted) and in many other applications that has propelled some of the most spectacular advances of basic research in molecular biology and genetics (Suzuki et al., 1989; Darnell, 1990). The methods of genetic engineering have become indispensable for studies in human, animal, and plant biology (Coldspring Harbor, 1986).

The techniques of genetic engineering are being used to alter animals and plants for commercial purposes, and to synthesize new drugs in the pharmaceutical industry. These applications, and applications of genetic engineering in the human genome project as well, raise vexing ethical, scientific, and legal questions about the patenting of life forms, questions that surpass the scope of this chapter (U.S. Congress, 1989). We would also need an entire chapter to cover current debates about forensic uses of tests resulting from genetic engineering. Use of these tests to identify criminals, from even minute samples of blood, sperm, or bodily tissue left at the scene of a crime, have come to be known as "DNA fingerprinting." These tests are currently the centre of intense controversy on the reliability and legitimacy of science-based evidence, and the rights of suspects who are presumed innocent (Neufeld, 1990; Chakraborty, 1991; Lewontin, 1991; Kirby, 1990; Lander, 1989).

This chapter will concentrate exclusively on issues relating to the genetic diagnostic tests and genetic therapies resulting from applications of genetic engineering, on the controversial prospect of applying genetic engineering to the human germ line (to ova and spermatozoa, and hence to future generations), and on uses of genetic technology to achieve the mapping and sequencing objectives of the human genome project.

The Objectives

Mapping and sequencing of the human genome have been underway now for many years. The particular *novelty* of the human genome project is its aim to map and sequence that genome *rapidly*, and in its *totality*. This chapter seeks *first* of all to situate the human genome project historically, to sketch the scientific developments leading up to the project, and to review the evolution of ethical concern that has followed closely upon the heels of these developments. *Second*, the human genome project itself will be described, and attention paid to some of the major methodological, social, and ethical issues it raises. *Third*, as Chapter 7 identified the major ethical issues associated with prenatal and preimplantation diagnosis, this chapter will introduce the social and ethical issues raised by *presymptomatic diagnosis and screening*. The ability to diagnose the presence of a genetic defect that will inevitably, or with varying degrees of probability, come to expression as severe and lethal disease only later in life, such as Huntington's disease, introduces novel and unique kinds of ethical conflicts into medical practice, and into society. The emerging practice of predictive and probabilistic medicine, which will be based on an ever-expanding set of presymptomatic tests of genetic susceptibility to monogenic and polygenic diseases, will shift issues of *discrimination, confidentiality,* and *privacy,* already socially dominant in the HIV epidemic, square into the predominant centre of social, legal, and ethical discourse over the next decade. This chapter will show why these issues acquire dramatic new importance, in the wake of the advancing human genome project. *Fourth, genetic therapy,* foreseen as a future possibility in ethical discussions of genetics in the 1950s and 1960s, is now being offered increasingly as experimental treatment for a number of diseases primarily caused by gene defects. Where gene therapy is now, and under what conditions this experimental therapy is ethically acceptable, are two questions we shall discuss in this chapter. *Fifth,* what some people fear most is that the powerful tools of genetic engineering may be used, one day, for purposes having little to do with therapy and much to do with the redesign of human structure and the modification of human behaviour. At the present time, that fear precipitates into intense discussions of the pros and cons of genetic modification of the human germ line. Germ-line intervention would introduce irreversible changes into the sex cells, into the ovum and spermatozoon, changes potentially beneficial or disastrous, that would be passed on to future generations. The chapter will close with a consideration of this debate, a debate that extends the discussion of eugenics opened at the end of Chapter 7.

The Assumptions

Basic assumptions set the direction, and shape the content of any discussion. The following are some of the key assumptions, those at least that we can most readily identify, that guide the discussion in this chapter.

First, developments in science and technology are continuous and cumulative. Apparently small advances in seemingly unrelated disciplines slowly, at times more rapidly, accumulate and evanesce into the critical mass required for an explosion of socially significant, and controversial, human applications.

Second, ethical complacency is a luxury people cannot afford in this era of high technology in the life sciences. Ethical, legal, and social responses to the multiple challenges, problems, and opportunities of new power are not ready-made. They have to be invented with the same height and breadth, and with the same vigour, of intelligence that is at work in scientific and technological innovation.

Third, of the two principal approaches one can observe at work in bioethics over the last twenty years or so, namely, *condition ethics* and *assumption ethics,* greater emphasis will have to be given to assumption ethics over the next decade. *Condition ethics* seeks to answer the pragmatic, or "how," question, "Under what terms and within what limits may a given project or course of action be undertaken, maintained, and accepted in society?" *Assumption ethics* is more radical. It is concerned with matters of principle, or with the "whether" question. It centres critical reflection on the governing beliefs, presuppositions, concepts, and language that control the practice of *condition ethics*. Whereas *condition ethics* tends to the conclusion, "Yes, this project may go ahead, but only if the following conditions are met!" *assumption ethics*, when it comes to the crunch, tends to the imperative, "It makes no sense to contribute to the best possible conduct of a project that should not be done at all!"

The relationship between these two approaches in bioethics is not binary, in the sense that it is not a matter of choosing one or the other. Quite the contrary! While both approaches are necessary, there is a tension to be honoured in the emphasis given to either, at any particular moment in the science/technology-society relationship. We believe now is the time to emphasize critical reflection on the language and metaphors (such as the terms "holy grail," "biological book on humankind," and "editing or rewriting the genes") used to interpret the meaning of new power in genetics, and to adjudicate the purposes that power will serve. Moreover, as technological power penetrates ever more deeply towards reductionist mastery over the genetic origins of life, questions about what is and what is not "distinctively human" will become increasingly inescapable. Philosophical neutrality in the face of these questions could become incompatible with the protection of the common good (Roy, 1986, 106). That is why greater emphasis on *assumption ethics* will be needed over the coming decade.

ASSEMBLAGE OF THE KNOWLEDGE AND TECHNOLOGY FOR THE HUMAN GENOME PROJECT

Three Fundamental Questions About Genes

Students throughout the world today know that genes, the carriers of hereditary information from one generation to the next, are made of deoxyribonucleic acid (DNA). Scientists did not know this in the early 1940s, nor did they know how genes are structured. This genetic code linking DNA to messenger RNA, and governing the synthesis of amino acids to form enzymes and proteins was also still a mystery at the end of World War II.

By the early 1950s, the work of scientists such as Oswald Avery, Alfred Hershey, Martha Chase, Erwin Chargaff, and others demonstrated definitively that genes are made up of long molecules of DNA, and that DNA is composed of units of adenylic, guanylic, thymidylic, and cytidylic acid, units that came to be known as nucleotides (Avery, 1944; Chargaff, 1951; Hershey, 1952).

In 1953, James Watson and Francis Crick proposed their now-famous double helix mode of DNA structure. They demonstrated that DNA is made up of two chains of nucleotides, intertwined in the form of a double helix, and the nucleotides adenine (A), thymine (T), cytosine (C), and guanine (G) are ordered by the complementarity principle that pairs A with T, and C with G (Watson, 1953).

By the mid-1960s, the combined work of many scientists had deciphered the genetic code. A few basic facts about the *chemical logic of life* (Murrell, 1989, 12) sketch the framework for understanding how this code works. That logic can be summarized in four interlinked steps, somewhat as follows: the properties of living organisms result from the proteins they contain, and the human organism contains an estimated 30,000 proteins; the proteins are determined by the sequence of the amino acids of which they are constituted; the amino acid sequence, in turn, is governed by the order of the nucleotides in messenger RNA; and that order is determined by the sequence of nucleotides in the DNA of the genes.

The various combinations of the twenty amino acids involved in the building of proteins are put together in a part of the cell called the cytoplasm, which surrounds the cell nucleus containing the chromosomes and genes. The chemical information determining which amino acids are combined to make which proteins comes from the DNA within the cell nucleus. This information is coded in the sequence of the nucleotides A, T, C, and G of the DNA, and is carried to the protein-building part of the cell, the cytoplasm, by messenger RNA (ribonucleic acid). The nucleotides of messenger RNA are similar to those of DNA, except that messenger RNA contains the nucleotide uracil (U) instead of thymine (T).

A code establishes a rule of correspondence between two sets of symbols. In the case of the genetic code, the correspondence is between two chemical "alphabets": the four-letter "alphabet" of messenger RNA, consisting of A, U, C, and G, and the twenty-letter "alphabet" consisting of the twenty amino acids. Groups of three nucleotides, for example, AUG, GGC, or CAG, called triplet codons, determine which amino acids will be assembled in what sequence to form the variety of proteins in the human organism. The very recent report (March 1993) of the discovery of the gene involved in Huntington's disease indicates that it is an excess of the triplet codon CAG that causes the protein disorder leading to the devastating physical and mental symptoms of this disease (Angier, 1993, A16).

The genetic code was not broken in one stroke of genius. The deciphering of that code emerged slowly from the work of many scientists, and the story is complex (Judson, 1979). However, by 1959, the two essential steps governed by the genetic code — the *transcription* of DNA into messenger RNA, and the *translation* of messenger RNA for assembling and combining the amino acids — had been worked out. The research of François Jacob and Jacques Minod in Paris was of central importance (Jacob, 1961). The answer to the question about which particular sequences of the nucleotides select which amino acid in the construction of proteins emerged from the work of Marshall Nirenberg and Heinrich Matthaei at the National Institutes of Health in the U.S (Nirenberg, 1961).

The question about the genetic code was basically answered by the mid-1960s. That code has 64 triplet codons (four nucleotides occupying any of three positions in the codon gives 4^3 or 64 possibilities), the majority of which select amino acids for the construction of proteins. Three of the 64 codons act as stop signals in the construction of the amino acid chains.

Recombinant DNA and Genetic Engineering Technology

The Gordon Research Conference on Nucleic Acids, held in June 1973, announced a technical innovation in molecular biology: the development of methods to fabricate biologically active or living hybrid molecules, by recombining genes from different forms of life. The techniques came to be known as recombinant DNA technology, or simply recombinant DNA. The power of this technology derives from its ability to manipulate the chemistry of life, to determine and modify precisely the nucleotide sequences defining the hereditary messages genes transmit from one generation to the other.

Recombinant DNA technology involved the *splicing of genes* from one form of life, for example, animals and humans, to another form of life, for example, bacteria, and the production of multiple copies of a gene or of a DNA fragment, a process called *molecular cloning.* Molecular cloning suggested the need to establish DNA libraries. Some of the world's oldest and best libraries possess only fragments, not complete texts, of the ancient writers. Diel's edition of the fragments of the pre-Socratic philosophers is an example. These fragments are all the world will ever know of these works, because the complete originals have been forever lost or destroyed. The DNA libraries now in existence contain copies, or clones, of genes or fragments of DNA from the human genome. The goal of the human genome project, as we shall see, is to provide the complete genetic text of human life.

Gene transfer and *directed mutagenesis,* tools in the genetic engineering kit, depend upon recombinant DNA technology. The methods of *gene transfer* enable scientists to splice specific genes into cells, not only into lines of cells cultured in the laboratory, but into the body cells and germ-line cells (the ova and spermatozoa from which new generations arise) of living animals. In one of the earlier gene transfer experiments, the rabbit gene for the protein beta-globin was microinjected into mouse eggs shortly after fertilization. The rabbit gene worked in the resulting adult mice and was transmitted to their offspring (Wagner, 1981). When scientists in another experiment transferred human growth hormone genes into fertilized mouse eggs, the resulting mice grew more rapidly than other mice and attained double their normal size (Palmiter, 1983). The creation of transgenic mice is now a routine procedure for research in molecular biology and genetics. *Directed mutagenesis* is the precisely targeted, nonrandom modification of the genome. Scientists now quite routinely use directed mutagenesis to create so-called "knockout" mice as models to study how the loss of a specific gene affects development and functioning of the animal organism, and of animal behaviour as well. Knockout mice — mice having a specific gene deleted from their genome — also serve as animal models for the study of human diseases, such as cystic fibrosis (Barinaga, 1992).

A map allows one to find one's way successfully to cities in a strange region or country, and then to locate a desired street in that city, and then to find the building or house where one's meeting is to take place. Analytical tables of contents and indexes in large books, are also maps of a kind, helping the reader to find a passage of interest among the thousands of other paragraphs bearing no relation to the purpose at hand. One also needs maps of a special kind to find genes within the nucleus of the cell. To map a gene, or *gene mapping*, means locating its precise position on a particular chromosome (McKusick, 1993).

Until the late 1970s, human gene mapping was a relatively slow process, with about four genes among the estimated 100,000 or so genes in the human genome being mapped per month. Applications of recombinant DNA technology accelerated the process. Nevertheless, since the discovery that the gene for Huntington's disease is somewhere on the upper arm of chromosome 4 (Gusella, 1983), it has taken ten years of grueling search to locate that gene precisely, to find the house on the street, as it were. The laborious search for the Huntington's disease gene, following upon quite recent location of the genes for Duchenne muscular dystrophy and for cystic fibrosis, may well mark the end of one era in gene mapping. The tracking down of the genes for specific diseases, one after the other, will now most likely give way to the increasing involvement of scientists in systematic gene mapping efforts of the human genome project (Angier, 1993, A16).

Ignorance of how the letters of the alphabet are arranged to form words is called illiteracy. *Gene sequencing*, another of the tools of genetic engineering, reveals how the nucleotides are arranged to form genes. It is the key to genetic literacy, to the ability to "read and write" genes.

Towards the end of the 1970s, Allan Maxam and Walter Gilbert at Harvard University, and Frederick Sanger and colleagues at Cambridge University, developed two methods for relatively rapid DNA sequencing, or to continue with the metaphor, for speed reading of genes (Maxam, 1977; Sanger, 1977). The genome of the human mitochondrion, a small rod-shaped structure in the human cell, was completely sequenced using the Sanger method. That work took quite a bit of time, and the mitochondrion genome is only 16,569 nucleotide pairs in length. If a thousand nucleotide pairs, called base pairs, is a kilobase, the human mitochondrion is about 16.5 kilobases. Sequencing the entire human genome, one of the objectives of the human genome project, will require the sequencing of approximately 3 million kilobases, or 3 billion base pairs. One of the preliminary steps of the human genome project, as we shall see, will be towards development of sequencing technology more rapid and efficient than the methods used in the late 1970s and early 1980s.

The proposal to launch the human genome project emerged from uses scientists all over the world were making of the tools of genetic engineering to map, clone, and sequence various bits of DNA in the human genome. We turn to that project, after examining briefly the emergence of ethical discourse on molecular biology, before the announcement of recombinant DNA technology and throughout the debate on this technology in the 1970s.

THE EMERGENCE OF ETHICAL DISCOURSE ON MOLECULAR BIOLOGY AND GENETICS

Over a period of twenty years, from the early 1940s to the mid-1960s, the powerful discoveries in genetics and molecular biology discussed above occurred largely in laboratories, insulated from public debate and controversy. The scientific moves, if not the ethical rules, of the game in molecular biology were set while the people were scientifically asleep or preoccupied elsewhere. There were few, if any, passionate expressions of concern or warnings of danger about genetics, during the two decades following World War II.

A literature of awakening began to appear in the 1960s and early 1970s, even before the 1973 Gordon Conference announcement of the recombinant DNA innovation, an innovation that provoked intense ethical and social controversy throughout the remainder of the 1970s. Scientists, such as Robert Sinsheimer and Salvador Luria, and people working in disciplines such as law, philosophy, ethics, sociology, and theology stood up to draw the attention of the general public to momentous happenings in the biological sciences (Roy, 1991, 3).

Ten years before scientists, accompanied by some lawyers and journalists, met at Asilomar in California to devise guidelines for laboratory work with recombinant DNA technology, Rollin Hotchkiss let his imagination probe the future. He envisioned that a programme of genetic engineering could be turned to frightful and mischievous ends, such as secret intervention on the genes of individual persons, or the establishment of farms of cultured human cells for producing markers, that could then be inserted into viruses for rapid copying and subsequent transfer, by viral infection, into deficient people (Hotchkiss, 1965). A decade or so later, viral vectors did come to be used for gene transfer and as one possible instrument for gene therapy. Although Hotchkiss was right on that point, his apocalyptic scenarios have, up to now, remained in the realm of his imagination.

In 1966, Robert Sinsheimer raised the theme of rational, that is, genetic control of human structure and function. After speaking about future possible genetic therapy and genetic control of growth and aging, he raised the spectre, some might say the dream, of genetic modification of the physique, emotions, and intelligence of human beings, all of which are, at least in part, the outcome of inheritance patterns (Sinsheimer, 1966).

In 1968, Martin Golding warned in the *UCLA Law Review* that it would be in the field of biological engineering that a crisis of confidence would roar between society and science, between ordinary people and scientists. He went on to invoke the possibility of employing that engineering for what he called "atypogenics," the creation of abnormal, weird, and bizarre organisms. He recognized these applications as being science-fictional at the time of his writing, but feared they could become reality on the basis of the principle, similar to the one of Medawar mentioned above, that any new technique discovered is generally put to use (Golding, 1968, 447).

Three years later, Salvador Luria's article, already cited, emphasized the awesome possibilities in the future of genetic surgery — the correction, replacement, removal, or addition of genes — and identified highly controversial potential future applications of molecular biology, such as the insertion of supposedly "desirable genes" in modifications of the human germ line (Luria, 1969, 407-408).

The literature of awakening of the 1960s and 1970s, sampled above, illustrates ethical reflection emerging as an early warning system about where science could be heading, and about the dangers against which society might have to prepare itself. Many of these essays used inflated, promethean, and even inflammatory language. The authors, as said above, stood up to awaken and warn the people. Some scientists, if one can judge from their strong criticism of this literature, seem to have believed that these "prophets" should have stayed sealed and silent (Thomas, 1977). Yet, this literary genre serves its societal purpose, if it mobilizes people to participate effectively in defining the public values, purposes, and corresponding new institutions needed to master the novel and deep powers of scientific and technological innovation (Roy, 1986, 112). The arrival of recombinant DNA technology offered the first major test, from the domain of molecular biology, of how society would respond to a new technology marked by risks of danger and promise of benefit that were, at the outset, largely conjectural.

Intense public debate preceded, accompanied, and followed the Asilomar meeting in 1975 (Watson, 1981). During these debates, Maxine Singer, a scientist, cited the failure of scientists to educate the people adequately, and emphasized that it should be not surprising "if deep fears and ambiguities arise in the minds and hearts of those who suddenly learn the depths of modern insights into the nature of living things."(Singer, 1977, 30)

The recombinant DNA debate propelled people to educate *themselves*. The Cambridge Experimentation Review Board, appointed by the City of Cambridge, Massachusetts, to consider questions of safety relative to recombinant DNA, was composed of nonscientists. The members met several hours each week for four months, and spent even more time on their scientific homework to prepare for the meetings. Though this review board recommended that research on recombinant DNA should continue, it also emphasized that decisions regarding potentially dangerous scientific inquiry must not be left to the inner circles of the scientific establishment (Nelkin, 1978, 191).

By the early 1980s, attention had shifted from discussions about the safety and regulation of recombinant DNA to discussions about patenting rights on new forms of life fabricated in the laboratory, an issue revisited in the early 1990s, in connection with the human genome project. Attention also centred on the propriety of emerging industrial-academic-corporate connections based on biotechnology's growing commercial power (Roy, 1986, 158-161). Controversy within the scientific-medical community at this time centred on an attempt, generally judged to be premature, at human gene therapy using recombinant DNA methods. Speculation in the early 1980s also centred on completing the total map of the human genome, an achievement that would be accomplished by the early 1990s, in the view of one expert (Williamson, 1982, 418). We have arrived at one of the main objectives of the human genome project.

THE HUMAN GENOME PROJECT: SCIENCE AND IDEOLOGY

An earlier section of this chapter has already introduced the concepts of *gene mapping* and *gene sequencing*. The *human genome project (HGP)* is the mammoth international undertaking to map and sequence the entire human genome over fifteen years, with 1990 taken as the starting point. France, Italy, Japan, the United Kingdom, the United States, Canada, the European Community, and Russia are involved in the project with genome programmes of their own. Institutions such as the Centre d'étude du polymorphidone humain (CEPH) in France, the Howard Hughes Medical Institute (HHMI) in the United States, the United Nations Educational, Scientific, and Cultural Organization (UNESCO), and the Human Genome Organization (HUGO) carry varying degrees of responsibility for coordinating the project (Yager, 1991, 454). It is estimated that the total cost of the project, over fifteen years, will be in the order of three billion U.S. dollars.

We refer readers to the selection of the literature published since 1987, on administrative, historical, and methodological aspects of this project, a discussion of which would far exceed the space of a chapter (National Research

Council, 1988; U.S. Congress, 1988; Kevles, 1992; Watson 1990). We shall limit our attention, in this section, to a succinct overview of the science of the project, including its goals, the logic linking these goals, and what may possibly result from its successful completion. Secondly, we shall briefly examine the claim that this project reflects a reductionistic and deterministic view of human life, health, and disease.

The Human Genome Project: An Overview of the Science

The human genome project really encompasses two closely related projects, one centring on the human genome, the other aiming at a complete understanding of the function of the genes in the genomes of four so-called *model organisms*: the bacterium *Escherichia coli (or E.coli)*, the nematode worm, *caenorhabditis elegans*, the fruit fly *drosophila melanogaster*, and eventually the *mouse*. We seek to understand the objectives of each project, and the logic linking them.

The complete sequencing of the DNA in the entire human genome is the ultimate objective of the human genome project. The entire DNA in the human genome is *not* set out in *one* long helical double chain, but is packaged into 46 such chains in the chromosomes. The chromosomes are paired, so there are 24 distinct chromosomes in the human cell, the 22 autosomes and the two sex chromosomes, the X and Y chromosomes. The genes of the human genome, generally estimated to number about 100,000 (estimated, because no one at this moment really knows exactly how many genes the human genome contains), are laid out along the length of the chromosomes. Before these genes can be sequenced, they have to be mapped so that they can be found. Consequently, complete sequencing of the human genome depends on the precise location of the genes on the 24 distinct chromosomes. Total mapping of the human genome, then, requires 24 maps, one for each of the chromosomes.

The first phase of the human genome project aims at mapping and locating the genes on each of the chromosomes. Two principal kinds of maps, called genetic-linkage maps and physical maps — the details of which need not occupy us here — are being used to achieve this goal. As of July 15, 1992, and as can be seen on the wall chart published in *Science* of the concurrent state of progression in gene mapping, 2,372 genes, 612 of these being disease-related genes, have been mapped on the 24 distinct chromosomes. For example, 225 genes, 111 of these disease-related, have been mapped on the X chromosome; 39 genes, 8 disease-related, have been mapped on chromosome 22. (Jasny, 1992).

Complete sequencing of the human genome, within the deadlines set for the project, will require the development of more rapid and efficient sequencing technology, one of the technical objectives of the HGP (Hunkapiller, 1991). The sequence of a gene, as said earlier, is the complete DNA text of the gene made up of the nucleotides A, T, C, G, set out in their proper order. For example, the gene for beta-globin, a protein of 146 amino acids, that forms part of the molecule carrying oxygen in the blood, has 1,500 nucleotides. The first line of the sequence of one of the two DNA strands of this gene, read from left to right, runs: *CCCTGTGGAGCCACACCCTAGGGTTGGCCA*, and there are 67 such lines of this length in the entire sequence text of the beta-globin gene (National Research Council, 1988, 21). Since the DNA in the entire human genome has about three billion of these nucleotides, the similar text of the total sequence of the human genome would probably fill a thousand thousand-page telephone books (Gilbert, 1992, 84), or something like 13 sets of the *Encyclopedia Britannica*.

Once the sequencing of the human genome is completed, how is that massive sequence text to be interpreted? Making sense of the sequence text means answering the question: what do all these sequence genes do? How do they function? What is the meaning or function of the particular ways these genes are ordered in the total sequence text?

The second of the projects of the HGP, namely, mapping, sequencing, and determining the function of the genes in the *model organisms* mentioned above is being undertaken to assist interpretation of the total sequence text of the human genome. The principle linking the *model organism* project to the *project of understanding the human genome* is found in the fact that many of the genes of these smaller organisms function in ways very similar to corresponding human genes, for example, the genes controlling development of nerve, muscle, and intestine tissues (Green, 1991, 1971). This principle even links human genes to genes in yeast, since the human genes controlling regulation of the cell cycle and cell growth can substitute for the corresponding genes in yeast (Lee, 1987). Of course, the mouse is much more closely related to the human organism than is yeast. The creation of transgenic and knockout mice, already mentioned in an earlier section, is a powerful and promising approach to achieving understanding of the function of genes in the human genome.

The Likely Impact of the Human Genome Project on Medicine

Though the human genome project is widely expected to facilitate and propel research and development in a diversity of scientific disciplines, such as developmental, evolutionary, and population biology, and in commercially related fields, such as agriculture and pharmacology, the more immediately challenging ethical impacts of the HGP are likely to be seen in medicine. Certain presymptomatic tests for highly catastrophic diseases already exist, and the HGP will very likely promote the proliferation of presymptomatic molecular diagnostic tests for susceptibility to a variety of common diseases, causing premature death and much suffering. Genetic therapy has already been experimentally undertaken on human beings for a number of diseases, the list of protocols for human gene therapy is already lengthening every year, and continuing advances in the HGP will quite surely stimulate the use of molecular therapeutics for an ever-expanding range of human diseases.

Since we shall consider some of the ethical challenges of the impact of the HGP on medicine in later sections of this chapter, we now turn to consider a critique directed against the HGP, namely, that it harbours a reductionistic, deterministic view of human life, health and disease (Lippman, 1992).

The Human Genome Project: An Ideology?

The information that will be accumulated from mapping and sequencing the entire human genome raises, in Walter Gilbert's view, three striking questions about the nature of human beings. *First*, how does a human being develop from an egg? This is a question for developmental biology. The *second* question, a question for population biology, is about how human beings differ from one another. The *third* question is about what actually specifies the human organism, and differentiates human beings from animals. Succinctly, what makes us human? In Gilbert's view, the human genome project answers this third question about what makes us human (Gilbert, 1992, 84). Does this way of understanding the question about what makes us human, and the power it attributes to the HGP in answering this question, harbour a reductionistic, deterministic view of human life, and of human health and disease, as well?

One expression of a reductionistic and deterministic view of life appears in the statement of a leading molecular biologist, cited by Lewontin, to the effect that if he had a powerful enough computer and the complete DNA sequence of an organism, he could, in principle, *compute* the organism: *compute the organism* meaning that he could totally describe its anatomy, physiology, and behaviour (Lewontin, 1992, 34). The *deterministic* component on this view of life is that for every action taken, there are causal mechanisms that preclude any other action. The *reductionistic* component would situate these causal mechanisms in the sequence of DNA. Some believe that mapping and sequencing the genome, *combined* with tracing the pathways linking genes to behaviour, will sketch a deterministic view of human life (U.S. Congress, 1988, 86). The implication of this view, as in the above idea of computing the organism, is that mastery of DNA causal mechanisms and of the contexts in which they operate would be equivalent to a power to predict human development and human behaviour.

This view is quite totally ignorant of the fact that living organisms, preeminently human beings, are complex adaptive systems (Waldrop, 1992). The development and behaviour of such systems, at any moment, is the expression of a unique history, resulting from the nonpredictable interaction of internal and external forces, of an organism and its environment. Moreover, the world in response to which an individual organism develops — these external forces — is also modified and shaped by the activities of the organism itself (Lewontin, 1992, 34). Those who view life in reductionistic, deterministic terms are using *linear models* of thought. Unfortunately for reductionism and determinism, living organisms, and certainly human beings, exemplify the workings of *nonlinear* dynamics. In linear dynamical systems, the whole really can be, and usually is, greater than the sum of its parts (Waldrop, 1992, 64).

The ideology of genetic and biological determinism has been, and may continue to be, a futile breeding ground for eugenic initiations, as we shall consider briefly in this chapter's last section.

PREDICTIVE GENETIC TESTING: PRIVACY, CONFIDENTIALITY, AND THE DANGER OF GENETIC DISCRIMINATION

Completion of the human genome project will extend prenatal, neonatal, carrier, and presymptomatic testing to entirely new orders of magnitude (Botkin, 1990). This extension will intensify the difficulties and the complexity of ethical problems relating to abortion (Post, 1991), privacy, confidentiality, and discrimination. In this section, we concentrate exclusively on presymptomatic testing, and on ethical issues relating both to privacy and confidentiality and to genetic discrimination.

Presymptomatic Genetic Testing

Chapter 7 of this book discussed the interest and direct methods of genetic diagnosis (also called molecular diagnosis or DNA diagnosis), in the context of prenatal diagnosis. Genetic testing is *diagnostically positive* when it verifies the presence of a genetic defect that is now expressing itself as a pathology or a disease. Genetic testing is *predictively positive* when it uncovers a genetic defect that will definitively, or with varying degrees of probability, express itself as disease in the future. Such testing is said to be presymptomatic, because it reveals that a person is destined, or is highly susceptible, for a disease long before, often years before, any symptoms appear or any disease can be clinically diagnosed. Those testing positive on genetic presymptomatic tests may, depending on the future disease in question, remain perfectly healthy and lead normal lives for years after being tested, regardless of whether the testing is done pre- or postnatally.

Huntington's disease, already discussed in Chapter 7, was one of the first of the disorders of genetic origin for which presymptomatic testing became available and was used, though in limited fashion until recently. Huntington's is a Mendelian dominant disorder, meaning that everyone who inherits the defective gene will eventually fall prey to this disease, a disease manifesting itself in uncontrolled movements, dementia, and then death. There is now no treatment available for this disease, which shows up later in life, usually between 30 and 45 years of age. The precise location of the Huntington gene in chromosome 4 has been found very recently. Presymptomatic testing will now be made more predictive, and may even be able to pinpoint more precisely the age in life when the disease will appear (Angier, 1993, A16).

Presymptomatic testing is also available (but with less reliability than the test for Huntington's disease) for another inherited dominant disorder, called familial adenamatous polyposis (FAP), which predisposes those with the gene to a form of cancer (Tops, 1989).

Advances in the human genome project will expand the number of presymptomatic tests available, not only for the relatively rare recessive and dominant Mendelian genetic disorders, but also for genetic susceptibility for the more common polygenic and multifactorial diseases, such as cancer, diabetes, atherosclerosis, cardiovascular disease, and psychiatric disorders (McGuffin, 1992; Alexander, 1992). When effective methods to prevent the appearance of these diseases, or to treat them when they do appear, are not available, particular ethical tensions may arise regarding who may and who should not have access to this presymptomatic information, information a number of people, other than the persons affected, may have great interest in obtaining.

Privacy and Confidentiality

The ability to anticipate reliably future dangerous trends, in the case at hand, to foresee and prepare for possible threats to privacy and confidentiality, depends in part on an accurate and comprehensive grasp of what has happened in the past, and of what is happening now.

Huntington's disease offers examples of how genetics can be dangerously abused. In 1916, Davenport viewed Huntington's disease in the U.S. as traceable to a few founding families emigrated from England. He mistakenly thought that if *those* families had been screened at the immigration port of entry and had been kept out of the country, Huntington's disease could have been largely avoided in the U.S.. He also proposed sterilization of all those who already had Huntington's disease, or showed premature signs of the disease (Davenport, 1916, 215).

Threats to the privacy of persons with HIV disease, and to the confidentiality of their medical files, have already been mentioned in an earlier chapter of this book. Similar threats have occurred in the present case, regarding the privacy and confidentiality of persons with Huntington's disease. These threats have taken several forms, such as requests for predictive testing of prisoners and persons committed to psychiatric hospitals; requests, in connection with life and health insurance, for the results of presymptomatic testing; and requests that children under consideration for adoption be presymptomatically tested (Harper, 1992, 463; Morris, 1988; Morris, 1989).

A survey commissioned by the March of Dimes Birth Defects Foundation, and conducted in the U.S. by Louis Harris and Associates, found a majority of Americans believing that spouses, other family members, and even insurance companies and employers would have a right to information about a person's genetic defects. Many, if would seem, believe that people with a genetic disease or with a gene defect discovered by presymptomatic tests have a right neither to absolute privacy nor to unequivocal confidentiality (Angier, 1992).

Benno Müller-Hill, a geneticist and ardent critic of the abuses of genetics, recently expressed his astonishment over the *laissez-faire* attitude of some people involved in the human genome project, regarding privacy of genetic information. He found a number of these people believing it was none of their business to declare that no one has a right to determine a person's genotype without that person's consent, and that insurance companies and employers do not even have the right to ask people about their genotypes (Müller-Hill, 1991, 470-471).

The Privacy Commission of Canada has stated that no surveillance technology is more threatening to privacy than that designed to unlock the information contained in human genes. The Commissioner's report also emphasized that people must have meaningful control over the communication of genetic information in the private sector and, especially, in governments (Privacy Commissioner, 1992, 2-3). A particular threat to privacy and confidentiality exists if and when genomic information on individuals is, or will be, stored in computerized genetic registers (Harper, 1992, 462). Protecting the privacy and confidentiality of genomic information is a matter of protecting the human dignity of people (Knoppers, 1991).

The Danger of Genetic Discrimination

Unravelling and revealing a person's genomic secrets may release the brakes societies have set on the social process of stigmatization and ostracism. This process need not, but could, accelerate, as the human genome project designs more and more molecular markers for presymptomatic testing and screening of individuals and families (Markel, 1992, 209). Stigmatization will occur if molecular markers become social markers, markers that may set those with gene defects off as different from other human beings, and provoke their exclusion from goods and services to which they have as much a right as everyone else.

Stigmatization leads to discrimination, as we have already discussed in Chapter 10 in the context of HIV disease. Unjust discrimination excludes persons on arbitrary, unreasonable grounds from benefits, goods, services, and opportunities to which they have a right equal to the rights of all others in society. The Billings study, conducted to collect samples of genetic discrimination in New England, distinguished *genetic discrimination* from *discrimination based on disabilities* resulting from a genetic disorder. The study set out to learn whether services and entitlements were being denied to individuals who have a genetic diagnosis, but who are asymptomatic or will never become significantly impaired. They consequently defined *genetic discrimination* as discrimination directed against an individual or family, solely because of their apparent or perceived variation from the "normal" human genotype (Billings, 1992, 476-477).

Ostracism of people and discrimination against them on the basis of their genotype is not merely a hypothetical or future potential danger. Only twenty years ago, carriers of the gene for some of the inherited hemoglobinopathies (blood disease), such as beta thalassemia, were socially ostracized in Greece, and considered to be less than desirable partners for marriage (Stamatoyannopoulus, 1974). These people were neither sick nor disabled, but they suffered socially when it was known that they were carriers. Discrimination thrives in ignorance, and the ignorant care little about the distinctions, explained in Chapter 7, between homozygosity and heterozygosity. In a similar fashion, African-Americans suffered stigmatization and exclusion from health and life insurance, and from employment, because they, though not sick themselves or disabled, were carriers of the gene for sickle cell anemia, a disease of the blood manifested in persons who are homozygous for the sickle cell gene. Genetic discrimination in these cases was compounded by racial discrimination, because the discrimination was often only directed against African-American sickle-cell carriers, even though people from other ethnic groups can also carry this trait (Markel, 1992, 213).

Genetic discrimination also occurs in the present. The Billings study received reports of 41 separate incidents of possible discrimination, from the 29 responses to their inquiry that could be evaluated. Most of these incidents involved discrimination in the form of denial of access, or restrictions on access, to employment and insurance (Billings, 1992, 478).

One of the benefits of presymptomatic testing is that early knowledge that one is predisposed to a disease will allow preventive treatment, when such is available, to block progression of the genetic disease and serious, irreversible deterioration of health. At times, treatments are available that will keep the genetic disease under control and allow people, who would suffer severe symptoms without treatment, to live healthy normal lives. The Billings study uncovered evidence suggesting that a very disturbing question of social ethics may become even more urgent in the wake of the human genome project than it is now. Will the benefits of presymptomatic genetic testing, such as prevention and timely treatment, exact the social price of stigmatization, ostracism, and discrimination? Could an expansion of presymptomatic genetic

testing, contrary to the noblest of therapeutic intentions, lead to the social creation of a new genetic underclass of people who are, on the basis of their
genotype alone, increasingly barred from education, insurance, employment,
and other opportunities and services that are supposed to be open to all in an
open society?

GENETIC THERAPY AND ENGINEERING: THE CURRENT STATE OF ETHICAL DISCUSSION

Genetic Therapy

Things move very quickly in the realm of genomic science and technology. A
new scientific journal, *Human Gene Therapy*, was launched in 1990. Writing in
the second number of that journal's first volume, T. Friedmann, one of the
pioneers whose publications on gene therapy go back to the early 1970s, could
state that, as of the summer of 1990, no effective therapeutic application of gene
therapy had yet taken place. Gene therapy, he wrote, does not yet exist
(Friedmann, 1990, 176).

The first attempt at gene therapy to be undertaken, after passing through a
rigorous process of ethical review, was initiated a few months after Friedmann's
statement. A deficiency in adenosine deanimase results from a single gene
defect, and causes severe combined immunodeficiency (SCID), an inability to
ward off infections. On September 14, 1990, a four year-old afflicted with
adenosine deanimase ADA deficiency received an infusion into her blood
stream of cells from her own immune system, cells that had been extracted
from her body and into which a normal adenosine deanimase gene had been
inserted. In December 1992, W. French Anderson, the physician-scientist who
led this first gene therapy experiment, wrote that two ADA-deficient girls, who
had received gene therapy for this deficiency since 1990, were now leading
essentially normal lives (Anderson, "End-of-the-Year," 1992, 617). A normal
life means many things, all resulting from the fact that they do not have to live
in a special protective and sterile environment, a kind of bubble room, as did
David, the child who came to be known as the "bubble boy," for eleven years.

If gene therapy did not exist in the summer of 1992, twenty gene therapy
protocols were listed as underway in the 1993 summary of the registry for gene
therapy. These therapies were initiated for treatment of a number of diseases,
such as the already mentioned severe combined immunodeficiency disease
(SCID); hemophilia B; familial hypercholesterolemia, a disease leading to high
levels of cholesterol and premature heart disease; and a number of cancers, such
as malignant melanoma (a skin cancer), several of the leukemias (cancers of the
blood), brain tumors, and breast cancer (Human Gene Marker, 1993).

Categories of Genetic Engineering

Human gene therapy represents one use of genetic engineering, of which there are *five categories* (Anderson, "Uses and Abuses," 1992, 1). *First, somatic-cell gene therapy*, such as the therapies mentioned above in the registry we have cited, aims to correct a defect in the body cells of individual patients. *Second, germ-line gene therapy* would, if and when undertaken, aim to correct a genetic defect in the spermatozoa or ova (the germ or reproductive cells) of an individual. If this therapy were successful, the individual's children and future descendants would be freed from inheriting the gene defect. *Third, enhancement genetic engineering* could be directed to body cells (somatic-cell genetic engineering), to improve or perfect a particularly valued physical trait, such as height or eye colour. Enhancement genetic engineering is already underway, in experiments conducted on laboratory and farm animals. Some of these experiments go back ten years or more. For example, a report in 1982 described the successful genetic modification of eye colour in the fruit fly. This genetic modification changed the eye colour of later generations of these fruit flies, not only the eye colour of the fruit fly embryos that were the immediate target of the genetic engineering experiments (Rubin, 1982). This genetic modification of a specific trait in future generations would be the objective of the *fourth* category of genetic engineering, namely, *enhancement genetic engineering of germ cells*. Fifth, *polygenic engineering for the purposes of positive eugenics* (the improvement of individuals or of the human species) would seek to perfect complex features of human beings, such as intelligence, personality, behaviour.

The Current State of Ethical Discourse

The fifth category of genetic engineering, *polygenic engineering for positive eugenics*, is so far beyond current technology that ethical discussion of the limits, conditions, and consequences of the perhaps future possible applications of genetic engineering to human beings is hardly possible or meaningful.

For all practical purposes, debate on the ethical acceptability of *somatic-cell gene therapy*, the first category listed above, is over. The ethical aspects of somatic-cell gene therapy have been extensively explored, and debated, over the last thirteen years, particularly since the widely criticized premature gene therapy experiment attempted by Dr. M. Cline and colleagues in 1980, without prior approval of the ethics committee or institutional review board (IRB) of their university (Roy, 1986, 130-132, 145-147). Numerous publications have traced this evolution of ethical discourse on gene therapy (Fletcher, 1990; Murray, 1990; Tauer, 1990; Walters, 1991; Friedmann, 1992). One end point of this evolution has been the achievement of wide consensus about the scientific, medical, and ethical conditions under which somatic-cell gene therapy for the treatment of diseases may proceed (Subcommittee on Human Gene Therapy, 1990; Medical Research Council, 1990; Juengst, 1990).

The centre of ethical controversy has now, early in the 1990s, shifted to the second of the above-mentioned categories, namely *germ-line gene therapy*. Many who would ethically approve genetic treatment of body cells would absolutely oppose genetic engineering of germ cells, the modifications of which would affect descendants.

Ethical controversy over germ-line genetic engineering goes back to the early 1970s. In 1970, B. Davis stated the view that predictable alteration of germ cells, were it ever to become possible, would be even more useful than somatic cure of monogenic diseases. Germ-line therapy would allow an individual with a defective gene to have children, without condemning them to inherit that gene (Davis, 1970, 1280). In 1978, R. Novick stated that he would rigidly interdict any intervention in the germ line, including attempts at correcting specific diseases (Novick, 1978, 76). In 1982, J. Becker cited a proposal that legislators at the European Human Rights Convention in Strasbourg should define a right to a genetic inheritance free from any form of engineering (Becker, 1982). Would this come down to enshrining a right to inherited genetic disease?

In its 1990 *Guidelines*, the Medical Research Council of Canada adopted a cautious approach to possible future attempts at germ-line genetic therapy. Though stating that there are no indications for undertaking germ-line therapy at present, the Council drew no absolute lines in the sand, emphasizing only that risks (of harm) and benefits would have to be weighed very carefully, were it to become reasonable to envision germ-line therapy in the light of scientific progress (Medical Research Council, 1990, 23). The European Research Council has asserted more strongly that germ-line gene therapy should not be contemplated (Danielson, 1988).

Ethical discussion of germ-line genetic therapy is now moving from what Whitehead, cited by Juengst, has called the romantic stage (1) of inquiry, to the stage (2) of precision in inquiry (Whitehead, 1929; Juengst, 1991, 587-588). Whitehead's romantic stage is where we find the prophetic, early-warning, and even promethean, apocalyptic kind of literature mentioned earlier in this chapter. Stage 2, the arena for precision in inquiry, displays careful construction and evaluation of arguments marshalled for and against a proposal, in this case, for and against germ-line genetic therapy. The 1991 issue of *The Journal of Medicine and Philosophy*, devoted to the theme of human germ-line engineering and edited by Juengst, cited above, catalogues and analyzes the main arguments featured in the current ethical controversy over germ-line genetic therapy. When ethical discussions enter Whitehead's third stage of inquiry, the stage of generalization, it will become increasingly necessary to shift from condition ethics to assumption ethics, as mentioned earlier in this chapter. Emergent proposals for enhancement genetic engineering (categories three and four, mentioned in the previous sub-section) will drive ethical inquiry back to clarification of the basic assumptions and beliefs, to the ethos, that should control the wielding of power over the human genome.

REFERENCES

Alexander J.R., Lerer B. and **Baron M.** "Ethical Issues in Genetic Linkage Studies of Psychiatric Disorders." *British Journal of Psychiatry* 1992;160:98-102.

Anderson W.F. "Editorial. End-of-the-Year Potpourri -1992." *Human Gene Therapy* 1992;3:617-618.

Anderson W.F. "Editorial. Uses and Abuses of Human Gene Transfer." *Human Gene Therapy* 1992;3:1-2.

Angier N. "Many Americans Say Genetic Information Is Public Property." *The New York Times,* September 29, 1992:C2

Angier N. "Team Pinpoints Genetic Cause of Huntington's." *The New York Times,* March 24, 1993:A1, A16.

Avery O.T., MacLeod C.M. and **McCarty M.** "Studies on the Chemical Nature of the Substance Inducing Transformation of 'Pneumococcal' Types." *Journal of Experimental Medicine* 1944;79:137-158.

Barinaga M. "Knockout Mice Offer First Animal Model for CF." *Science* 1992;257:1046-1047.

Becker J. "Rights on DNA." *Nature* 1982;295:545.

Billings P.R. et al. "Discrimination as a Consequence of Genetic Testing." *American Journal of Human Genetics* 1992;50:476-482.

Botkin J.R. "Ethical Issues in Human Genetic Technology." *Pediatrician* 1990;17:100-117.

Chakraborty R. and **Kidd K.K.** "The Utility of DNA Typing in Forensic Work." *Science* 1991;254:1735-1739.

Chargaff E. "Structure and Function of Nucleic Acids as Cell Constituents." *Federation Proceedings* 1951;10:654-659.

Coldspring Harbor Laboratory "Molecular Biology of Homo Sapiens." *Coldspring Harbor Symposia on Quantitative Biology* 1986;51:1-1229.

Danielson H. "Gene Therapy in Man: Recommendations of the European Medical Research Councils." *Lancet* 1988;1:1271-1272.

Darnell J., Ludish H. and **Baltimore D.** *Molecular Cell Biology.* 2nd Edition. New York: W.H. Freeman, 1990.

Davenport C.B. and **Muncey M.D.** "Huntington's Chorea in Relation to Heredity and Insanity." *American Journal of Insanity* 1916;73:195-222.

Davis B. "Prospects for Genetic Intervention in Man." *Science* 1970;170:1279-1283.

Fletcher J.C. "Evolution of Ethical Debate about Human Gene Therapy." *Human Gene Therapy* 1990;1:55-68.

Friedmann T. "A Brief History of Gene Therapy." *Nature Genetics* 1992;2:93-98.

Friedmann T. "The Evolving Concept of Gene Therapy." *Human Gene Therapy* 1990;1:175-181.

Gilbert W. "A Vision of the Grail." In: D.J. Kevles and L. Hood, eds. *The Code of Codes. Scientific and Social Issues in the Human Genome Project.* Cambridge, Mass.: Harvard University Press, 1992:83-97.

Golding M.P. "Ethical Issues in Biological Engineering." *UCLA Law Review* 1968;15:443-479.

Green E.D. and **Waterston R.H.** "The Human Genome Project. Prospects and Implications for Clinical Medicine." *Journal of the American Medical Association* 1991;266:1966-1975.

Gusella J.F. "Polymorphic DNA Marker Genetically Linked to Huntington's Disease." *Nature* 1983;306:234-238.

Harper P.S. "Huntington's Disease and the Abuse of Genetics." *American Journal of Human Genetics* 1992;50:460-464.

Hershey A.D. and **Chase M.** "Independent Functions of Viral Protein and Nucleic Acid in Growth of Bacteriophage." *Journal of General Physiology* 1952;36:39-56.

Hotchkiss R.D. "Portents for a Genetic Engineering." *Journal of Heredity* 1965;56:197-202.

"Human Gene Marker/Therapy Patient Registry - Summary." *Human Gene Therapy* 1993;4:123.

Hunkapiller T. et al. "Large-Scale and Automated DNA Sequence Determination." *Science* 1991;254:59-67.

Jacob F. and **Minod J.** "Genetic Regulatory Mechanisms in the Synthesis of Proteins." *Journal of Molecular Biology* 1961;3:318-356.

Jasny B.R. "Genome Maps III." *Science* 1992;258:87-102.

Judson H.F. *The Eighth Day of Creation: Makers of the Revolution in Biology.* New York: Simon & Schuster, 1979.

Juengst E.T. "Germ-Line Gene Therapy: Back to Basics." In: E.T. Juengst, issue ed. "Human Germ-Line Engineering." *The Journal of Medicine and Philosophy* 1991;16:587-592.

Juengst E.T. "The NIH 'Points to Consider' and the Limits of Human Gene Therapy." *Human Gene Therapy* 1990;1:425-433.

Kevles D.J. and **Hood L.**, eds. *The Code of Codes. Scientific and Social Issues in the Human Genome Project.* Cambridge, Mass.: Harvard University Press, 1992.

Kirby L.T. *DNA Fingerprinting. An Introduction.* New York: Stockton Press, 1990.

Knoppers B. *Human Dignity and Genetic Heritage: A Study Paper.* Ottawa: The Law Reform Commission of Canada, 1991.

Lander E.S. "DNA Fingerprinting on Trial." *Nature* 1989;339:501-505.

Lee M.G. and **Nurse P.** "Complementation Used to Clone a Human Homologue of the Fission Yeast Cell Cycle Control Gene cdc2." *Nature* 1987;327:31-35.

Lewontin R.C. and **Hartl D.L.** "Population Genetics in Forensic DNA Typing." *Science* 1991;254:1745-1750.

Lewontin R.C. "The Dream of the Human Genome." *The New York Review of Books* 1992;XXXIX(May 28):31-40.

Lippman A. "Led (Astray) by Genetic Maps: The Cartography of the Human Genome and Health Care." *Social Sciences in Medicine* 1992; 35:1469-1476.

Luria S.E. "Modern Biology: A Terrifying Power." *Nation* October 20, 1969:406-409.

Markel H. "The Stigma of Disease: Implications of Genetic Screening." *The American Journal of Medicine* 1992;93:209-215.

Maxam A.M. and **Gilbert W.** "A New Method for Sequencing DNA." *Proceedings of the National Academy of Sciences of the United States of America* 1977;74:560-564.

McGuffin P. and **Thapar A.** "The Genetics of Personality Disorder." *British Journal of Psychiatry* 1992;160:12-23.

McKusick V.A. and **Amberger J.S.** "The Morbid Anatomy of the Human Genome: Chromosomal Location of Mutations Causing Disease." *Journal of Medical Genetics* 1993;30:1-26.

Medawar P.B. *The Threat and the Glory. Reflections on Science and Scientists.* New York: HarperCollins, 1990.

Medical Research Council of Canada *Guidelines for Research on Somatic-Cell Gene Therapy in Humans.* Ottawa: Minister of Supply and Services, 1990.

Morris M. et al. "Problems in Genetic Prediction for Huntington's Disease." *Lancet* 1989;2:601-603.

Morris M., Tyler A. and **Harper P.S.** "Adoption and Genetic Prediction for Huntington's Disease." *Lancet* 1988;2:1069-1070.

Müller-Hill B. "Psychiatry in the Nazi Era." In: S. Bloch and P. Chodoff, eds. *Psychiatric Ethics.* 2nd Edition. New York: Oxford University Press, 1991:461-472.

Murray T.H. "Human Gene Therapy. The Public and Public Policy." *Human Gene Therapy* 1990;1:49-54.

Murrell J.C. and **Roberts L.M.** *Understanding Genetic Engineering.* Chichester, New York, Toronto: Hulstead Press (John Wiley & Sons), 1989.

National Research Council, Committee on Mapping and Sequencing the Human Genome *Mapping and Sequencing the Human Genome.* Washington, D.C.: National Academy Press, 1988.

Nelkin D. "Threats and Promises. Negotiating the Control of Research." *Daedalus* 1978;107/2:191-209.

Neufeld P.J. and **Colman N.** "When Science Takes the Witness Stand." *Scientific American* 1990;262/5:46-53.

Nirenberg M.W. and **Matthaei J.H.** "The Dependence of Cell-Free Protein Synthesis in E. Coli Upon Naturally Occurring or Synthetic Polynucleotides." *Proceedings of the National Academy of Sciences of the United States of America* 1961;47:1588-1602.

Novick R. "The Dangers of Unrestricted Research: The Case of Recombinant DNA." In: J. Richards, ed. *Recombinant DNA: Science, Ethics, and Politics.* New York, San Francisco, London: Academic Press, 1978:71-102.

Palmiter R.D. et al. "Metallothionein-Human GH Fusion Genes Stimulate Growth of Mice." *Nature* 1983;222:804-814.

Post S.G. "Selective Abortion and Gene Therapy: Reflections on Human Limits." *Human Gene Therapy* 1991;2:229-233.

Privacy Commissioner of Canada *Genetic Testing and Privacy.* Ottawa: Minister of Supply and Services Canada, 1992.

Roy D.J. and **de Wachter M.A.M.** *The Life Technologies and Public Policy.* Montréal: The Institute for Research in Public Policy, 1986.

Roy D.J., Wynne B.E. and **Old R.W.** "Introduction." In: D.J. Roy, B.E. Wynne and R.W. Old, eds. *Bioscience - Society.* Chichester: John Wiley & Sons (Schering Foundation Workshop), 1991:1-7.

Rubin G.M. and **Spradling A.C.** "Genetic Transformation of Drosophila with Transposable Element Vectors." *Science* 1982;218:348-353.

Sanger F., Nicklen S. and **Coulson A.R.** "DNA Sequencing with Chain-Terminating Inhibitors." *Proceedings of the National Academy of Sciences of the United States of America* 1977;74:5463-5467.

Singer M. "The Involvement of Scientists." In: *Research with Recombinant DNA. An Academy Forum, March 7-9, 1977.* Washington, D.C.: National Academy of Sciences, 1977:24-30.

Sinsheimer R. "The End of the Beginning." *Engineering and Science* 1966;30/3:7-10.

Stamatoyannopoulos G. "Problems of Screening and Counseling in the Hemoglobinopathies." In: A.G. Motulsky and F.J.G. Ebling, eds. *Birth Defects: Proceedings of the Fourth International Conference.* Vienna: Excerpta Medica, 1974:268-276.

Subcommittee on Human Gene Therapy, Recombinant DNA Advisory Committee, National Institutes of Health "Points to Consider in the Design and Submission of Protocols for the Transfer of Recombinant DNA into the Genome of Human Subjects." *Human Gene Therapy* 1990;1:93-103.

Suzuki D. and **Knudtson P.** *Genethics. The Clash Between the New Genetics and Human Values.* Cambridge, Mass.: Harvard University Press, 1989.

Suzuki D.T. et al. *An Introduction to Genetic Analysis.* New York: W.H. Freeman, 1989.

Tauer C. "Does Human Gene Therapy Raise New Ethical Questions?" *Human Gene Therapy* 1990;1:411-418.

Thomas C.A. "The Fanciful Future of Gene Transfer Experiments." *Brookhaven Symposium in Biology,* 1977. Quoted here from the reprint in: Watson J.D. and Tooze J. *The DNA Story. A Documentary History of Gene Cloning.* San Francisco: W.H. Freeman, 1981.

Tops C.M. et al. "Presymptomatic Diagnosis of Familial Adenamatous Polyposis by Bridging DNA Markers." *Lancet* 1989;2:1361-1363.

U.S. Congress, Office of Technology Assessment *Mapping Our Genes. The Genome Project: How Big, How Fast?* Washington, D.C.: U.S. Government Printing Office, 1988.

U.S. Congress, Office of Technology Assessment *New Developments in Biotechnology. Patenting Life.* New York, Basel: Marcel Dekker, 1989.

Wagner T.E. et al. "Microinjection of a Rabbit Beta-globin Gene Into Zygotes and Its Subsequent Expression in Adult Mice and their Offspring." *Proceedings of the National Academy of Sciences of the United States of America* 1981;78:6376-6380.

Waldrop M.M. *Complexity. The Emerging Science at the Edge of Order and Chaos.* New York, Toronto: Simon & Schuster, 1992.

Walters L. "Human Gene Therapy: Ethics and Public Policy." *Human Gene Therapy* 1991;2:115-122.

Watson J.D. and **Crick F.H.C.** "Molecular Structure of Nucleic Acids. A Structure for Deoxyribase Nucleic Acid." *Nature* 1953;171:737-738.

Watson J.D. and **Tooze J.** *The DNA Story. A Documentary History of Gene Cloning.* San Francisco: W.H. Freeman, 1981.

Watson J.D. "The Human Genome Project: Past, Present, and Future." *Science* 1990;248:44-49.

Whitehead A.N. *The Aims of Education.* New York: MacMillan, 1929.

Williamson R. "Gene Therapy." *Nature* 1982;298:416-418.

Yager T.D., Nickerson D.A. and Hood L.E. "The Human Genome Project: Creating an Infrastructure for Biology and Medicine." *Trends in Biomedical Sciences* 1991;16:454-458.

19

THE FUTURE OF BIOETHICS

Throughout this book, our primary intention has been to present an accurate picture of the current state of bioethics in Canada. Now, in conclusion, we wish to speculate on its future. Speculation is the appropriate term, since, at the present time, it is quite uncertain how bioethics will develop during the next ten, twenty, or thirty years. It may continue to thrive and expand, as it has during the past three decades. Or it may prove to be a passing fad, and be replaced by greater attention to the economic, political and legal dimensions of health care.

Are there any sources of information that can enable us to predict the future of bioethics? We believe that there are. Just as traditional medical ethics changed in response to social, political, scientific, legal, and ethical developments in the 1960s, 1970s, and 1980s, to become bioethics as it has been described in this book, so now is it likely that current bioethics will change in response to comparable developments in the 1990s and beyond. To predict the future of bioethics, it is necessary first to identify and describe the major factors of change in society in general, and the health care system in particular, that are already underway in the 1990s.

The plan of this chapter is as follows: we shall first review the origins of contemporary bioethics, in order to answer the question: where has it come from? Next, we will describe the main features of bioethics to determine: where is it now? Finally, we shall examine current trends in health care and ethics, to provide an answer to the question: where is bioethics going?

THE ORIGINS OF BIOETHICS

In Chapter 1, we stressed the importance of history for an understanding of contemporary bioethics. We outlined three major stages in the historical development of this field: (1) pre-1900, (2) 1900-1960s, and (3) 1960s to 1990s. Throughout most of the book, we have concentrated on Stage 3, with references to Stage 2 where appropriate, for example, in the chapter on research ethics. Although Stage 1 may seem far removed from the present, it too is of central importance for understanding both current and future bioethical issues. Why is this?

In Chapter 2, we saw that many conflicts in bioethics arise at the levels of ethos and morality. The principal sources of these ethos and moralities are religions, philosophies, and professional identities, most of which extend far into the past. The Hippocratic tradition in medicine is just one example. It has guided medical ethics for centuries, and is still a source of inspiration for many physicians. However, it has long been associated with a paternalistic approach towards patients, and can therefore conflict with philosophical traditions that stress patient autonomy. Unless the historical sources of such conflicts can be identified, it is often very difficult, if not impossible, to reach satisfactory solutions.

Whereas the transition from Stage 1 to Stage 2 in the history of bioethics was gradual, the move from Stage 2 to Stage 3 was nothing less than revolutionary. The emergence of bioethics in the 1960s was due to several factors that made this decade radically different from those that preceded it. In Chapter 2, we characterized the changes that took place during the 1960s in terms of "breakthrough" and "breakdown." The principal breakthroughs were in medical science and technology. Advances in understanding life forms, and the development of diagnostic, surgical and pharmaceutical treatments offered unprecedented opportunities for combating diseases. Other major breakthroughs during this period were the recognition and implementation of human rights, including those of patients and research subjects, and a new social awareness and acceptance of death and dying.

These breakthroughs occurred at a time of breakdown of the social consensus on values and principles, in countries such as Canada. An important aspect of this consensus was respect for authority, whether political, legal, ecclesiastical, or professional. The 1960s witnessed numerous challenges to previously accepted patterns of authority, in the name of individual autonomy or on behalf of disadvantaged groups. Protest movements attracted many participants, but were often strongly resisted by those in power. The result of this breakdown was a growing moral pluralism in society, with no single individual or group able to state authoritatively what is right and what is wrong. Into this void entered bioethics, which attempted to establish standards of behaviour in health care that would be acceptable to all reasonable persons, regardless of their political, religious, philosophical, or professional status.

The early development of bioethics took place at a crucial period in the history of the Canadian health care system. As we saw in Chapter 4, the consolidation of the national health insurance programme, Medicare, occurred during the late 1960s. This programme has provided the context, the source, and the focus of discussion for bioethics in this country, and increasingly, in the U.S.A. as well. Although the bioethical issue most directly affected by the health care system is allocation of resources, there are few, if any, issues that can be discussed in isolation from the way in which health care is financed and delivered. Changes in the health care system that are being introduced in the 1990s will have no less profound an impact on the future of bioethics in Canada.

THE CURRENT STATE OF BIOETHICS

Between the 1960s and the 1990s, bioethics gradually developed and matured into the form that has been described throughout this book. The following summary of its principal features will give a basis for predicting how it is likely to develop in the future.

- Bioethics can be defined as the study of right conduct in medical and biomedical interventions into life; into human life in particular.

- Bioethics attempts to answer the questions: what must we do, what should we permit, what can we tolerate, and what must we prohibit, among all the new and often untested things that can be done to and for human beings, as a result of advances in medicine and the life sciences?

- Bioethics is not a morality, nor a professional ethics, nor a theological or philosophical ethics, nor applied ethics.

- Bioethics is not law, although law deals with many of the same issues, and bioethics must take into account the legal status of medical interventions.

- Bioethics is ethics, that is, the working out of the judgments that have to be made, the compromises that have to be struck, and the guidelines and policies that have to be devised when individuals and groups in a pluralistic society clash on the levels of ethos and morality, in matters of medicine and the life sciences.

- Bioethics has become both an academic discipline and a profession. There are philosophers, theologians, legal scholars, physicians, nurses, and social scientists who list bioethics as their academic specialty. There are an increasing number of students doing master's and doctoral degrees in bioethics, and a significant number of bioethicists are employed either full or part-time in hospitals, research centres, and professional associations.

- Bioethics has three major fields: research, clinical, and public policy ethics. Each of these fields has its own specialties and subspecialties, for example, psychiatric research ethics, geriatric clinical ethics, reproductive public policy ethics.
- Bioethics deals with conflicts. In Chapter 2, we identified no fewer than seven types of conflicts for bioethics, each of which requires a different strategy for its resolution.
- Bioethics deals with issues. During the past three decades, some of these issues have been resolved, for example, whether patients can refuse life-prolonging treatments; others have been clearly defined, even though no consensus has been reached, for example, abortion; a third group includes those that are still being clarified, and about which many people have yet to make up their minds, for example, physician-assisted suicide; and finally, there are issues that are just beginning to be identified and discussed, for example, genetic modifications of the human germ line.
- Bioethical issues arise in, and are dependent upon, a particular context, namely, each country's health care system.
- In virtually all countries of the Western world, the growth of bioethics during the past three decades was accompanied by significant increases in health care spending. In the early 1990s, this growth in spending slowed to a crawl, if not to a complete stop.

Each of these statements is important for an overall understanding of what bioethics is in the early 1990s. In the years to come, it will probably retain many of these features, but it is even more likely to undergo significant changes. These changes will be determined by factors both internal and external to bioethics. Identifying and analyzing these factors will help predict the future of bioethics.

INTO THE FUTURE

There is little doubt that one of the most significant differences between the 1960s and the 1990s is the economic climate. The health care system, like all other government budget categories, is undergoing cutbacks, which are unlikely to be reversed in the foreseeable future. The questions this raises for bioethics are: is bioethics part of the health care funding problem, something that can no longer be afforded? Or should it be part of the solution, one of the elements of better, and more efficient, health care? Its proponents will naturally choose the latter response. However, they are not necessarily the ones who will make the ultimate decision. Funding for bioethics, as for other elements of the health care system, will be determined by government officials, research funding agencies, university presidents and deans, and hospital administrators, who will have to be convinced that bioethics is valuable enough to deserve a share of their budgets.

As important as it is, the economy is only one of the factors that will determine the future of bioethics. A list of other significant factors must include the following:

- Medical science and technology, one of the primary influences on the early development of bioethics, continue to advance at an ever-increasing rate. Most of these discoveries carry a very high price tag, and as a result, there is a continual widening of the gap between the potential supply of health care resources and the funds needed to pay for them. A major challenge for bioethics in the future is to determine what types of scientific and technological research and development should even be considered; this may result in decisions not to search for cures for conditions such as aging, whose elimination would likely have serious social and economic consequences.

  It is also possible that medical science will achieve major breakthroughs in the prevention or cure of illness and disease. As we saw in the previous chapter, recent advances in medical genetics have engendered great hopes that genetically caused abnormalities can be detected and neutralized early in their development. If these hopes bear fruit, the overall cost of health care may decrease significantly in the future.

- Health care itself is undergoing significant rethinking and redefinition. The vast majority of health care efforts, during the past thirty years, were directed towards curing illness and disease, such as infections, heart malfunction, hypertension, and cancers. There have been some notable successes in preventing diseases through the use of vaccines and, more recently, through emphasis on lifestyle and environment, but the funds directed towards prevention have been minuscule, in comparison to those for curative medicine (especially surgery and drugs).

  In the 1990s, there is growing recognition that curative medicine, while important, should be deemphasized in favour of health promotion. This emerging model of health care has several characteristic features: it considers health to be not just the absence of disease, but part of overall personal well-being (the "holistic" concept of health); it encourages individual responsibility for health, especially regarding lifestyle (diet, exercise, avoidance of smoking, etc.); it sees an inseparable link between the health of individuals and of their social surroundings ("healthy communities").

- Another major determinant of the future of bioethics is the environmental crisis. Although it has been in the making throughout the developmental period of bioethics, it was not a significant factor in bioethical reflection during this time. Now, however, it can no longer be ignored. Not only does it have a direct impact on health, for example, the rapidly growing incidence of skin cancers, due at least in part to the thinning of the ozone layer, but it is likely to have many indirect effects, as nations are forced to choose between expensive cleanup programmes and higher rates of environmentally caused diseases.

- Closely related to the environmental crisis is another crisis, which is not new but which has been largely neglected by bioethics, namely, world poverty. The link between poverty and ill health has been known for years, but the responsibility of the wealthier nations, provinces, and individuals for the underprivileged is only now emerging as a fundamental issue for bioethics.

- Canada is a nation of immigrants, and its multicultural character is becoming more evident with each passing year. During its developmental phase, bioethics has been clearly monocultural, reflecting the values of the white, largely Anglo-Saxon, professional class that has dominated Canadian society, including its science and medicine. The inadequacy of this approach has been alluded to throughout this book. If bioethics is to be relevant to Canadian society in the future, it must develop a multicultural sensitivity. This must include a growing recognition of, and respect for, aboriginal culture and health care practices. More specifically, bioethics in Canada will have to take account of the role and status of aboriginal herbal and psychiatric medical practices, and of the priority given, in traditional cultures, to community entitlements over individual or autonomous rights.

- Canada is also an aging society. The ethical issues described in Chapter 12 are certain to become more prominent in the years to come, as the proportion of elderly persons increases and the proportion of the wage-earning population decreases.

These are some of the external factors that are likely to influence the future development of bioethics. Among them, some are certain (the environmental crisis, world poverty, our aging population); others are probable (the continually increasing gap between demand and supply of health care resources, greater emphasis on preventive health care); and still others are at least possible (new means of preventing or curing diseases). If bioethics does not soon begin to take these factors into consideration, it will quickly become obsolete.

There are also some internal characteristics of bioethics that may undergo change in the future. One of these is the priority that has been given to individual autonomy. The passage of the *Canadian Charter of Rights and Freedoms* in 1982 contributed greatly to the protection and enhancement of individual rights, and bioethics has been among the principal defenders of these rights, especially with regard to informed choice in health care. However, it may well be that autonomy and self-determination, important as they are, have been overemphasized, and that the pendulum may swing back towards a less individualistic, and more communitarian, foundation for ethical decision-making. The euthanasia debate may be a crucial test of the rights of the individual versus the rights (or interests) of society. If autonomy continues to be given paramount importance, then it is likely that euthanasia will be legalized. However, if social values are recognized as at least equal to individual needs and desires, then society may well say no to euthanasia, even when it seems to be in an individual's own best interests.

Another potential battleground for individual versus collective rights is Canada's publicly financed health care system. The five principles of Medicare, especially equality of access, are threatened by cuts in government funding. There are suggestions that the shortfall be covered by private contributions, but this will inevitably discriminate against the poorer members of society. Since bioethics is rooted in the health care system, any such changes will have profound effects on how both clinical and public bioethics function.

Another feature of bioethics that may undergo significant change in the future is its professionalism. During the past thirty years, professional bioethicists in increasing numbers have dominated the field, whether as teachers, researchers, consultants, or clinical ethicists. Many of these individuals have felt all along that the real work of bioethics has to be done by physicians, nurses, and other health care professionals as part of their everyday care of patients, and that patients and their families also have a significant role to play. As the number of caregivers and patients who have been exposed to bioethics teaching continues to increase, and as these individuals grow more confident about their ability to make good ethical decisions, the domination of the field by professional bioethicists may well diminish. There will still be need for specialists in the field, to function as teachers, researchers, and consultants, but the bulk of the work will probably be done by nonspecialists.

BIOETHICS: A PERMANENT PROJECT

The future of bioethics will, indeed, depend on how well it deals with the changing factors in health care and ethics that have just been outlined. In the end, though, the greatest contribution that bioethics can make is to help humans think about some of their most basic questions: what is life? what is health? how should we live?

Although these questions need to be asked anew in the 1990s, they are very much part of human history. They take us back to the Judaeo-Christian origins of our culture, back to the high cultural period of ancient Greece, to the thought of Socrates, Plato, and Aristotle, and forward into a culture in which the great ideas will have to be thought through again by people throughout the world, if the perils of great power are not to become the realities of intolerable abuse.

The ancient Greeks spoke of "making humanity." Their process was called *paideia*, a process of transcendental education. The goal was to shape people according to the *universal* laws of human nature, common to all human beings. The Greeks viewed medicine as a paradigm of *paideia*, because it offered a model of how to meet *paideia*'s central challenge: the concrete realization of a universal pattern or standard in highly individual and varied lives. Medicine was seen as governed by the same objective as *paideia*: to bring human beings into harmony with the *logos*, that is, the meaning and purposes of human nature. Human nature, in the thought of ancient Greece, served as a *normative principle* for the practice of medicine and for *paideia*.

Contemporary medicine remains a profession and an art, as was medicine in the period of the great Greek thinkers. But today, medicine, hand in hand with advanced specializations in biomedicine and the life sciences, has vastly amplified the modest scientific initiatives of ancient Greek medicine into a massive project of research. Human nature, once the normative principle of medicine, has now become the object and the target of ever more precise, penetrating, and methodical inquiry. Human nature, once a principle for ancient cultures, is for our culture a question, an as-yet-unanswered question.

Furthermore, science today, biomedicine and the life sciences included, is closely interlocked with the development of technology and power. Human nature is now not only a target of scientific inquiry, but also increasingly an object of technological manipulation. Human nature, once the guiding principle of human activity, has now become its project.

Modern medicine, linked to high science and technology, now occupies centre spot in our cultural stage. The drama enacts hope, but fear, anxiety, and uncertainty as well. The uncertainty is manifest in the ethical dilemmas we have discussed throughout this book. These ethical dilemmas and uncertainties will increase in number and difficulty as scientific insight into the nature of living things deepens, and the technological power to modify life expands.

Down the road of scientific-technological advance, we may come face to face with the most difficult question of all. If the *logos*, the meaning and purpose immanent in human nature that guided the ancients, falls subject to scientific and technological change, where shall we then turn to discover a new *logos* and a higher order of guidance? Bioethics will remain, throughout this century and into the next, as the expression of our common search for a wisdom equal to our growing scientific and technological power over life.

Appendix A

The Canadian Medical Association Code of Ethics

Principles of Ethical Behaviour for all physicians, including those who may not be engaged directly in clinical practice.

I

Consider first the well-being of the patient.

II

Honour your profession and its traditions.

III

Recognize your limitations and the special skills of others in the prevention and treatment of disease.

IV

Protect the patient's secrets.

V

Teach and be taught.

VI

Remember that integrity and professional ability should be your best advertisement.

VII

Be responsible in setting a value on your services.

GUIDE TO THE ETHICAL BEHAVIOUR OF PHYSICIANS

A physician should be aware of the standards established by tradition and act within the general principles which have governed professional conduct.

The Oath of Hippocrates represented the desire of the members of that day to establish for themselves standards of conduct in living and in the practice of their art. Since then the principles established have been retained as our basic guidelines for ethical living with the profession of medicine.

The International Code of Ethics and the Declaration of Geneva (1948), developed and approved by the World Medical Association, have modernized the ancient codes. They have been endorsed by each member organization, including The Canadian Medical Association, as a general guide having world-wide application.

The Canadian Medical Association accepts the responsibility of delineating the standard of ethical behaviour expected of Canadian physicians.

An interpretation of these principles is developed in the following pages, as a guide for individual physicians and provincial authorities.

RESPONSIBILITIES TO THE PATIENT

An Ethical Physician

Standard of Care

1. will practise the art and science of medicine to the best of his/her ability;
2. will continue self education to improve his/her standards of medical care;

Respect for Patient

3. will practise in a fashion that is above reproach and will take neither physical, emotional nor financial advantage of the patient;

Patient's Rights

4. will recognize his/her professional limitations and, when indicated, recommend to the patient that additional opinions and services be obtained;
5. will recognize that a patient has the right to accept or reject any physician and any medical care recommended. The patient having chosen a physician has the right to request of that physician opinions from other physicians of the patient's choice;
6. will keep in confidence information derived from a patient or from a colleague regarding a patient, and divulge it only with the permission of the patient except when otherwise required by law;
7. when acting on behalf of a third party will ensure that the patient understands the physician's legal responsibility to the third party before proceeding with the examination;
8. will recommend only diagnostic procedures that are believed necessary to assist in the care of the patient, and therapy that is believed necessary for the well-being of the patient. The physician will recognize a responsibility in

advising the patient of the findings and recommendations and will exchange such information with the patient as is necessary for the patient to reach a decision;

9. will, upon a patient's request, supply the information that is required to enable the patient to receive any benefits to which the patient may be entitled;

10. will be considerate of the anxiety of the patient's next-of-kin and cooperate with them in the patient's interest;

Choice of Patient

11. will recognize the responsibility of a physician to render medical service to any person regardless of colour, religion or political belief;

12. shall, except in an emergency, have the right to refuse to accept a patient;

13. will render all possible assistance to any patient, where an urgent need for medical care exists;

14. will, when the patient is unable to give consent and an agent of the patient is unavailable to give consent, render such therapy as the physician believes to be in the patient's interest;

Continuity of Care

15. will, if absent, ensure the availability of medical care to his/her patients if possible; will, once having accepted professional responsibility for an acutely ill patient, continue to provide services until they are no longer required, or until arrangements have been made for the services of another suitable physician; may, in any other situation, withdraw from the responsibility for the care of any patient provided that the patient is given adequate notice of that intention;

Personal Morality

16. will inform the patient when personal morality or religious conscience prevent the recommendation of some form of therapy;

Clinical Research

17. will ensure that, before initiating clinical research involving humans, such research is appraised scientifically and ethically and approved by a responsible committee and is sufficiently planned and supervised that the individuals are unlikely to suffer any harm. The physician will ascertain that previous research and the purpose of the experiment justify this additional method of investigation. Before proceeding, the physician will obtain the

consent of all involved persons or their agents, and will proceed only after explaining the purpose of the clinical investigation and any possible health hazard that can be reasonably foreseen;

The Dying Patient

18. will allow death to occur with dignity and comfort when death of the body appears to be inevitable;

19. may support the body when clinical death of the brain has occurred, but need not prolong life by unusual or heroic means;

Transplantation

20. may, when death of the brain has occurred, support cellular life in the body when some parts of the body might be used to prolong the life or improve the health of others;

21. will recognize a responsibility to a donor of organs to be transplanted and will give to the donor or the donor's relatives full disclosure of the intent and purpose of the procedure; in the case of a living donor, the physician will also explain the risks of the procedure;

22. will refrain from determining the time of death of the donor patient if there is a possibility of being involved as a participant in the transplant procedure, or when his/her association with the proposed recipient might improperly influence professional judgement;

23. may treat the transplant recipient subsequent to the transplant procedure in spite of having determined the time of death of the donor;

Fees to Patients

24. will consider, in determining professional fees, both the nature of the service provided and the ability of the patient to pay, and will be prepared to discuss the fee with the patient.

RESPONSIBILITIES TO THE PROFESSION

An Ethical Physician

Personal Conduct

25. will recognize that the profession demands integrity from each physician and dedication to its search for truth and to its service to mankind;

26. will recognize that self discipline of the profession is a privilege and that each physician has a continuing responsibility to merit the retention of this privilege;

27. will behave in a way beyond reproach and will report to the appropriate professional body any conduct by a colleague which might be generally considered as being unbecoming to the profession;

28. will behave in such a manner as to merit the respect of the public for members of the medical profession;

29. will avoid impugning the reputation of any colleague;

Contracts

30. will, when aligned in practice with other physicians, insist that the standards enunciated in this Code of Ethics and the Guide to the Ethical Behaviour of Physicians be maintained;

31. will only enter into a contract regarding professional services which allows fees derived from physicians' services to be controlled by the physician rendering the services;

32. will enter into a contract with an organization only if it will allow maintenance of professional integrity;

33. will only offer to a colleague a contract which has terms and conditions equitable to both parties;

Reporting Medical Research

34. will first communicate to colleagues, through recognized scientific channels, the results of any medical research, in order that those colleagues may establish an opinion of its merits before they are presented to the public;

Addressing the Public

35. will recognize a responsibility to give the generally held opinions of the profession when interpreting scientific knowledge to the public; when presenting an opinion which is contrary to the generally held opinion of the profession, the physician will so indicate and will avoid any attempt to enhance his/her own personal professional reputation;

Advertising

36. will build a professional reputation based on ability and integrity, and will only advertise professional services or make professional announcements as

regulated by legislation or as permitted by the provincial medical licensing authority;

37. will avoid advocacy of any product when identified as a member of the medical profession;

38. will avoid the use of secret remedies;

Consultation

39. will request the opinion of an appropriate colleague acceptable to the patient when diagnosis or treatment is difficult or obscure, or when the patient requests it. Having requested the opinion of a colleague, the physician will make available all relevant information and indicate clearly whether the consultant is to assume the continuing care of the patient during this illness;

40. will, when consulted by a colleague, report in detail all pertinent findings and recommendations to the attending physician and may outline an opinion to the patient. The consultant will continue with the care of the patient only at the specific request of the attending physician and with the consent of the patient;

Patient Care

41. will cooperate with those individuals who, in the opinion of the physician, may assist in the care of the patient;

42. will make available to another physician, upon the request of the patient, a report of pertinent findings and treatment of the patient;

43. will provide medical services to a colleague and dependent family without fee, unless specifically requested to render an account;

44. will limit self-treatment or treatment of family members to minor or emergency services only; such treatments should be without fee;

Financial Arrangements

45. will avoid any personal profit motive in ordering drugs, appliances or diagnostic procedures from any facility in which the physician has a financial interest;

46. will refuse to accept any commission or payment, direct or indirect, for any service rendered to a patient by other persons excepting direct employees and professional colleagues with whom there is a formal partnership or similar agreement.

RESPONSIBILITIES TO SOCIETY

Physicians who act under the principles of this Guide to the Ethical Behaviour for Physicians will find that they have fulfilled many of their responsibilities to society.

An Ethical Physician

47. will strive to improve the standards of medical services in the community; will accept a share of the profession's responsibility to society in matters relating to the health and safety of the public, health education, and legislation affecting the health or well-being of the community;

48. will recognize the responsibility as a witness to assist the court in arriving at a just decision;

49. will, in the interest of providing good and adequate medical care, support the opportunity of other physicians to obtain hospital privileges according to individual personal and professional qualifications.

"The complete physician is not a man apart and cannot content himself with the practice of medicine alone, but should make his contribution, as does any other good citizen, towards the well-being and betterment of the community in which he lives."

Appendix B

The Canadian Nurses Association Code of Ethics

CLIENTS

I
A nurse is obliged to treat clients with respect for their
individual needs and values.

Standards

1. Factors such as the client's race, religion, ethnic origin, social status, sex, age or health status may not be permitted to compromise the nurse's commitment to that client's care.

2. The expectations and normal life patterns of clients are acknowledged. Individualized programs of nursing care are designed to accommodate the psychological, social, cultural and spiritual needs of clients, as well as their biological needs.

3. The nurse does more than respond to the requests of clients, by accepting an affirmative obligation to aid clients in their expression of needs and values within the context of health care.

4. Recognizing the client's membership in a family and a community, the nurse, with the client's consent, attempts to facilitate the participation of significant others in the care of the client.

II
Based upon respect for clients and regard for their right to control
their own care, nursing care should reflect respect
for the right of choice held by clients.

Standards

1. The competent client's consent is an essential precondition to the provision of health care. Nurses bear the primary responsibility to inform clients about the nursing care that is available to them.

2. Consent may be signified in many different ways. Verbal permission or knowledgeable cooperation are the usual forms in which clients consent to nursing care. In each case, however, a valid consent represents the free choice of the competent client to undergo that care which is to be provided.

3. Consent properly understood is the process by which a client becomes an active participant in care. All clients should be aided in becoming active participants in their care to the maximum extent that circumstances permit. Professional ethics may require of the nurse actions that exceed the legal requirements of consent. For example, although a child may be legally incompetent to consent, nurses should nevertheless attempt to inform and involve the child in treatment.

4. Force, coercion and manipulative tactics must not be employed in the obtaining of consent.

5. Illness or other factors may compromise the client's capacity for self-direction. Nurses have a continuing obligation to value autonomy in such clients, for example, by creatively providing them with opportunities for choices, within their capabilities, thereby aiding them to maintain or regain some degree of autonomy.

6. Whenever information is provided to a client, this must be done in a truthful, understandable and sensitive way. It must proceed with an awareness of the individual client's needs, interests and values.

7. Nurses should respond freely to their client's requests for information and explanation when in possession of the knowledge required to respond accurately. When the questions of the client require information beyond that of the nurse, the client should be informed of that fact and referred to a more appropriate health care practitioner for a response.

III
The nurse is obliged to hold confidential all information
regarding a client learned in the health care setting.

Standards

1. The rights of persons to control the amount of personal information that will be revealed applies with special force in the health care setting. It is, broadly speaking, up to clients to determine who shall be told of their condition, and in what detail.

2. In describing professional confidentiality to a client, its boundaries should be revealed:

   a) Competent care requires that other members of a team of health personnel have access to or be provided with the relevant details of a client's condition.

   b) In addition, discussions of the client's care may be required for the purpose of teaching, research or quality assurance. In this case, special care must be taken to protect the client's anonymity. Whenever possible, the client should be informed of these necessities at the onset of care.

3. An affirmative duty exists to institute and maintain practices that protect client confidentiality, for example, by limiting access to records.

Limitations

The nurse is not morally obligated to maintain confidentiality when the failure to disclose information will place the client or third parties in danger. Generally, legal requirements to disclose are morally justified by these same criteria. In facing such a situation, the first concern of the nurse must be the safety of the client or the third party.

Even when the nurse is confronted with the necessity to disclose, confidentiality should be preserved to the maximum possible extent. Both the amount of information disclosed and the number of people to whom disclosure is made should be restricted to the minimum necessary to prevent the feared harm.

IV
The nurse has an obligation to be guided by consideration
for the dignity of clients.

Standards

1. Nursing care should be carried out with consideration for the personal modesty of clients.

2. A nurse's conduct at all times should acknowledge the client as a person. For example, discussion of care in the presence of the client should actively involve or include that client.

3. As ways of dealing with death and the dying process change, nursing is challenged to find new ways to preserve human values, autonomy and dignity. In assisting the dying client, measures must be taken to afford as much comfort, dignity and freedom from anxiety and pain as possible. Special consideration is given to the need of the client's family to cope with their loss.

V
The nurse is obligated to provide competent care to clients.

Standards

1. Nurses should engage in continuing education and in the upgrading of skills relevant to the practice setting.

2. In seeking or accepting employment, nurses should accurately state their areas of competence as well as limitations.

3. Nurses who are assigned to work outside of an area of present competence should seek to do that which, under the circumstances, is in the best interests of their clients. Supervisors or others should be informed of the situation at the earliest possible moment so that protective measures can be instituted. As a temporary measure, the safety and welfare of clients may be better served by the best efforts of the nurse under the circumstances than by no nursing care at all.

4. When called upon outside of an employment setting to provide emergency care, nurses fulfill their obligations by providing the best care that circumstances, experience and education permit.

Limitations

A nurse is not ethically obliged to provide requested care when compliance would involve a violation of her or his moral beliefs. When that request falls within recognized forms of health care, however, the client should be referred to a more appropriate health care practitioner. Nurses who have or are likely to encounter such situations are morally obligated to seek to arrange conditions of employment so that the care of clients is not jeopardized.

VI
The nurse is obliged to represent the ethics of nursing
before colleagues and others.

Standards

1. Nurses serving on committees concerned with health care or research should see their role as including the vigorous representation of nursing's professional ethics.

2. Many public issues include health as a major component. Involvement in civic activities may afford the nurse the opportunity to further the objectives of nursing as well as to fulfill the duties of a citizen.

VII

The nurse is obligated to advocate the client's interest.

Standards

1. Advocating the interests of the client includes assistance in achieving access to quality health care. For example, by providing information to clients privately or publicly, the nurse enables them to satisfy their rights to health care.

2. When speaking to public issues or in court as a nurse, the public is owed the same duties of accurate and relevant information as are clients within the employment setting.

VIII

In all professional settings, including education, research and administration, the nurse retains a commitment to the welfare of clients. The nurse bears an obligation to act in such a fashion as will maintain trust in nurses and nursing.

Standards

1. Nurses accepting professional employment must ascertain that conditions will permit provision of care consistent with the values and standards of the Code. Prospective employers should be informed of the provisions of the Code so that realistic and ethical expectations may be established at the beginning of the nurse-employer relationship.

2. Accurate performance appraisal is required by a concern for present and future clients and is essential to the growth of nurses. Nurse administrators and educators are morally obligated to provide timely and accurate feedback to nurses, and their supervisors, student nurses and their teachers.

3. Administrators bear special ethical responsibilities that flow from a concern for present and future clients. The nurse administrator seeks to ensure that the competencies of personnel are used efficiently. Working within available resources, the administrator seeks to ensure the welfare of clients. When competent care is threatened due to inadequate resources or for some other reason, the administrator acts to minimize the present danger and to prevent future harm.

4. An essential element of nursing education is the student-client encounter. This encounter must be conducted in accordance with ethical nursing practices, with special attention to the dignity of the client. The nurse educator is obligated to ensure that nursing students are acquainted with and comply with the provisions of the Code.

5. Research is necessary to the development of the profession of nursing. Nurses should be acquainted with advances in research, so that established results may be incorporated into practice. The individual nurse's competencies and circumstances may also be used to engage in, or to assist and encourage research designed to enhance the health and welfare of clients.

The conduct of research must conform to ethical nursing practice. The self-direction of clients takes on added importance in this context. Further direction is provided in the Canadian Nurses Association publication entitled, *Ethical Guidelines for Nursing Research Involving Human Subjects.*

HEALTH TEAM

IX

Client care should represent a cooperative effort, drawing upon the expertise
of nursing and other health professions. Acknowledging personal
or professional limitations, the nurse recognizes the perspective
and expertise of colleagues from other disciplines.

Standards

1. The nurse participates in the assessment, planning, implementation and evaluation of comprehensive programs of care for clients. The scope of a nurse's responsibility should be based upon education and experience, as well as legal considerations of licensure or registration.

2. The nurse accepts a responsibility to work with others through professional nurses' associations to secure quality care for clients.

X

The nurse, as a member of the health care team, is obliged to take steps
to ensure that the client receives competent and ethical care.

Standards

1. The first consideration of the nurse who suspects incompetence or unethical conduct should be the welfare of present clients or potential harm to future clients. Subject to that principle, the following should be considered:

    a. The nurse is obliged to ascertain the facts of the situation in deciding upon the appropriate course of action.

    b. Institutional mechanisms for reporting incidents or risks of incompetent or unethical care should be followed.

c.   It is unethical for a nurse to participate in efforts to deceive or mislead clients regarding the cause of their injury.

d.   Relationships in the health care team should not be disrupted unnecessarily. If a situation can be resolved without peril to present or future clients by direct discussion with the colleague suspected of providing incompetent or unethical care, that should be done.

2.   The nurse who attempts to protect clients threatened by incompetent or unethical conduct may be placed in a difficult position. Colleagues and professional associations are morally obliged to support nurses who fulfill their ethical obligations under the Code.

3.   Guidance concerning those activities that may be delegated by nurses to assistants and other health care workers is found in legislation and policy statements. When functions are delegated, the nurse should be satisfied regarding the competence of those who will be fulfilling these functions. The nurse has a duty to provide continuing supervision in such a case.

THE SOCIAL CONTEXT OF NURSING

XI

Conditions of employment should contribute to client care and to the professional satisfaction of nurses. Nurses are obliged to work towards securing and maintaining conditions of employment that satisfy these connected goals.

Standards

1.   In the final analysis, the improvement of conditions of nursing employment is often to the advantage of clients. Over the short term however, there is a danger that action directed toward this goal will work to the detriment of clients. Nurses bear an ethical responsibility to present as well as future clients and so the following principles should be noted:

a.   The safety of clients should be the first concern in planning and implementing any job action.

b.   Individuals and groups of nurses participating in job actions share this ethical commitment to the safety of clients. However, their responsibilities may lead them to express this commitment in different, but equally appropriate ways.

c.   Clients whose safety requires ongoing or emergency nursing care are entitled to have those needs satisfied throughout the duration of any job action. Members of the public are entitled to know of the steps that have been taken to ensure the safety of clients.

d. Individuals and groups of nurses participating in job actions have a duty of coordination and communication to take steps reasonably designed to ensure the safety of clients.

RESPONSIBILITIES OF THE PROFESSION

XII

Professional nurses' organizations recognize a responsibility to clarify, secure and sustain ethical nursing conduct. The fulfillment of these tasks requires that professional organizations remain responsive to the rights, needs and legitimate interests of clients and nurses.

Standards

1. Sustained communication and cooperation between the Canadian Nurses Association, provincial associations and other organizations of nurses, is an essential step towards securing ethical nursing conduct.

2. Professional nurses' associations must at all times accept responsibility for assuring quality care for clients.

3. Professional nurses' associations have a role in representing nursing interests and perspectives before non-nursing bodies, including legislatures, employers, the professional organizations of other health disciplines and the public media of communication.

4. Professional nurses' associations should provide and encourage organizational structures that facilitate ethical nursing conduct.

    a. Changing circumstances may call for reconsideration and adaptation of this Code. Supplementation of the code may be necessary in order to address special situations. Professional associations should consider the ethics of nursing on a regular and continuing basis and be prepared to provide assistance to those concerned with its implementation.

    b. Education in the ethical aspects of nursing should be available to nurses throughout their careers. Nurses' associations should actively support or develop structures designed towards this end.

Index